Assertive Outreach
in Mental Health

Dedication

This book is dedicated to Reg Burns who always put the social workers' perspective, and to Markus 24.01.01.

Assertive Outreach in Mental Health
a manual for practitioners

Tom Burns

Professor of Social and Community Psychiatry
Department of Psychiatry,
St George's Hospital Medical School,
London

and

Mike Firn

Team Leader
Wandsworth, ACT Team,
London

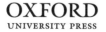
OXFORD
UNIVERSITY PRESS

OXFORD

UNIVERSITY PRESS

Great Clarendon Street, Oxford OX2 6DP

Oxford University Press is a department of the University of Oxford.
It furthers the University's objective of excellence in research, scholarship,
and education by publishing worldwide in

Oxford New York

Auckland Cape Town Dar es Salaam Hong Kong Karachi
Kuala Lumpur Madrid Melbourne Mexico City Nairobi
New Delhi Shanghai Taipei Toronto

With offices in

Argentina Austria Brazil Chile Czech Republic France Greece
Guatemala Hungary Italy Japan South Korea Poland Portugal
Singapore Switzerland Thailand Turkey Ukraine Vietnam

Oxford is a registered trade mark of Oxford University Press
in the UK and in certain other countries

Published in the United States
by Oxford University Press Inc., New York

© Oxford University Press, 2002

A catalogue record for this title is available from the British Library

Library of Congress Cataloging in Publication Data
(Data available)

ISBN 0 19 851615 0 (pbk.) 978 0 19 851615 6

10 9 8 7 6 5 4

Typeset in Minion
by Integra Software Services Pvt. Ltd., Pondicherry, India
www.integra-india.com
Printed in Great Britain
on acid-free paper by Biddles Ltd., King's Lynn, Norfolk

Preface

We wrote this book because our team (and that includes us) needed it. We have been working as an assertive outreach team for individuals with severe mental illness since the beginning of 1994. Establishing the Wandsworth assertive community treatment (ACT) team was prompted by a trip to examine some of the model ACT teams in the US, set up after Stein and Test's (1980) landmark publication. These US teams were as marked by their differences from one another as by their similarities—hardly surprising, as America is a diverse society with dramatic variations in health and social care. If the approach could make a difference despite all those differences in context, then the model would probably survive translation to the UK.

When the team was set up it seemed a useful service development, worth trying out for a few years before deciding whether to continue. Its success was far from guaranteed. Much of what our American colleagues considered characteristic of ACT (continuity of care, outreach, integrated multidisciplinary working) was well established, even taken for granted, in our local generic community mental health teams (CMHTs). Would the smaller case loads and explicitly targeted work practices make such a noticeable difference as to justify the costs?

Since then, the context of mental health care in the UK has changed almost out of all recognition. Practice has become much more explicitly accountable. The upside of this has been a noticeable raising of standards and consistency—but a price has been paid. This price includes a shift to a greater emphasis on risk management and a sense of a 'blame culture', with inevitable effects on staff recruitment and morale. We have also witnessed a quite astounding increase in the prescription of service models and structures. Assertive outreach (encompassing ACT) has been one of these prescriptions, albeit one based on sound evidence-based practice. What started out seven years ago as a local initiative (though not an isolated one) is now national policy.

When we started, our relative obscurity was a benefit. It meant that we were free to develop a viable way of working, trying out different configurations and styles and learning new skills. It was not always an easy time—we made several mistakes and often had to retrace our steps and start again. It took time even to discover what sort of staff liked this way of working (not everybody will!) In particular, tolerance and persistence was necessary to establish effective relationships with all the other components of mental health care. Our team did not develop in a vacuum, and it had its critics.

Newly established assertive outreach teams will find themselves exposed to intense scrutiny from their colleagues. This scrutiny will not always be supportive or even neutral. And why should it? Proposing a change in practice, no matter how diplomatically phrased, implies a deficiency in existing practice. We hope that this book will help members of such newly established teams to identify what needs to be done differently, where the evidence for this originates, and how to get on with it.

Evolution or revolution?

It will be clear from this book that we consider ACT or assertive outreach to have more in common with current CMHT practice than differences. Indeed, we think that overstating the differences has been in nobody's real interests. It sets up false conflicts and risks the abandonment of effective strategies that have evolved over time to accommodate local needs. Our view of assertive outreach is that it is best understood as a refining and targeted application of evidence to a part of CMHT practice rather than a new practice.

It is like the distinction between a *technological development* and a *new technology*. This is a fine distinction, and one that may be unstable over time. Developments can go both ways. For instance, that core feature of ACT teams—'a defined maximum case load per worker'—was a clear distinction for us seven years ago. A consequence of working with it, however, is that we have imported the principle into our CMHTs. The level is higher (currently a maximum of 35 patients per key worker) but the principle, which once clearly differentiated the two ways of working, is now the same in both types of teams.

Who is this book for?

We have aimed this book at multidisciplinary staff who work in any form of community mental health team which moves out beyond the clinic. It takes assertive outreach teams as its starting point, but we hope that most of it is relevant to practice within a whole range of teams and to a whole range of disciplines. The middle section of the book on 'Health and social care practice' will be useful to anyone working with community patients suffering from major psychotic illness.

How did we choose what to leave out?

No book can be perfect. We are conscious that some will criticize us for leaving out more detailed information on specific treatments or for not summarizing all the available scientific and research evidence. Others will criticize us for putting in too much about research and, still others, that there is no obvious logic in how much space we have accorded various topics. (Why so much on schizophrenia and so little on obsessive-compulsive disorder or anorexia nervosa?)

We have tried to reflect the reality of our day-to-day work in the book. This work is with a highly targeted group of individuals trying to survive in society despite severe and enduring mental illness. They are individuals for whom the alternative is, too often, hospital admission. We have focused on those things that keep coming up in our team discussions. Issues that are rare or peripheral are mentioned but not described in detail. We have no other excuse for our choice.

Some readers may be incensed that we have often given our own opinions on contentious or unresolved matters. We hope we have made it clear when we are expressing an opinion that it is just that—an opinion. However, we would defend the importance of opinions based on long clinical experience. There is a risk in this era of evidence-based practice that clinical experience can be too easily dismissed. There is no shortage of opinion and prejudice masquerading as 'proven fact'. We hope we have been honest about ours.

'Patient' or 'client'?

One such issue of opinion was whether to use the term 'patient' or 'client' throughout the book. We do not think this is a big issue, and in our team meetings we use both terms interchangeably. But for a book you need to be consistent. As explained in Chapter 2, we chose 'patient' eventually because of a survey that suggested that that is the term that patients themselves prefer. It is not a political point and does not imply allegiance to some outmoded form of medical model. We hope it does not give offence, and if it does we are sorry.

Thanks

This book arises from the discussions that the Wandsworth ACT team engages in every day when we review our patients, plan care and problem solve. It has also been shaped by the many questions raised by visitors to the 'Beacon' days we held in 2000 and 2001. The main stimulus to write the book, however, came from the needs expressed by patients and team members, and its contents reflect those preoccupations. Were it not for them sharing their skill, hard work, optimism, and tolerance we would never have had the energy or time to write it.

Since we cannot name our patients, it would not be fair to name all our colleagues. Several colleagues, however, have helped develop our ideas and establish the team over the years—Chris May and Dr Andy Kent in the early years, Caroline Ridley and Mike Fleet throughout, and Drs Rob Bale and Louise Guest at significant periods in between. Coping with a research study was no easy task and Matthew Fiander deserves a mention in this respect. As for the legion of colleagues who have invested time and careers on behalf of all our patients, we, the patients, and you, know who you are, and we thank you.

A very special thanks is due to Geraldine Bowers who typed and reshaped successive drafts with her unwavering good humour, her organizational flair, and her ability to read our awful handwriting.

Tom Burns and Mike Firn   London, September 2001

Contents

Part III **Structural issues**

Part I

Conceptual issues

Chapter 1

Origins of assertive outreach

Outreach in the UK and Europe

Assertive outreach is not new in mental health practice in the UK. The publication of Stein and Test's landmark paper in 1980 (Stein and Test 1980) is often taken as its starting point, and certainly led to increased international attention. However, the practice of taking services to severely mentally ill patients rather than requiring them to attend hospitals and clinics had been long established in the UK and in several European countries. Querido in Amsterdam had started his mobile clinic in the 1930s (Querido 1968). The French developed their 'secteur' approach, which involved limited home visiting, in the 1960s (Kovess *et al.* 1995). In the US, Pasamanick had explored the value of home visiting in discharged schizophrenia patients (Pasamanick *et al.* 1964).

Community psychiatric nurses

In the UK, the community psychiatric nurse (CPN) has been the backbone of outreach in mental health practice. T.P. Rees, the physician superintendent at Warlingham Park Hospital in Croydon, first introduced CPNs in 1954 (Moore 1961). As with Pasamanick's study, his team were originally concerned with the follow-up of schizophrenia patients recently discharged from hospital and their primary purpose was to encourage them to continue medication.

CPNs have developed exponentially since these first early steps in Croydon. Like social workers, they have always considered their brief to be broad, covering both patient and family, and, also in common with social workers, have conducted the greater part of their work in patients' homes. Over three-quarters of CPN services were established in the 1970s (White 1991) and the first CPN training course in 1974. By the end of the 1980s they outnumbered consultant psychiatrists and, between 1990 and 1996, their numbers rose from 4000 to 7000 in England and Wales (White 1999) and they became fully integrated within community mental health teams (CMHTs).

The 1959 Mental Health Act in England

The 1959 Mental Health Act set the scene for the expansion of CPNs and of outreach more broadly. The Act required any mental hospital that accepted compulsorily detained patients to provide an out-patient service. While this may seem unremarkable now it was extremely prescient then and ensured a tradition of comprehensive mental health care and the development of the multidisciplinary team. The same group of clinicians who were responsible for in-patient care were also responsible, in collaboration with the patient's general practitioner, for their care after they were discharged from hospital.

The 1959 Act was promulgated soon after the Welfare State was developed and was infused with recognition of the need for co-ordinated health and social care. It mandated collaboration between health and social care authorities. At its most basic it required social workers to be involved in the process of compulsory detention but, in practice, led to close working relations. Social workers, unlike doctors, had never been particularly institution-based, often visiting and assessing clients and their families in their homes. The integration of social workers into CMHTs has been much more variable than that of CPNs. Some teams were fully integrated in the late 1960s and some are only achieving this now with the advent of single management.

The joint influence of social workers and CPNs has dominated the style of CMHTs so that virtually all would provide some form of home visiting or 'outreach'. The benefits of home visiting, not just for follow-up but also for assessment, have become clear to medical members of the team (Burns *et al.* 1993*a*; Jones 1982).

Social influences on the course of mental illness

Home visiting in pioneer services such as Dingleton Hospital in the Scottish borders (Jones 1982), and in social work generally, was not simply a response to the problems experienced by many long-term patients in terms of unreliability, lack of motivation, or difficulty in getting to the hospital. Its rationale was also to obtain a broader, richer understanding of the context of the patient's problem and of how social influences affected the outcome in severe mental illness.

The therapeutic community movement at the end of the Second World War had emphasized how a patient's relationships and social pressures could impede or encourage recovery from breakdown (Jones 1952). Studies of long-term patients in mental hospitals, such as the famous 'Three Hospitals Study' (Wing 1968), demonstrated dramatically that the progress of even very serious illnesses such as schizophrenia could be improved by careful attention to the social environment. Applying this awareness to out-patients, if social stressors were to be reduced and social supports strengthened then staff had to know about the patient's situation. The most effective way of doing this was obviously for them to go and see for themselves. The whole mental health team in these early pioneer services began to invade the traditional territory of the social worker.

Deinstitutionalization

The fledgling developments in social care in mental health were to receive a massive boost from the recognition of the negative impact of some aspects of mental hospital care. Russell Barton introduced the concept of 'institutional neurosis' (Barton 1959). He pointed out that much of the apathy and self neglect in long-term schizophrenia patients (traditionally attributed to an inherent deterioration in the illness) was a demoralized response to the monotony and disempowerment of hospital existence. While we would now consider this an oversimplification, there were undoubtedly significant numbers of patients who had recovered but whose recovery went unnoticed in these vast hospitals and who flourished once they were discharged. The ease with which many of these 'forgotten' patients adapted to life outside hospital led to an over-optimism about the redundancy of mental hospitals, speeding their run-down. This over-optimism was challenged in the 1980s and 90s when much more disabled patients were being discharged.

Irving Goffman's book, *Asylums*, is probably the most influential text on the damaging effects of prolonged mental hospital care (Goffman 1960). This extraordinarily eloquent book was the result of the sociologist, Goffman, spending several months 'under cover' in a large Washington mental hospital where he worked as an aide. His conclusion was that such hospitals were 'total institutions' (environments where all an individual's needs—food, shelter, recreation, company—were provided from a single source). He argued that total institutions were inherently damaging to humans, disempowering them and robbing them of their individuality and vigour—precisely the qualities they needed to recover from a mental illness. His vivid portrayal of the toxic effects of unvarying routines and procedures, applied with no accommodation for individual variation, on the inmates' fragile sense of self had a worldwide impact on the status of mental hospitals and hastened their demise.

A series of damning reports of degrading and cruel conditions within mental hospitals (Committee of Inquiry 1969) accelerated the public's desire to see them abandoned. This feeling is well encapsulated in Enoch Powell's now famous 'Water Tower' speech, as Health Minister, in which he referred to their ominous and looming presence (Powell 1961). Since the 1960s there has been a dramatic reduction in the number of beds in mental hospitals and, recently, the closure of most of the large Victorian institutions. Britain, along with most developed nations, has now less than a third of the psychiatric in-patient beds that it had in the mid-1950s. This run-down in institutional care means that out-patient services have been dealing with increasingly disabled patients for the last 30 years. As the pressure has increased on these services, the need for multidisciplinary working (to meet the complex and varied needs of such patients), and the need for outreach, have become inevitable.

Community mental health teams (CMHTs)

CMHTs are the service model which has evolved in the UK, and much of Europe, to meet this challenge. In the UK they serve over 90% of the population (Johnson and Thornicroft 1993). Though there is no simple, universally accepted definition of a CMHT they are fairly easy to recognize. They are multiprofessional teams who work closely together to provide comprehensive care to individuals requiring secondary mental health services, usually in a defined catchment area. The definition of that catchment area can vary—several CMHTs may fall within a hospital's catchment area or each CMHT may have its own tightly defined sector. Increasingly, CMHTs are defining their catchment areas with reference to groups of general practitioners in order to improve liaison and shared care (Burns and Bale 1997).

What constitutes a multiprofessional team? Most workers in the area consider that there has to be a minimum of three professions—nursing, medicine, and social work are the commonest. In addition most CMHTs also include clinical psychologists and occupational therapists. The last few years have also witnessed the increasing inclusion of mental health support workers who have no specific relevant professional training, although many have relevant experience or an undergraduate degree.

CMHTs developed in the UK alongside the therapeutic community movement and share important characteristics with that approach (Burns 2000*a*; Jones 1952). These include a recognition that many mental health interventions can be delivered by several members of the team, not all of whom require a dedicated professional training. This has led to a 'blurring' of roles (e.g. either a nurse or a social worker may take responsibility for organizing accommodation, and a doctor or psychologist may provide psychotherapy).

Most CMHTs contain a healthy tension around the balance between 'generic' and 'specific' interventions. This tension is generally productive and creative when well managed, and evidence of this is the gradual evolution of cross-disciplinary responsibilities within the team. A team may identify an individual with special skills and responsibilities not restricted to their own profession (e.g. an occupational therapist may be the team expert in family management and a nurse the expert in work placement).

Within CMHTs there is a wide range of operation. Most are exclusively providers of secondary care (taking all their referrals from general practice, social services, and hospitals), but some offer degrees of direct access. In the 1980s direct access was encouraged but most teams now restrict it to known patients. Open access often resulted in the skewing of the team's activity towards less ill (and often not ill at all) individuals who were more vocal and demanding than the more seriously mentally ill. The most disabled patients were thus further disadvantaged. In addition, it was often unrewarding for staff, who were unable to use many of their skills. It also caused confusion about responsibility for primary care (providers of which were often short-circuited) and led to the duplication of work.

Increasingly, CMHTs have had to introduce tighter procedures such as a single point of entry, systematic care programme reviews (Department of Health 1990), and active case load management in order to maintain capacity while targeting the severely mentally ill. CMHTs have evolved slowly and pragmatically and, despite their apparent success, surprisingly little has been written about their functioning. Very few research studies have been conducted in which they are the experimental condition (Tyrer *et al.* 1999; Tyrer 2000*a*). This is in sharp contrast to the development of case management in the US.

Case management in the US

Case management evolved in the US during the 1970s and 1980s to deal with the problems facing patients discharged from mental hospitals which were downsizing and closing (Intagliata 1982). Deinstitutionalization in the US was ushered in by President Kennedy's 'New Deal for the Mentally Ill' initiative which launched the Community Mental Health Center Movement (Talbott *et al.* 1987). It started later in the US than in the UK, but followed a more rapid course. The lack of general social provision (such as affordable housing, support, and medical care) for previously long-term patients was strikingly obvious. Where in the UK the patient's general practitioner or local social services office would naturally shoulder overall responsibility for organizing and delivering care, there was no obvious US equivalent. Case managers (originally described as 'service agents') arose to meet this need.

The case manager was charged with the responsibility of co-ordinating (and often purchasing) necessary services for the individual. Initially, they had no clinical training, offering a predominantly administrative role of 'brokering' care. The role of the case manager in co-ordinating the care of individuals with complex disabilities and needs, discharged into a confusing and unwelcoming world, made obvious sense. For individuals with mental handicap, and for those suffering from dementia, the results of this approach were encouraging. Unfortunately, research into its efficacy for individuals with severe mental illness made sobering reading (Braun *et al.* 1981). By the time the research studies into brokerage case management were being published, the penny had already dropped and clinical practice had changed.

Clinical case management

Effective care for the severely mentally ill needs to be embedded in a supportive and trusting relationship. Establishing such a relationship is a core skill acquired in most mental health professionals' training. The central role of the case manager in organizing and co-ordinating the total care needs of the patient remained but, increasingly, the case manager was a trained mental health professional who provided much of the care personally. This approach has been referred to as 'full support' or, more often, 'clinical case management' (Holloway *et al.* 1995). It has been compared favourably with brokerage case management which has persisted in the UK as 'care management' in social services (Lancet 1995; Marshall *et al.* 1995).

Direct patient care from the clinical case manager is an efficient care system; most patients are well supported and need no input from other staff. Where their needs are more complex, direct care will often have cemented the therapeutic relationship with the case manager and the patient will be more likely to accept other input. Such close working also generally yields a better-tailored assessment of need.

Case management became well established in the US in the late 1970s and fits the plurality and complexity of that country's health and social care provision. Further development came with assertive community treatment which 'supercharged' the research and policy agendas and has led to a veritable industry in community psychiatry research (Mueser *et al.* 1998).

Assertive community treatment

Stein and Test's 1980 paper ushered in a new era in the practice of outreach in mental health. They operated within the context of a large, isolated mental hospital surrounded by office-based private practitioners. Frustrated by the lack of continuity of care (which resulted in the rapid readmissions of discharged patients over whose treatment they had no control) they took advantage of a ward closure to conduct their, now famous, experiment. Stein and Test studied a more intensive form of clinical case management in which the case managers had small case loads (10 patients each) and a vigorous commitment to following up and treating patients in their own neighbourhoods.

Initially, Stein and Test called their service 'training in community living' (TCL). They emphasized its role in teaching patients how to cope with chronic mental illness in the community rather than treating the illness. They randomized 130 patients with established psychotic illness, at the point of potential readmission, to either their TCL service or standard care (Stein and Test 1980).

The model of TCL care was comprehensive, with an emphasis on stabilizing the patient's living situation, monitoring and ensuring medication compliance, crisis resolution (including 24-hour availability to prevent rehospitalization), and training and supporting the patient in activities of daily living in their own environment. Each case manager was expected to develop at least a minimal competence across all these areas and to involve other team members routinely in the care and support of their patients. Professional flexibility was essential—the case manager did what was most necessary to keep the patient well and out of hospital even if this lay outside their normal professional priorities. For instance, it may be more immediately necessary to clean up the flat to prevent the patient being evicted than to increase medication to control symptoms. Contact was routinely several times per week, dependent on need.

This approach resulted in a dramatic reduction in hospital readmission and in-patient care and even in costs of care (Weisbrod *et al.* 1980). Patients also demonstrated an improvement in clinical status (they had fewer symptoms) and in social functioning (more were employed or engaged in structured daily activities) (Test and Stein 1980). However, when the funding for the new service ran out after 14 months it had to be abandoned. Stein and Test followed up their patients for a further 14 months and noted that all the advantages to the experimental group faded completely during this time. This brought home to them that the service they had developed was needed as an ongoing support, not simply a training. They consequently abandoned the term 'training in community living' and renamed it the 'programme in assertive community treatment' (PACT).

Replications of ACT

The PACT approach has become the most widely replicated model of case management in mental illness (Marshall and Lockwood 1998). It has become the accepted model for assertive outreach—although not the only one by a long way (Mueser *et al.* 1998).

There is controversy around which aspects of the PACT model are essential. For example, is a 'team approach' or 24-hour availability a requirement for ACT to function? What constitutes 'frequent contact' or 'an emphasis on medication'?

Despite there being a specific scale to measure 'ACTness'—the Dartmouth ACT scale (Teague *et al.* 1998), agreeing when a team should be classified as ACT remains contentious. There are furious academic debates about whether some forms of case management are ACT or not (Marshall 1996; Marshall *et al.* 1999). The change in practice of case management over time (Holloway *et al.* 1995) and the tendency of Europeans to use the term 'intensive case management' where ACT is used in the US provide fertile ground for confusion and conflicting interpretation of studies.

Conclusions

The last 50 years have witnessed a revolution in the care of the mentally ill. The locus of activity has shifted from an essentially in-patient service to one where most care is delivered outside hospitals or in out-patient departments. This shift has reflected a reaffirmation of the importance of relationships in mental health. Whether they are a patient's relationships with family and friends or the therapeutic relationship with staff members, they are the bedrock of successful treatment. In-patient care remains an essential provision for times of severe disorganization (when patients may need constant monitoring and care) but is simply one option among many over the patient's illness career.

For the severely mentally ill a flexible and broadly constituted approach has evolved in which both health and social care can be delivered and co-ordinated by trained individuals working within teams.

From two quite different health care cultures (the US and the UK), two approaches to outreach have evolved and have been converging—the CMHT approach and ACT. Despite historical and organizational differences these two approaches have much in common and they meet around the concept of assertive outreach with which this book is concerned. Assertive outreach is already an area scarred by dogma and vested interest and we do not intend to continue such empty arguments. Current practice has been informed by both CMHTs and by discrete assertive outreach teams. Although the 'functional' team approach is the one behind this book, we anticipate that much of that discussed should be equally applicable in a generic CMHT as in a dedicated assertive outreach team.

Chapter 2

Current context and aims

Modernization of mental health services

The rate of change in provision in mental health services has been gathering pace for the last 20 years. As outlined in Chapter 1 this has been driven by the shift in emphasis from long-term care in mental hospitals to support in the community, with only episodic admissions to hospitals for acute breakdowns. This shift has been accompanied by the process of deinstitutionalization and the closure of the large, old mental hospitals. Such a picture is, of necessity, an oversimplification. There remains a significant minority of long-term patients who have not been able to transfer to community care. For some this is because their illnesses are so severe, or their behaviour so unacceptable, that psychiatric hospital remains the only tolerant and safe environment for them. Others have remained in hospital because their mental illness has been compounded by age and infirmity. They are often referred to as 'graduate long-stay' because their original psychotic illness has become overshadowed by cognitive impairment.

There is also a group of 'new long-stay' patients who, despite care within modern services, remain in hospitals for several years. These are usually younger patients with psychotic illnesses, often complicated by substance abuse and personality difficulties. Failure to allow for their slowly increasing numbers has led to serious underestimates of bed needs in the past (Hirsch 1988). The new long-stay population includes some with offending behaviour who may constitute a risk to those around them and require extended periods of secure care. The 1990s saw an acknowledgement of this patient group's needs with the expansion of medium secure forensic units (Butler 1975; Reed 1992) and a range of longer-term provision for behaviourally disturbed and resistant patients. While an important and high-profile patient group, they remain a very small proportion of those who need secondary mental health care.

Changes in mental health care are not solely due to deinstitutionalization. There have been other important developments which have converged to produce the current climate. Among these has been the rise of consumerism in health care, the increasing importance of evidence-based medicine, improved treatments, individual professional developments, the rise to prominence of health services research with its international perspective on practice, and, more recently, a vigorous interventionist approach by governments. It would be impossible to rank these for their importance. There is considerable overlap between some of them (e.g. consumerism and government intervention) but each will be considered individually in some more detail.

Consumerism in mental health care

Informed patients

The era of 'doctor knows best' is long dead in health care in much of the developed world. While the challenge to professional authority may seem particularly extreme in the field of mental health it is in no way restricted to it. Nor indeed is it restricted to medicine. The Western world has experienced a profound re-evaluation of its relationship to professions and 'experts' alike. Scientists, doctors, lawyers are all questioned in ways that would have seemed unthinkable only 30 years ago. As the population has become better educated, individuals want to know about the possible courses of action open to them. They also want to influence that choice.

When the medical sociologist, David Tuckett, called his book on the doctor–patient consultation *Meetings between experts* he meant that the doctor was the expert on the treatment and the patient, the expert on him or herself (Tuckett *et al.* 1985). Now, the patient, with access to libraries and the internet, may arrive at the consultation better informed about their illness than the doctor or nurse. Access to their own case notes has helped emancipate patients and mould their view of the relationship they have with staff—even if not that many insist on reading them (Kosky and Burns 1995). The management of disorders (especially chronic disorders) is improved when the patient is as fully informed as possible. Evidence from a wide range of studies—from terminal care (Hinton 1967), through diabetes (White *et al.* 1996), to the discussion of side-effects and risks of antipsychotic medication (Chaplin and Kent 1998)—demonstrates that better-informed patients, who are actively involved in their treatment decisions, do better.

'Patient' or 'client'?

Even the term 'patient' has been criticized for implying a passive, dependent role in a paternalistic relationship. Social workers and some nurses prefer the term 'client' to emphasize both the breadth of the relationship (extending beyond the purely medical) and also the fact that it is the client who should be able to control what services they receive. Further emphasizing the consumerism of the relationship, some people insist on the term 'service user' (often shortened to 'user' as in 'users and carers'). Presumably this stresses a power relationship in which the professional is the junior partner. Taken to extremes, some radical patient groups use the term 'survivor' to express their antipathy to mental health services. This attention to terminology indicates a real concern with the nature of the therapeutic relationship and a wish to see the status of the two players in it altered.

We have chosen to use the term 'patient' throughout this book; it could possibly have been 'client'. We rejected 'survivor' because we considered it unnecessarily confrontational. It is, however, important to remain alert to the ambivalence many members of the public feel towards mental health in general and psychiatry in particular. 'User' poses special problems. While it expresses the consumerist preference well, it is confused in US writings with drug users and seems clumsily non-specific, even when expressed as the cumbersome 'service user'. 'Carer' also seems wilfully vague in mental health where carers are almost invariably family members, who we feel should be acknowledged. It also requires involved constructions to avoid confusing informal and formal carers in systems.

We preferred 'patient' to 'client' because it registers that this is, first and foremost, a therapeutic relationship. We welcome its specificity and the fact that it is 'state-dependent'—an individual is a patient only for as long as they are receiving treatment (just as one ceases to be a passenger when one gets off a bus). It is not a life-long characteristic, is not stigmatizing (few of us will not be patients at some time in our lives), and does, surely, shake off any last vestiges of paternalistic passivity. Lastly, and perhaps most importantly, we chose 'patient' because that is what patients wish to be called! The only systematic studies of 'patient/client' preference (Ritchie *et al.* 2000) confirms this emphatically, with 77% of those asked preferring 'patient' over 'client'. Even healthy women attending antenatal clinics prefer the term 'patient' (Byrne 2000).

Our choice of the term 'patient' does not deny the increasing importance of consumerism in mental health. Well-informed patients are a powerful force for improvement in services. They will enquire about, and insist on, the best up-to-date treatments, and demand ease of access and respectful, polite care. Consumerism will, however, inevitably introduce tensions into traditional relationship. For instance, patients who are well aware of the best treatments according to the evidence may not want them and insist on alternative approaches (Laugharne 1999). These tensions are manifest not only in individual treatment choices (e.g. in preferences for 'talking' treatments over medication or vice versa) but also in service structures. A particularly pressing example is the debate over 24-hour crisis access. While strongly advocated by patient and family groups (Department of Health 1999*a*), there is little evidence of its value and strong evidence of its impracticability (Cooper 1979).

Planning and delivering outreach services are currently strongly influenced, both for good and ill, by the rise of consumerism. The views of all relevant stakeholders must be carefully considered and the rationale behind choices fully explained or even the best of services will come to grief.

Treatment improvements

A paradox of the increasingly critical attitude and general scepticism towards medicine is that it should be occurring now, just when we are delivering more effective, and less dangerous, treatments. There is now a range of pharmacological treatments for many of the more severe mental illnesses. For depression there is a choice between several different tricyclic antidepressants or the selective serotonin reuptake inhibitors (SSRIs), plus mood stabilizers such as lithium and carbamazepine for resistant patients and maintenance in bipolar affective disorder. In schizophrenia and delusional disorders the traditional phenothiazines can now be substituted with the newer 'atypical' antipsychotics and, in resistant cases, the superiority of clozapine has been well-demonstrated (Kane *et al.* 1988).

Treatment improvements extend beyond pharmacotherapy with the refining and testing of structured psychotherapies such as cognitive behaviour therapy (CBT), cognitive analytical therapy (CAT), and interpersonal therapy for depression, anxiety states, and some persistent personality problems. Behavioural therapies in family work with schizophrenia patients and in obsessive compulsive disorders have also been vastly improved, operationalized, and their effectiveness confirmed by research studies (Mari and Streiner 1994*a*).

This increasing therapeutic armamentarium has influenced the context of practice enormously. Mental health staff are now also judged predominantly on their skills and knowledge, not just their wisdom and personality. Services have to be delivered in the recognition that patients are increasingly informed, and informed about an increasingly wide range of treatments. Not all these treatments may be available locally and it is important to be able to explain this and why. Neither will all the treatments be equally well established or appropriate. A willingness to engage in an honest discussion of this is now part of the job. The media often transmit misleading and exaggerated impressions of new treatments (currently, for example, the efficacy of CBT for delusions in schizophrenia) which can often make such discussions difficult. We need to remember that the patient may, understandably, be anxious and clutching at straws. While there has been a remarkable improvement in the treatments we have on offer, unfortunately this improvement has been far exceeded by the rise in the public's expectations from us.

Evidence-based practice and clinical governance

Evidence-based practice and clinical governance are major current preoccupations in health care. With an exponential increase in research findings about different treatments, the decisions about which are appropriate for which patient should result from a rational weighing of the evidence rather than simply from personal preference. Not surprisingly many clinicians form preferences for particular interventions (e.g. one psychiatrist might favour a more psychological approach for depressed patients while another vigorously tests a whole range of antidepressants). Evidence-based practice aims to even out such variations. It requires us to look regularly at all that is currently known about the subject and base treatment decisions on that knowledge.

Levels of proof

Evidence-based practice favours certain forms of 'proof' above others and has established a hierarchy of evidence (Sackett *et al.* 1997). In particular it stresses the random controlled trial (RCT) and so-called meta-analyses. RCTs are studies to establish the relative effectiveness of treatments and they involve randomly allocating half the patients to the treatment under investigation and the other half either to no treatment (placebo) or to a current standard treatment. In drug trials great efforts are taken to ensure that neither patient nor researcher know which group the patient is in (double blind), but this is rarely possible in psychological or treatment structure studies. RCTs are not the only method of researching treatment efficacy but they are subject to fewer problems in interpretation. Other types of studies include *cohort* studies (following a group of patients over time) or *case control* studies (matching patients who receive the treatment with patients of, for example, similar age and diagnosis who do not).

Meta-analysis involves collecting together a series of RCTs, where there is enough data given about the patients and their outcomes, and treating the collected data as if they were one big study. This is very useful in psychiatry because studies often have quite small numbers. With the meta-analysis of the larger sample one can place greater confidence in the conclusions. A good example of this is the meta-analysis of behavioural family management in schizophrenia (Mari and Streiner 1994*a*). Here, data from a series of small studies was added together, allowing the number of family treatments required to prevent a relapse to be calculated (the 'number needed to treat') and for trends in efficacy to be demonstrated. The number needed to treat got higher in later studies, requiring seven family treatments to prevent one relapse compared to only five family treatments in the earlier studies.

A very common misunderstanding about evidence-based medicine is that where there is no conclusive evidence of the success of a treatment based on RCTs and meta-analyses, then that treatment is ineffective. This is not the case. Many treatments were well established before RCTs or even structured research trials became the norm. There are more ways of accumulating knowledge than conducting scientific research studies. Many things we do have no firm basis in formal research but are founded on established clinical practice (e.g. providing close monitoring for suicidal patients, ECT for severe delusional depression) and few would question their value. However, where there is established, strong evidence in favour of one form of treatment (e.g. lithium as prophylaxis in bipolar disorder (Cookson 1997) or clozapine in resistant schizophrenia (Kane *et al.* 1988)), then one needs a good reason for not using it.

Clinical governance and the need for judgement

Clinical governance is the regular monitoring of health care practice to ensure that the best evidence-based practices are being followed and that they are being applied correctly and competently. For assertive outreach staff, evidence-based medicine and clinical governance set the scene of practice but pose very special problems. There is generally little ambiguity about the evidence base for individual treatments (e.g. CBT in depression, maintenance antipsychotic medication in schizophrenia) but real controversy surrounds the evidence base for alternative service structures. Strongly contradictory positions are held by researchers on the benefits of service configurations such as case management (Marshall 1996; Marshall *et al.* 1999), ACT (Marshall and Lockwood 1998; Tyrer 2000*b*; UK700 Group: Burns *et al.* 1999*a*), and home treatments (Burns 2000*b*; Pelosi and Jackson 2000; Smyth and Hoult 2000).

There is a real discrepancy between the methodological rigour of treatment studies and of care systems studies. Treatment studies have a long history of well-established methodologies to reduce bias. However, research methodologies in service evaluations are much newer and the subject matter inherently more complex. Despite this the evidence is that service studies are probably more influential on practice than the more robust treatment evidence (Burns 1997a). As assertive outreach is such a highly politicized issue (see below) it is crucial for exponents to develop critical research appraisal skills. Only then can they reach informed opinions about the strength of evidence and not accept blindly the statements of politicians or health service managers. This will be returned to more below and in Chapter 29, 'Research and development'.

Health services research and the international perspective

Studying the organization of health care delivery is often referred to as health care research. In mental health the realization that how care was delivered impacted on the outcome was dramatically demonstrated in the process of deinstitutionalization. The specific treatments offered out of hospital were no different but the outcomes were very different. Early studies of home-based care (Hoult *et al.* 1984) soon showed a reduction in the need for hospitalization (taken as a proxy measure for relapse). Because of the enormous financial implications of reducing hospital care, studies of alternative community-based services have been encouraged and funded by governments and health service managers to support this downsizing. As outlined in Chapter 1, the volume of such research expanded enormously after the publication of a cost-benefit analysis of Stein and Test's 1980 study (Weisbrod *et al.* 1980). The study of mental health care services is now big business and there is a confusing range of study types and outcome measures.

Interpreting health services research

There are particular problems with studying mental health services for severely mentally ill individuals which matter for interpretation. In the first instance, most disorders are phasic. Studies tracking the changes in clinical state before and after the introduction of a new service are notoriously misleading. Patients are commonly recruited into the study when they are most ill and so improvement is not surprising and it is risky to attribute this to the intervention. In a large, multisite RCT of intensive case management, the UK700 study, (UK700 Group: Burns *et al.* 1999b; UK700 Group: Creed *et al.* 1999) both the experimental *and* the control patients had significantly reduced hospital care in the two years of the study compared to the two years before. Hence the importance of RCTs in this patient group. Excluding difficult patients can also mislead as these are precisely the patients who soak up most care (Coid 1994). Similarly misleading are studies of newly set-up services that often comprise the most able, enthusiastic staff.

Importance of context

Perhaps the most complicated aspect of interpreting mental health services research is that of context. Health service research has fostered a healthy internationalism in mental health planning. With some notorious exceptions most countries are keen to examine practice in other parts of the world and import them if they seem beneficial. In the 1980s, Italian community psychiatry attracted the limelight for its radical approaches. Currently, research from the English-speaking US and the UK dominates the field, with the US a clear leader. Most of the early studies into case management and ACT stemmed from the US and these have influenced thinking about assertive outreach in Europe and elsewhere. A problem with importing services research across cultures is that the context in which they operate may have a significant impact on the relative advantages they confer.

Current arguments about the failure of European studies to replicate the US advantages for case management and ACT fall into two camps. One argues that implementation of the service differs (the Europeans fail to replicate the American ACT, a failure in 'model fidelity') (Marshall *et al.* 1999). The other argues that the main difference is that the control services in Europe are very different to the US (being more like the experimental case management service or ACT) and also that the social welfare provision modifies the impact (Tyrer 2000*b*). There is probably some truth in both positions. Practice does differ somewhat and routine services in Europe are more likely to contain many of the elements of ACT thought to be effective. Clearly what is needed is greater attention to characterizing the context when such studies are reported (Burns and Priebe 1996; Thornicroft and Tansella 1999)—but this is far in the future. For the time being care should be exercised in importing conclusions across different health care cultures.

Importance for assertive outreach teams

These issues are not simply academic for staff working in assertive outreach. Early US studies, such as Stein and Test's, were set against a very rudimentary control service indeed, consisting of only hospital care or isolated, office-based private psychiatrists, with no multidisciplinary working. These studies demonstrated enormous reductions in the need for hospital care. Later US studies (Drake *et al.* 1998; Mueser *et al.* 1998) and European ones (Holloway *et al.* 1995; Holloway and Carson 1998) did not show anything like the same reductions.

Unfortunately, the belief that assertive outreach will empty wards is a very strongly held one. Teams need a realistic understanding of what is, and what is not, possible. If not, then disappointment and demoralization will follow.

Professional developments

Mental health care is no longer a case of doctors making diagnoses and nurses providing direct patient care. The range of disciplines involved has broadened to include social workers, clinical psychologists, occupational therapists, vocational counsellors, drug and alcohol counsellors, and many more. Not only is the range extended but the training, skills, and expectations of individual staff are barely recognizable from 30 years ago. Occupational therapists have moved out from the wards to be integral members of teams and expect to key work patients and provide psychotherapy as well as their traditional assessments of disabilities and structuring of activity and rehabilitation. Similarly, clinical psychologists have all but abandoned their traditional activities of psychometric testing and are busy delivering and evaluating more operationalized forms of psychotherapy (often renamed 'psychological treatments') and developing a high profile in staff supervision and training.

Changes in mental health nursing

Nursing has probably experienced the most radical changes. CPNs led the move into the community and have come increasingly to view themselves as an independent profession. Graduate entry into nursing and the reconfiguration of basic nurse training away from its traditional practical apprenticeship to a university degree with increased emphasis on academic achievement have profoundly altered the style of the profession. This has been reflected in the development of nurse specialist posts and, more recently, nurse consultants.

Outreach has been a driving force in this development—nurses visiting patients at home must, inevitably, take full professional responsibility. There is no one there to observe and supervise. This sense of independence, allied with the nurses' focus on holistic assessment, has forged an enormously strong professional identity around the nurse–patient relationship. While the multidisciplinary team has encouraged joint working, role blurring, and peer supervision, the newly acquired self-confidence of the constituent professions has generally led to a more equal, productive dialogue. Such levels of professional self-determination require a commitment to life-long learning. Increasingly, continuing professional education is cross-disciplinary. Assertive outreach has only become possible with such levels of skill and self-monitoring.

Government intervention

Mental health care, once the proverbial neglected 'Cinderella' service, is now high up the agenda of most Western governments. The severely mentally ill are cared for within state-sponsored health care programmes throughout the developed world. Despite market approaches to health care this is one group of patients who don't find their way into private or insurance-based services. Mental health care is also very expensive because of the long duration of the disorders and the complexity of needs. Community care has made the issues very visible. The public is concerned about perceived failures of such care, such as vagrancy and homicide, despite clear evidence that there has been no significant contribution of community care to these problems (Leff 1993; Taylor and Gunn 1999).

The result is that mental health care operates within a highly politicized framework which may distort rational service planning and certainly makes life difficult for staff.

Nowhere is this more obvious than in community support and outreach to psychotic patients. Ever the optimists, politicians remember and quote the most successful and dramatic study results and service developments. They rarely take note of the more balanced or negative findings. Neither their training nor their interest lies in the dusty academic pursuit of weighing up all the available evidence and forming a balanced judgement. They are guided by advisors who know that what politicians want to hear are positive messages (they get enough negative ones from the media). As a result they expect assertive outreach to improve engagement with services in disenchanted patients (particularly in the homeless and ethnic minorities), reduce in-patient care (thereby generating financial savings), and, last but not least, prevent homicides and suicide by the mentally ill.

Reviewing current practice

This book is a handbook for mental health professionals working predominantly out-side hospitals—whether as members of assertive outreach teams or providing home-based support for their patients from within generic CMHTs. The emphasis of the book is practical, focusing on procedures that can be carried out to help individuals. Inevitably such a practical approach carries the risk of redundancy as treatments change. It is important to be aware of this when using the handbook.

This book does more than simply present a litany of current treatments. As empha-sized in these first two chapters this is a rapidly changing and often confusing area of practice. We aim to encourage a critical approach to reviewing current practice. It really is not enough just to know of a research study and its published results. A careful evalu-ation needs to be made of such studies which should be tested against a set of questions to establish their relevance.

Assessing a research study

- How robust was the methodology? Was the sample big enough to prove its findings?
- Is the difference in outcome clinically important? Is it sufficient to justify the potential upheaval of retraining or even restructuring services to achieve it?
- Was the study carried out with patients who are like those you work with? This is particularly important beyond diagnosis—were offender patients, drug- and alcohol-abusing patients, or homeless patients excluded? If so, how transferable are the results to your practice?
- How similar is the service context to your own? Do the control and support services seem sufficiently similar so you can anticipate similar gains?
- How feasible is the approach locally? Do you have similar staff and resources or will an attempt at replication just lead to frustration and disarray?

In each of the practical chapters these questions will be articulated. Only by paying serious attention to them can it be possible to ensure that services meet our patients' needs and are not structured according to political and financial imperatives. While the intense public attention focused on outreach can be a nuisance it does, however, provide the opportunity to improve services. For this to be a reality clinicians (albeit in collaboration with patients and families and health service planners) must take a very active role in the setting of aims and objectives in service development.

Chapter 3

Who is assertive outreach for? Referrals and discharges

The wrong question!

Which patients an assertive outreach team should target is the first question usually asked when the decision is made to establish such a service. Various proposals are made, some based on evidence, some on wishful thinking, and some on simple desperation—'revolving door patients', 'dual-diagnosis patients', 'personality disorder patients', 'offender patients', 'the homeless', etc. A local needs' assessment promptly follows which identifies the number of potential patients who meet the agreed profile. From this calculations are made about the size of the team and the resource implications.

This is the wrong question to start off with. The fundamental question should be 'what is assertive outreach for?' In other words, 'what treatments and procedures, of proven worth, can we not provide currently that we could with an assertive outreach service?' From the answer to this question comes the answer to 'who is it for?'.

What is assertive outreach for?

Len Stein, one of the major driving forces in the establishment of assertive outreach, is fond of saying that the purpose of ACT (his form of assertive outreach) is to:

1. maintain regular and frequent contact *in order to*
2. monitor the clinical condition *in order to*
3. provide effective treatment and rehabilitation.

Note that there is no inherent virtue suggested for regular contact in its own right; no magical, healing properties are attributed to engagement. It is a tool, a prerequisite, for making a competent clinical assessment in order to offer effective treatment for an illness or disorder. This in no way devalues the prolonged efforts that may have to be spent in engagement or the wide-ranging support that may be necessary for a patient's precarious social survival (dealt with at some length in later chapters). What it emphasizes is that assertive outreach exists to provide treatments. If those treatments can be provided equally well by current services then there is little reason to establish a specific assertive outreach team.

This is an important point. We have been involved in discussions about setting up assertive outreach teams where it has become clear that they are either not needed or not viable. Patients who match the usual descriptions of candidates for this service can be identified, but local circumstances can profoundly affect the likely benefit of an assertive outreach service. For instance, in some rural areas excellent general practice and district nurse services, along with low morbidity and well-functioning CMHTs may meet many of the service objectives of a traditional assertive outreach team. Similarly, we have known proposals for assertive outreach to be hopelessly compromised by local 'political' complications (for example, where there are entrenched, local territorial conflicts between health and social services or between different components of a health care service). In these cases, although the patients and the need can be identified and the team recruited, the consequent complex accountability arrangements may prohibit the joint, flexible working that is essential to achieve the added benefits of assertive outreach.

We would also question the establishment of assertive outreach teams, as such, where there is no consensus on the existence of psychiatric illnesses or disorders. (A fuller discussion of this issue is beyond the scope of this book.) Even within teams that do broadly accept their reality there is continuing ambiguity surrounding the concepts of mental illness and the limits and extent of the 'medical model'. The relative prominence of such issues will also vary. For teams who are specifically targeting homeless or 'hard-to-engage' individuals, for example, the 'treatment' component may take a very secondary place to 'engagement'. There does, however, need to be some agreement on what will be offered when engagement has been achieved. This will vary according to the patient's needs, but a core of skills and therapeutic aspirations is required within the team.

For some social service based teams there is an important purpose served in attempting to make contact with isolated and vulnerable individuals, to determine whether they have significant unmet needs (for treatments, social support, financial aid, etc). Although these teams are assertive in the sense that they may repeatedly approach patients uninvited (and are often colourfully resisted!), they rarely aim at the high frequency contact which is usually considered an essential feature of assertive outreach as the term is currently used. These services, which assess needs and then organize appropriate provision to meet those needs, have more in common with assertive brokerage case management (Holloway *et al.* 1995). They rarely require the structure and approach addressed in this book.

Clinical opinion or evidence-based?

Clinical experience has gradually identified those patients whose care seems to be significantly improved by assertive outreach, and this has been supported by research evidence. Clinical experience and research have also helped identify subgroups of patients who are significantly more responsive and those who are likely to be less responsive to assertive outreach.

There is such a current preoccupation with evidence-based practice that clinical impressions and experience tend to be dismissed. It is important to remember that research findings invariably *follow after* clinical opinion. Experimental studies are conducted to test hypotheses, and hypotheses arise from clinical practice. Thus, the first major assertive outreach study (Stein and Test 1980) arose from Len Stein's conviction that patients with unstable psychotic illnesses would experience fewer relapses with this approach.

Major clinical studies involve considerable disruption and cost. They are not undertaken unless their protagonist is convinced that there is a significant likelihood of proving his or her point or of disproving a commonly held one with which they disagree. It is a common mistake to believe that where no formal research evidence is available for a treatment then that treatment is not justified. This is not true. The absence of research evidence does not negate clinical evidence for the effectiveness of a treatment. Where evidence and experience contradict one another, however, then we will give evidence precedence. This is not always straightforward. As detailed in Chapter 2 the applicability of research to your local situation needs to be carefully judged.

Which patients do benefit from assertive outreach?

Indicators from research studies

The weight of evidence favours the use of assertive outreach with *psychotic* patients and, in particular, those who relapse frequently, requiring hospital admission (Mueser *et al.* 1998). This may be somewhat circular as most of the research into assertive outreach has used hospitalization as the primary outcome measure. Consequently, only patients likely to relapse and be admitted during the trial period are usually studied. Patients with psychotic illnesses are those most studied and there is considerable clinical support for the belief that it is the *unstable*, often somewhat chaotic, younger psychotic patients who have most to gain. Within this psychotic group patients who are *poorly engaged* with services are also targeted, along with those with established patterns of *poor compliance* with previous treatment. As a consequence of poor compliance and poor engagement they often have an extensive history of *compulsory admissions*. Although it is hard to operationalize, most teams also try to prioritize patients who match the above description and have relapses that are 'more severe'. This usually means relapses associated with *high risk*—those who harm themselves or relatives or, for example, bipolar patients whose hypomanic episodes particularly threaten their social survival.

The above group of characteristics broadly defines the target population of most assertive outreach services. They are young psychotic patients, usually in the first 10–15 years of the illness, where relapses and positive symptoms predominate over negative symptoms and social disabilities. They are disproportionately male (often reflecting poor engagement and poor compliance) and are often impulsive and threatening when ill. Not surprisingly, many often have fearsome reputations within the service. Clinical experience, not supported as yet by strong research evidence, helps focus the patient target group more.

Ethnic minorities

Ethnic minority patients and, in particular (in the UK), many young black African–Caribbean patients may fit the above description. Controversy rages around whether these patients are poorly engaged and poorly compliant because services fail to meet their needs adequately or as a result of more fundamental and widespread cultural forces. Whichever is the case there is no doubting the difficulties encountered by mentally ill patients in ethnic minorities (Littlewood and Lipsedge 1997) and many assertive outreach services explicitly target them (UK700 Group: Creed *et al*. 1999).

Bipolar affective disorder

Severe bipolar affective disorder probably results in more social disruption than almost any other psychotic condition. It also has several other characteristics that fit it for assertive outreach. The mental state is fragile and markedly unstable, often with poor insight and poor medication compliance. The consequences of relapse can be quite disastrous (e.g. sexual disinhibition in an otherwise devout Muslim wife). This is a group of patients who often only have contact with the services when they are very ill and rapidly absent themselves when recovered. This disengagement from services is driven partly by the fact that the patient does make a significant and abrupt recovery, with little residual deficit, and afterwards feels embarrassed and ashamed of his or her behaviour during the manic episode. Getting to know these patients in depth, as real people, is only possible between episodes—hence the benefits of assertive outreach.

Psychosis and borderline learning disability

Although there have been no published studies of assertive outreach services deliberately targeting individuals with learning disability, such services are being created. The model fits well with traditional clinical practice with this group. A secondary analysis of the UK700 Intensive Case Management Trial demonstrated a preferential advantage to intensive outreach to patients with psychotic illness and lower IQ (UK700 Group: Tyrer *et al*. 1999). This finding emphasizes the benefits of targeting assertive outreach on individuals with multiple or complex needs.

Features of patients who benefit from assertive outreach

Agreed characteristics:

- A psychotic illness
- Fluctuating mental state / social functioning
- Poor compliance with prescribed treatment

> **Features of patients who benefit from assertive outreach** (*Continued*)
>
> ◆ Poor engagement with services / poor relationships
> ◆ Severe consequences of relapse
>
> **Emerging indicators**
>
> ◆ Ethnic minority patients
> ◆ Severe bipolar affective disorder patients
> ◆ Borderline intellectual disability

Which patients do not benefit from assertive outreach?

Starting up an assertive outreach team is often associated with an understandable surge of optimism. Now we will be able to really help all those patients where, up to now, we have been limited by time constraints! This is true of most patients who fit the characteristics outlined above, but there are some groups of patients who, despite the best intentions, do not seem to gain extra benefit.

Personality disorder patients

The selection of psychotic patients for assertive outreach focuses heavily on those who comply poorly with treatment and are difficult to engage. Not surprisingly, they are often patients who have been labelled as suffering from personality problems or even personality disorder in addition to their psychosis. Assertive outreach is an approach that targets individuals who have difficulty in forming and trusting relationships. Extrapolating from this, attempts have been made to use assertive outreach for individuals with a primary diagnosis of personality disorder. There are no scientific studies of these attempts yet. The accumulating clinical impression, however, is that it is not successful beyond the initial goals of engagement.

'Personality disorder' is a vague term, covering a mixed bag of problems, and there is no consensus on effective treatment. Treatments are usually targeted on individuals diagnosed with borderline personality disorder and are very intensive and institution-based rather than community-based (e.g. behavioural dialectical therapy) (Shearin and Linehan 1994). However, there are likely to be developments in this area and our current scepticism may soon be outdated.

Individuals with predominantly negative symptoms

Most CMHTs carry a significant number of individuals with long-term psychotic illnesses who lead a very restricted existence with poor quality of life. They are often characterized by negative symptoms of their psychosis with few, if any, productive symptoms such as hallucinations or delusions. We often think that assertive outreach will significantly improve the quality of their lives by introducing more structure, activity, and company, and that the consequence will be more motivation and self care. Experience has, however, been disappointing.

There are real benefits from structure and activity, as demonstrated by the original Three Hospitals' Study (Wing and Brown 1970), but assertive outreach does not seem to be any more successful in engaging such demotivated patients than CMHTs. It is likely that the level of contact already achieved by CMHTs is more a result of what the patients will tolerate than a capacity or operational issue for the team.

Forensic and offender patients

The clinical profile of a standard ACT team is likely to contain a number of patients with extensive offending behaviour. Just under 30% of those in our team have criminal convictions and a further 15% have offences without convictions. Attempts to target a purely forensic population have not been successful in the past and Solomon found that intensively managed forensic patients spent longer in prison (Solomon and Draine 1995*a* and *b*). To some extent this is circular if hospitalization is taken as the outcome measure. This is a patient group where decisions about discharge from hospital are likely to be determined more by restriction orders and the opinions of the courts than local clinical judgements.

We have had positive experience with offender patients but this is dependent on the severity of the offences. Serious offences such as arson and dangerous assaults impose severe restraints on community support. Forensic assertive outreach teams are being developed and evaluated currently and there should soon be better evidence on which to base decisions.

Nuisance crimes (such as repeated petty theft) are not uncommon and frequently pose ethical and treatment dilemmas. Police will often not press charges where the patient is known to be in receipt of intensive psychiatric care. Without legal sanctions to hold them to account (before delinquent behaviour escalates to dangerous crimes), patients are deprived of a normal and often necessary learning opportunity.

Which patients may benefit from assertive outreach?

Dual diagnosis: psychosis and substance abuse

An inevitable consequence of community care of severely mentally ill individuals is that they are not protected from the normal problems within society. The massive increase in drug and alcohol consumption which has affected Western societies since the Second World War has equally affected those with mental illness. Young men particularly acquire the bad habits of their peers and drink and abuse intoxicants to excess. This appears to be more of a problem in the US than in the UK, but still a significant minority of people with psychotic illnesses report a lifetime incidence of alcohol and drug abuse (Drake and Wallach 1993; Menezes *et al.* 1996; Scott *et al.* 1998).

Schizophrenia patients are marginally less likely to drink and use drugs to excess than the general population because they tend to be shy and generally less sociable.

The impact of drug and alcohol abuse on their long-term outcome is also complex. Some researchers have suggested that it is always worse, whereas others have been surprised to find similar or even better outcomes (UK700 Group: Laugharne *et al.* 2002). The speculation about these better results is that the patients who abuse drink and drugs are the less ill, less disabled individuals.

There is no doubt that in the short term substance abuse leads to a more chaotic existence for the patient and for his or her carers. It is highly likely that this is due to fluctuations in mental state as a direct consequence of episodic intoxication and, more importantly, of poor compliance with treatment resulting from a chaotic existence (Owen *et al.* 1996; Teague *et al.* 1995). Cannabis and alcohol are the two substances most widely used among young psychotic patients. Opiates and hallucinogens appear to be very rare in the UK, although heroin is reported as a significant problem in the US. Crack cocaine is still rare in the UK but invariably disastrous when it is used. The result is usually a highly unstable mental state and an equally unstable and highly charged series of manoeuvres dodging police and unpaid drug dealers.

Assertive outreach has been recommended as a preferred treatment option for dual diagnosis patients with substance abuse (Drake *et al.* 1989, 1993, 1998). Most published work has been from Drake's team in New Hampshire, where the substance abused is alcohol and the social environment relatively stable. Their results strongly emphasize an integrated assertive outreach approach with the same team dealing with both mental health and substance abuse problems, and a less forceful, slower style of substance abuse counselling. Their results are positive but not overwhelming. Currently, the balance of evidence would encourage ongoing work with dual diagnosis patients in assertive outreach teams, although whether they require a dedicated separate team is far from established.

First onset psychosis patients

First episode patients (often called 'first break' patients in the US) were not usually included in early assertive outreach services. This was partly because assertive outreach focused on frequently relapsing patients who absorbed a disproportionate amount of routine care. First episode patients also often make a good clinical recovery and there is understandable concern about not 'over-medicalizing' what may be a one-off breakdown.

More recent research has tended to suggest that although there is good clinical response in this first episode (hallucinations and delusions recede quickly when medicine is taken), there are other important, though subtle, changes occurring. These cause educational and vocational decline, loss of social supports, family stress, and possibly even cognitive impairment (McGlashan 1998; Szymanski *et al.* 1995). Although there is doubt about the consistency of these findings (Barnes *et al.* 2000), they have been very influential. One consequence has been to initiate public education programmes in a number of countries (e.g. Norway) (Johannessen 1998) to encourage general awareness in schools and families about psychosis and, through that, earlier detection and treatment.

Because of the range of health and social care needs identified in this group, and also because of the understandable reluctance of young patients to be involved in institutional care, assertive outreach has been the model most widely promoted. Some of the clinical teams reported from Australia have been very ambitious and include modules for medication management, psychoeducation, individual psychotherapy, coping skills training, etc. (Birchwood *et al.* 1997; Jackson *et al.* 1998). The UK National Service Framework (Department of Health 1999*a*) encourages the establishment of first episode teams and these are likely to be assertive outreach in form. Their aims are, in some important ways, different to those of routine assertive outreach teams. These are not necessarily 'revolving door' patients and, even when compliance and social stability has been achieved, there are pressing clinical and social problems still requiring their retention in the team.

Unlike dual diagnosis patients, where the question of including them in a general assertive outreach team or providing a separate service is debatable, there is nothing to be gained by including first episode patients in a general assertive outreach team. They will need their own team if it is to work.

The referral process

Assertive outreach is targeted on patients during the stormy, first half of their illness career. It is in the nature of both schizophrenia and bipolar disorder that, for those very severe ill patients, the first 10–15 years are often the worst and then things settle (Kendrick *et al.* 2000). To what extent this is a 'biological' process or one of adapting to the illness is unclear. There is nothing new about it however. The slogan 'once a patient, always a patient' was popular in the 1980s to emphasize the value of follow-up and continuity of care. We would dispute this anyway, but it is certainly not the case for assertive outreach.

If this expensive resource is to be efficiently targeted then patients should only be on the case load during that turbulent phase of their illness when stabilizing social and clinical functioning requires intensive input. When they have settled they can, and should, move back to CMHT care and possibly, eventually, GP care. Patients stay with our team an average of about 5–6 years. Obviously this is very much an average—some hardly engage with us and leave early, a few have been with us from the very start. A 6-year average means that key workers (with a case load of 12) expect two new patients a year. A well thought-through process to select and accept new patients into the service is necessary. Even more important, a rational approach must be developed for discharging patients back to routine CMHT care. This 'handing back' has been almost totally ignored in the literature.

Explicit criteria

It is vital to have basic, explicit criteria for accepting patients into the assertive outreach team. There are three important reasons for being so specific. Firstly, if the target patient group is not explicit colleagues will not know who to refer and the team is likely to 'drift'. We have suggested above the characteristics of this target group as derived from the research literature and our experience. There may be local reasons for modifying this. For instance, some areas of London, because of local population characteristics, are focusing on black African and Afro-Caribbean men; some central metropolitan areas prioritize the homeless and socially mobile. We would stress the need for this to be clearly stated and written down in the team's operational policy and any literature that it distributes about itself. It is both unfair on patients and a frustrating waste of time to receive lots of inappropriate referrals.

Secondly, there is also that natural human tendency to accept patients you like and get on with—even if these are not those whose unmet needs have been the reason for setting up the team. Similarly, if the definitions are not clear it is possible to exclude perfectly appropriate, though uncomfortable, candidates. There are many patients, such as those with stable, restricted lives, who are often emotionally rewarding to work with, grateful for the contact, and with ostensibly impressive gains (such as better benefits and keeping the flat cleaner), but who hardly justify this level of input. Unclear criteria can be used to discriminate against unattractive patients—'too dangerous', 'not motivated', 'a drinker', etc.

Thirdly, without explicit criteria the performance of the team cannot be monitored nor can the comparative needs of patients waiting for acceptance and those possibly nearly ready for discharge be balanced.

Who refers?

Despite explicit 'admission' criteria the decision to take on a patient is a clinical one. We always meet with the patient and undertake the assessment, either on the ward prior to discharge or in their home along with their current key worker. The assessment is by the team leader and one of the other clinical case managers (CCM). Obviously, the team leader has to have the final say as he or she is responsible for the appropriate allocation of the team's resources and knows its capacities. Involving another CCM ensures that there is discussion and also that they understand the process. Most often the CCM selected is the one who is most likely to take on the patient and the assessment is an opportunity to start the handover and engagement process. As well as being the best one to understand the team's capacity, the team leader is usually the one most aware of local political considerations which can have some bearing on selection, and certainly on prioritization. Familiarity with individual patients is essential when dealing with pressures from different referring teams for urgent action.

Diagnosis is rarely a controversial issue, so the assessment does not necessarily need a medical input. Where there is real uncertainty, involvement of a doctor may help. Patients who only suffer brief psychotic episodes when intoxicated with drink or drugs may need careful diagnosis and are probably best redirected towards addiction services. There has also been the odd case where a patient has been labelled as suffering from a psychosis after some brief disorganized episode although the overall history is one of a personality disorder. It is questionable that they have much to gain from an assertive outreach team.

Case study

One of our first patients suffered from a reclusive schizoid personality (later to be rediagnosed as a mild form of Asperger's syndrome). His notes carried forward a diagnosis of schizophrenia made years previously when his difficulties in explaining his problems had been taken as evidence of thought disorder. Not surprisingly he found regular contact unbearable and was successfully settled in a supportive but unintrusive hostel.

A waiting list?

Should an assertive outreach team have a waiting list? In truth it is rarely possible to operate without at least some delay in taking on new patients. It sometimes seems impossible to generate the impetus to discharge patients back to CMHTs unless there are at least one or two patients known to be waiting for the service. Given a turnover of about two patients per CCM (equivalent to 10–20 a year for a team, dependent on size), most teams will be accepting at least one new patient a month.

We would argue for a maximum waiting list of 3–4 months. There is no science to this but it seems to make sense. Long waiting lists are unwieldy and things can change rapidly. If there are 6–8 patients on the waiting list and it is known that, for example, nothing will happen for at least six months, then teams may simply not refer. More needy patients than those on the waiting list may be denied the consideration of referral. It is almost impossible to take someone off the waiting list once accepted, so keeping the list short helps to ensure that the assessment process is rigorous.

Where patients are currently in the ward there is a strong case for being involved in the discharge process and taking over care promptly. This inevitably means delays for those patients in the community. These difficult decisions about prioritization must pay due attention to each individual clinical case and should be taken by the team leader.

A minimum period of engagement

How long should one struggle with a patient before accepting that assertive outreach is not working? No system can guarantee to work with all the patients who meet its intake criteria. Some patients will simply not engage with us, any more than they will with the CMHT, and it becomes a waste of resource to continue abortive visits. Some show no improvement (either in clinical stability or community tenure) despite intensive contact. We offer all patients 12 months of engagement and support before we allow ourselves to make the decision that we have failed. Clinical experience is that this is longer than necessary but, although there are few 'breakthroughs' in the second half of the year, staff may otherwise begin to 'ease off' earlier if the target period is only 6 months.

We have refined this for patients accepted directly from the ward. Sometimes difficult patients, with fairly intractable relapses and behavioural difficulties, are discharged from hospital before they are really fit. Heavy medication allows them to tolerate a brief period outside hospital but, following their quick transfer to the assertive outreach team, they still have to return to hospital ultimately for a prolonged admission. For ward-based patients we have introduced a requirement for the CMHT to accept them back if they relapse immediately on discharge (within 2 months) and we see that we have no real opportunity of successfully engaging them. This does not mean that they *have* to be handed back but allows us the option if we judge that our assessment was hopelessly wrong.

Case study

A young African man with a 6-year history of schizophrenia was referred to the team. He had recently experienced his longest admission—on the ward for 8 months. Affective features, made much worse by heavy cannabis use, dominated his clinical picture. In his brief stable periods he revealed that he was intelligent, quite charming, and artistically gifted. At the time of his discharge to his flat and acceptance by the assertive outreach team he was on depot neuroleptics and high doses of benzodiazepines. He immediately increased his cannabis use and was threatening to both the CCMs and his girlfriend. He had to be compulsorily readmitted 10 days later after a vicious attack on his girlfriend. It then became clear that these attacks had been escalating for the last two years and that a charge for rape was being pursued against him, which had been 'inexplicably' overlooked in the referral. We agreed we would reassess him when he was really fit for discharge.

Discharge back to CMHTs

The need for throughput

Psychiatrists have described extensively the natural history of schizophrenia and the psychoses—perhaps best in the era before the introduction of effective treatments (Ciompi 1988). There is considerable variation—from a single episode followed by total recovery to chronic, unremitting deterioration. Most patients fall in the middle ground with an episodic course comprising periods of illness interspersed by longer periods of full or partial recovery. The most turbulent period is in the first 10–15 years and most patients settle after that. Assertive outreach is not necessary once this period is passed and it would be an inefficient use of resources (not to mention an unwelcome intrusion into patients' lives) to continue with it. Assertive outreach teams need to target their limited resources on those who need them most and this means that they must actively monitor their case loads and assess whether patients might not be equally well served by discharge back to CMHTs. Only by being alert to the need to discharge back to CMHTs when the patient's condition improves will the team maintain a capacity to care for those who need it.

Throughput is also important to refresh staff perspectives. The experiences of the large mental hospitals should warn us of the risks that staff can become 'institutionalized'. Without the constant challenge of new patients and new problems it is very easy to develop a narrow, sterile professional approach. It can be very difficult to distinguish recovery (when the illness has receded) from improved functioning as a consequence of continued, effective treatment. Only when a patient remains well even with reduced clinical input, can we be absolutely sure of recovery. We should not attribute all improvement to our ongoing input.

Currently our team experiences about 10% turnover per year. This means that with our case-load of 100 we discharge and accept about one new patient per month. For individual CCMs it represents a new patient each year and for individual patients it represents a potential time with the team of 10 years. These turnover targets are probably a bit low—case loads should perhaps change by 15–20% and the average time a patient spends with the team should be about 5 years. It is too early to be dogmatic about this matter since nothing has been published internationally on these matters and our own experience is restricted by the lifetime of the team.

Explicit criteria

While much is written about the criteria for acceptance into assertive outreach, very little is published about when to discharge patients. In our team we have agreed that any patient whose mental state and social functioning have been stable for two years (i.e. no admissions and no serious indications of relapse) should always be considered for discharge. This consideration takes place in the routine formal Care Programme Approach (CPA, DOH 1990) reviews and is usually initiated by the team leader when the CCM reports continuing stability. The criterion is for 'review for discharge', not for 'discharge'. There is an important difference. We know from past experience that some patients are only stable as long as they get intensive support. Where a previous attempt at withdrawal of support has resulted either in a rapid deterioration or in potentially dangerous situations then a longer period of stability may be decided upon.

Case study

A 50-year-old Afro-Caribbean woman with a 15-year history of severe bipolar affective disorder had been stabilized by the team using a regime of high-frequency but low-ambition contact—visits varying between daily and three times per week. Visits were short and the emphasis was on medication. All previous relapses had resulted in compulsory admissions, with the police having to break in; there had been a serious assault on the GP on one occasion and a policeman on another.

She is a very private woman who only grudgingly accepts our contact and rejects any expansion of our role. After 30 months of stability an attempt at reducing the frequency of contact was initiated as a precursor to discharge. She immediately refused access and rapidly deteriorated, requiring compulsory admission. She has now been stable for a further 3 years but we have decided to wait for evidence of a qualitative change in the relationship with us or her functioning before considering discharge again.

Where there is a total failure of engagement—defined simply as an inability to have face-to-face contact at least once a week—we consider discharge. A minimum of 12 months attempted engagement is our usual requirement, although in exceptional circumstances this may be short-circuited. We recently had a patient with whom we had not been able to achieve a second contact in 4 months; we agreed that there was nothing to be gained by continued fruitless visits to an empty flat.

Discharge, or transfer to another service, may be considered if, on balance, we judge that the team is not improving the patient's outcome. We would expect to take 1–2 years to come to this decision. Usually these are patients who made contact with us but do not accept treatments or continue to have a totally unchanged relapse pattern. On rare occasions we have to simply accept that we cannot support a patient out of hospital or that the costs of doing so are too great for the patient and his or her carers and those living around them. These are the 'new long-stay' or offender patients already referred to. It is important for an assertive outreach team to acknowledge that it will not always succeed with all patients.

The process of discharge

Handing patients back to CMHTs is not a simple process. Careful liaison is required, particularly when the assertive outreach team has not been successful. Before the patient can be handed back as 'successfully stabilized' it is essential that the level of support offered by the assertive outreach team has reduced to that which the CMHT would routinely offer. We make sure that the patient has been stable for at least 3 months on one contact a month. The 'step down' process of reducing to one contact a month usually takes about 3 months, so the discharge process takes a total of 6 months. During this time there is ample opportunity to work through issues of dependency and loss. CMHTs will not thank you for handing over patients who feel 'dumped' or who are utterly bereft at the loss of their long-term CCM. Discussion and education with the patient (and carers) is required to effect a successful transfer.

Where the discharge is because the assertive outreach team has not been successful, the issues are different. Here it is essential that the CMHT are not left feeling that they are being expected to achieve, with less resources, what the assertive outreach team failed to achieve with much greater resources. Often it is a matter of agreeing that there are some patients who cannot be engaged and may simply have to be admitted and treated when they present in relapse. Obviously this can change over time, but sometimes patients have to learn the benefits of continuing care the hard way. This is particularly true of some young manic patients. Paradoxically, being able to share the sense of defeat with the CMHT can sometimes help professional relationships—especially if the assertive outreach team is viewed as specially privileged.

Conclusions

Assertive outreach in one form or another has been a component of UK mental health practice for several decades. The introduction of assertive outreach teams, however, marks a major step forward in what has been, until now, a steady evolutionary process. Our view is still one of evolution rather than revolution, although the pace of change has radically altered. Two other factors have marked this 'faultline' in development. Firstly, the introduction of explicitly capped case loads (both individual and team). Secondly, a deliberate attempt to shape the service from the evidence base rather than local consensus and evolving practice. Both these features focus attention much more clearly on selecting the appropriate target patient group than has ever been the case before in CMHTs.

The referral and discharge processes are central to establishing the style and effectiveness of the team (or in CMHTs, the choice of patients for high-contact outreach). Evidence drives us towards patients with psychotic illnesses and histories of high service use—so called 'revolving door patients'. We have emphasized the importance of being clear which *effective treatments* the outreach offers that could not otherwise be delivered. We have followed the evidence and therefore selected a group of patients with long-standing, unstable psychotic illnesses with prominent symptoms for our service. It should not be forgotten, however, that research can only follow practice, not lead it. It may well be that assertive outreach is effective with other groups (e.g. personality disorders, substance abuse) and we simply do not have the evidence. A healthy respect for evidence-based practice should not lead to a slavish obedience. We have allowed a few patients into our service who do not meet our referral criteria and we will draw clinical conclusions over time.

Any border creates border disputes. If assertive outreach services are to remain targeted on those who need them most then they must maintain their boundaries. They must not only resist taking on those for whom there is little evidence of added value but must also discharge back to CMHTs those who have improved and no longer need intensive work. The same process occurs between CMHTs and GPs. Anticipate that secondary health care colleagues will inevitably gripe about this—either when you cannot take on someone ('Typical elitist new team!') or when you hand back ('We would have thought they could cure her!'). Managing referrals and discharges is, however, probably the most important long-term influence on how well the team works. Ducking the issues or, even worse, letting others determine them for you, will please no one ultimately.

Chapter 4

Ingredients and standards (model fidelity)

The ACT model of assertive outreach

Assertive outreach is one of the most argued about forms of mental health practice. This is because there is a highly prescriptive model of how one form of it (ACT) should be practiced (Allness and Knoedler 1998; McGrew et al. 1994; McGrew and Bond 1995; McHugo et al. 1999; Teague et al. 1998). People do not argue about whether or not a day hospital is a 'real' day hospital or not, but they do argue fiercely about whether or not an ACT team is 'a real assertive outreach team'.

ACT, as first implemented by Stein and Test (1980), has been taken as gospel. Because it was so successful it has been assumed that all aspects of their innovative approach are 'essential'. This belief has been strengthened by the often-quoted study by McHugo and colleagues (1999) in New Hampshire, which showed that 'high-fidelity' assertive outreach teams achieved better outcomes than 'low-fidelity' teams. Fidelity was assessed by measuring the degree to which the teams' performances matched the ACT standards (e.g. frequency of contact, *in vivo* practice) that they had all agreed to follow.

It will be clear from the content of this book that we do not accept this interpretation. Firstly, there has been little work conducted to identify which individual components of the ACT package are the effective ingredients. Which could be modified or even abandoned without affecting efficacy? The UK700 study (UK700 Group: Creed et al. 1999) is one of the first such studies designed to address this question by varying only one element of the ACT model (case load size). We would argue that each of the assumed essential ingredients has to be subjected to some form of testing, even if this does not need the rigour of a large multisite RCT. Secondly, the instruments used to measure ACT fidelity, such as the Dartmouth ACT scale (DACT, McHugo et al. 1999), have poor 'psychometric' properties. They are the result of 'expert opinion' rather than any attempt to test the proposition. Such expert opinion tends to be rather circular—experts are those who agree with the model and are committed to its implementation. There is nothing wrong in itself with collecting expert opinion but the papers published, and the measures derived, are often quoted as if they reflected empirical knowledge. They do not. They are opinions—good opinions for the most, but only opinions.

Perhaps we should think more in terms of indicators of good practice in assertive outreach rather than absolute standards. Indicators would include a clearly defined target group of patients and a model that emphasized engagement and individualized, intensive, and comprehensive care.

The failure to implement a model of care faithfully may tell us something about the individuals providing that care. It has been shown in psychotherapy research that poor adherence to a range of accepted practices is associated with poorer outcomes, without that necessarily meaning that a specific model is inferior. Exploratory therapists who follow closely the principles of exploratory therapy do better than exploratory therapists who do not; interpersonal therapists who stick to the rules do better than those who do not (Rounsaville *et al.* 1988); and so on. But we have no evidence that exploratory therapy is better than interpersonal therapy.

Comparative studies may tell us more about the therapists than the treatments. Therapists who deviate from their model do less well—it is the deviation that matters. Such deviation presumably indicates casual practice or lack of focus and, therefore, it is not surprising that the results are poorer. Until individual components of assertive outreach practice have been demonstrated to effect outcome significantly then the claims made about the central need for model fidelity should be taken with a pinch of salt. There is every reason to continue to explore and develop the model. Purists who treat Len Stein's model as holy writ, hewn on tablets of stone, are doing neither him nor ACT a service.

Components of assertive outreach

The components of assertive outreach have been described in many ways and at different conceptual levels. Tyrer has suggested that it is primarily a way of thinking (Tyrer *et al.* 1999) and Len Stein has stated clearly that it is only a vehicle for delivering effective treatments and that it is these treatments that matter (Chapter 3). Assertive outreach is an effective vehicle for delivering these treatments, so getting it right does matter. A good starting point is to describe the organizational and process features that define it (Kent and Burns 1996). These are the features that are used to measure model fidelity. Most will be without controversy even if supporting evidence is lacking, but not all. We will highlight individual components where there doubt about their importance.

Key elements of the PACT model

- A core services team is responsible for helping the patient meet all of his/her needs and provides the bulk of clinical care.
- Improved patient functioning (in employment, social relations, and activities of daily living) is a primary goal.
- The patient is directly assisted in symptom management.
- The ratio of trained staff to patients should be small (no greater than 10–15:1).

> **Key elements of the PACT model (*Continued*)**
>
> - Each patient is assigned a key worker responsible for ensuring comprehensive assessment, care, and review by themselves or by the whole team (note Chapter 5).
> - Treatment is individualized between patients and over time.
> - Patients are engaged and followed up in an assertive manner.
> - Treatment is provided *in vivo*, in community settings—skills learnt in the community can be better applied in the community.
> - Care is continuous both over time and across functional areas.
>
> Adapted from Test (1992)

In vivo practice

Whatever else it does, assertive outreach requires staff to leave their offices to visit and treat patients in their homes and neighbourhoods. Assertive outreach is not an office-based or out-patient, clinic-centred practice. At the very least, three out of every four contacts need to be on the patient's territory if it is to match current UK practice by CPNs with their psychotic patients (Burns *et al.* 2000). The PACT program standards (Allness and Knoedler 1998) quantify a modest 75% or more of the services to be delivered outside the office—a figure comparable to standard care in the UK.

There are several reasons for this core aspect of the approach. Stein and Test originally considered their approach to be 'training in community living'—a recognition that a skill learnt in one setting was often not easily transferable to the most relevant situations for the patient. Training in daily living skills (e.g. using a washing machine) in an institutional setting was of little value if the machine in the patient's local laundrette had a totally different set of controls. These difficulties in transfer of learning in patients with psychotic illness (originally called 'concrete thinking') have been long recognized. *In vivo* practice enables appropriate skills to be learnt where they will be applied. Whether this is primarily a learning process or a support process will be dealt with later (Chapter 24).

In vivo practice is also invaluable in ensuring that the ongoing assessment of patients' disabilities, needs, and strengths is comprehensive. It is only in the individual's personal situation that accurate assessments can be made—it is not unusual to find that somebody who appears quite helpless in the hospital has well-developed routines and survival strategies at home (Perkins and Burns 2001). Only in the patient's home and neighbourhood can stressors and strengths be fully appreciated.

Outreach is also of great importance because people with severe mental illnesses are poor at attending appointments. At the very least they tend to lead disorganized lives and often lose letters and forget the date or become distracted by some other event. They are very unlikely to have a car and the hassle of getting to a clinic by bus or walking may seem insuperable when they are feeling low or unwell. Many may simply not

Case study

A middle-aged woman with long-standing paranoid illness was noted at out-patients to be anxious and losing weight. She said that she was lonely but could not get to the shops to buy food and found her neighbourhood threatening. Initially her antipsychotics were increased.

On a home visit, however, her CPN tried to take her shopping to 'confront and desensitize her anxiety'. She found that the route from the flat to the shop was past a very rough school where the patient was taunted and harassed by teenage boys. It was this that frightened her. The CPN worked out an alternative (though somewhat longer) route while approaching the headmaster about the boys (in vain).

During her visit a neighbour approached her and commented that she had known of the patient for several years and would love to help but 'did not want to interfere'. An introduction was arranged and soon the patient was regularly walking the older neighbour's dog and occasionally spending the evening in her flat watching TV together. Both seemed to really enjoy the company.

believe they need to keep appointments, either lacking insight that they have an illness at all or having little appreciation of the importance of their treatment (or wanting to avoid it because of side-effects!). For such individuals outreach, or *in vivo* practice, is the only way of successfully maintaining contact, developing effective engagement, and thereby having the opportunity of delivering effective treatments. The need to keep patients successfully engaged is one of the most consistent findings of assertive outreach studies (Marshall and Lockwood 1998): there is no controversy about its central importance.

Reasons for *in vivo* practice

- Maintaining contact
- Poor transfer of learning
- Comprehensive assessment

Small case loads

ACT teams usually insist that case loads should be small and fixed. In the US a maximum of 10 patients per full-time CCM is usually quoted (Allness and Knoedler 1998), although in clinical practice this often rises to 12–15 when a number of the patients are well settled. Experienced CCMs in established ACT teams warn against too rigorous an insistence on very small case loads. The work can become monotonous or (even worse for the patient) over intense and emotionally claustrophobic. A small case load is deemed essential, however, so that staff can maintain regular and frequent contact, and also so that they have the time to provide a wide range of inputs. These might include supporting a patient's leisure activities (e.g. going together to a football match, organizing a cinema visit or an outing), which is not possible without adequate protected time.

Frequent and flexible contacts (see below) require small case loads. In the UK a contact frequency of twice per week is hardly possible with case loads of over 1:12 per full-time worker. While there is no experimental evidence about what is the optimal case-load size, few would argue that the benefits of assertive outreach over routine CMHT practice can be achieved with case loads of over 12–15 per worker.

Frequent and flexible contact/crisis response

Patients' needs vary over time and assertive outreach staff need to be able to vary (or 'titrate' as it is often called) their input. This applies to both the focus of the visit and frequency. A basic routine of visiting, perhaps at a regular time once or twice a week, can be reassuring. But changes in mental state, crises in relationships, or times of stress (such as a flat being decorated or repair works being carried out) require increased visiting. A hallmark of good teams is that they can easily visit a patient daily for extended periods of time and, similarly, can provide joint visits with team colleagues at a moment's notice (for instance, if the patient is hostile). Staff must ensure that they have enough spare capacity in their schedules to respond immediately and with good grace. Team leaders have to see that CCMs do not overbook their schedules—if they have too many routine visits planned they can neither respond to their own patients' changing needs or to other team members.

Learning to 'back off' for a time is also an important part of good assertive outreach working. Maintaining contact that is not immediately clinically driven can be an essential part of engagement (Chapter 10). Similarly, patients often like to have some breathing space when things are going well. We often drop to weekly contact when things are going smoothly. Falling below this (which does sometimes happen) needs team agreement. The research evidence supporting the frequency and content of contacts is well summarized by Charles Rapp of the University of Kansas:

> Three conclusions seem warranted: first, frequency of case manager/client contact rather than hours of contact makes a difference; the use of the telephone may be a helpful supplement not a replacement. Second, frequency of contact and hospital outcomes will never be truly linear since those who are most ill will often receive the most contact but may also have higher rates of hospitalisation (even if reduced compared to similar control subjects). The third conclusion is that the quality of contact, not just frequency, may be a mitigating factor. For example, small caseloads employing ineffective methods or skill-deficit case managers would probably be ineffective.
>
> (Rapp 1998)

Crisis work has been a central tenet of assertive outreach since Stein and Test's original paper. Organizing the team so that an immediate response can be mobilized is crucial. A rapid response to failing compliance with daily supervised medication is one measure of flexibility and is a crisis response well worth the investment. Such flexibility needs to be at team level, not just a feature of individual case manager functioning. Even if crises have been well spotted in advance, situations can arise where a rapid intervention can modify if not prevent unwanted outcomes.

Case study

Robert is a patient the team considers we have done well with—admissions down from twice a year to about one every two years and of shorter duration. He has his own flat but refuses any form of structured daily activity. All relapses are characterized by increased cannabis use, withdrawal from services (often sleeping away), and eventual violence. This results in admission either by police on Section 136 or a Section 3 requiring the tactical support squad.

He had been out of contact for nearly three weeks and arrived back home aroused, threatening, and psychotic; he attacked his brother. Police and a social worker were rapidly on the scene and admission was both inevitable and welcome. Two team members went to the scene to take part in the admission process. This helped moderate the potential conflict with the police (who had genuine cause to be worried) and, also, one could stay behind and reassure and support his distraught mother.

As teams become longer established they find that the emphasis on crisis work is less. Staff know their patients better, are aware of stressors, and become increasingly sensitive to early warning signs of relapse. The emphasis shifts more to crisis prevention than crisis intervention. It is important, however, not to become complacent—crises will occur. The ability of the team to respond rapidly and coherently is an important measure of its effectiveness.

Comprehensive care (health and social)

Assertive outreach teams have a style of working that could be characterized as a form of 'one-stop shopping' in the care of the severely mentally ill. Wherever the team judges that it can meet the patient's need for care it endeavours to do it without requiring them to get involved with other care agencies. In this way assertive outreach is a response to fragmented and discontinuous services. The team offers continuity of care across functional and service boundaries as well as over time (Test 1992).

In recognition of the difficulties that most of our patients have in asking for what they need and in trusting authority figures we attempt to provide a broad-ranging health and social care service to them. Stabilization of both mental state and social supports go hand in hand. It is not possible to contain anxiety if you are facing possible eviction or if you are moving around from temporary accommodation to temporary accommodation.

Costed care and benefits

Care management (the provision of costed social care such as hostels and meals) which is provided by local authority social workers has to be assessed, justified, and accounted for through borough finances. This has traditionally involved structured, bureaucratic processes. Health care, on the other hand, has traditionally been left to professional discretion and funded from within an amorphous NHS budget.

Assertive outreach teams have to learn quickly how to access the most common social care components. This means that case managers with backgrounds in nursing or occupational therapy need to familiarize themselves with the complexities of the benefits procedures and become skilled in applying for the range of financial supports for which individuals with severe mental illness are eligible (Chapter 20). Optimally, the assertive outreach team should contain at least one social worker, as this eases enormously such negotiations with the local authority. Failing that there is often a need for clear arrangements to ensure that the local authority, benefits agencies, and housing departments will accept the assessments conducted by health care workers for such provision.

Although many case managers initially do not like the idea of all this form filling, they quickly learn that patients appreciate their efforts. Getting a community care grant for furniture or an increase in disability benefit for a new patient is often a very successful step in supporting engagement. It certainly makes clear to the patient that you are on their side. We have found virtually all the organizations that we have had to work with are very obliging. Apart from applications for very expensive, longer-term accommodation it has been very rare for us to be asked for the social worker's opinion in preference to the key worker's. Those organizations with which we have little contact may still require a doctor to fill out an application. Obviously, some introduction of the team is essential at the start and staff have to accept that they will often be referred to as the patient's CPN or social worker—although this is happening less.

Role of social workers

Initially, the establishment of assertive outreach teams generated some concerns in social work as the level of what is traditionally social work activity conducted by case managers is very high and very prominent. This concern has receded—social workers are as hard pressed as any of us! Inevitably, if social workers are recruited as case managers, the reverse situation will also arise. Social workers find themselves assessing mental states, delivering medicines, and even examining patients for side-effects of drugs. In truth, this is not that radical—psychiatric social workers have always done this. In the assertive outreach team, however, it is explicit and visible. The recognition of the value of generic work and the need to cross the health and social care divide routinely ensures that this causes no problem in assertive outreach teams. Indeed, this breaking of stereotypes often strengthens team identity. The social worker insists that the patient needs an increase in his anti-psychotics, the nurse asserts that the medicines are not going to do that much good until we can find some useful structured daytime activity for the patient.

A recent systematic review of home-based mental health care (Burns *et al.* 2001*a*) suggested that provision of health and social care from within the same team is a core feature of successful services. Its effect on outcome probably derives from efficient co-ordination of the essential components of care. It is also likely that the shift of focus from predominantly medical assessments and treatments makes the case manager much more acceptable to the patient. The latter feels that he or she is being treated as a person—not just a set of problems.

Mainstreaming

This emphasis on comprehensive care should not detract from the importance of 'mainstreaming' (i.e. encouraging patients to use non-mental health facilities where possible, thereby promoting their reintegration). Often, as the patient makes progress, the case manager may actively encourage them to seek social services support through routine channels. This is both to promote the patient's increasing independence and also to reduce the burden on the assertive outreach team. The guiding principle is that the patient should get comprehensive input to his health and social care needs from the team. The decision to access alternative sources of support should be a clinical one made in consultation with the patient, not one driven by restrictive professional practices.

Multidisciplinary care/team working

Successful assertive outreach requires close multidisciplinary working. Early brokerage studies in the US with non-clinical staff (Curtis *et al.* 1992; Franklin *et al.* 1987) and some intensive home-based approaches by exclusively nursing teams (Muijen *et al.* 1994) quickly demonstrated the limitations of such approaches. Our patients have complex and varied needs and it requires a range of skills to keep them well. Case managers can learn many of these skills and indeed do so. It is one of the attractions of working in such teams that there is such opportunity for skill sharing and learning. But in order to share skills there has to be someone in the team with those skills!

Perhaps the breadth of perspective is just as important as the range of skills that comes from a multidisciplinary team. Case reviews in such teams usually involve a discussion that touches on several differing points of view and differing ways of conceptualizing the problem. Sometimes these differences are more of language than fundamental disagreement about approach (see Chapter 26 on 'Managing the team'). However, it reminds everyone that there are alternatives, and that the process of discussion is in itself valuable. Teams composed of simply doctors and nurses often become sterile and rigid in their thinking as there are not sufficient differences in their approaches or in their conceptual models.

How many disciplines constitutes 'multidisciplinary'?

It is generally accepted that there needs to be at least three professions represented in a mental health team for it to be multidisciplinary. Some would argue that UK CMHTs should have a minimum of four disciplines, as three of them (medicine, nursing, social work) are statutory 'essentials' in the team. The doctor could restrict himself to assessments, prescribing, and mental health act duties; the nurse to delivering direct care and treatment; and the social worker to care management and mental health act work. Of course it rarely happens like this, but the addition of one of the non-mandatory professions (e.g. occupational therapy, clinical psychology) radically alters the dynamic. Their role is to add value—to improve the basic care. They must, if they are to achieve this, promote wider clinical discussions and broader reviews.

The weight of current opinion (Teague *et al.* 1995, 1998) is that psychiatrists are an essential part of the assertive outreach team, or indeed of any home-based care team for mental illness (Burns *et al.* 2001*a*). It would be impossible to run such a service without nurses, given the central importance of delivering and monitoring medications for psychotic patients, and they are the backbone of any UK team. In the US and Germany, social workers tend to dominate, with a nursing presence to ensure adequate medication. In the UK, a social worker is desirable. Assertive outreach teams have, however, managed without them, by drawing on duty social workers and CMHT social workers. Most team members quickly acquire a basic competence in social care.

Occupational therapists have proved themselves invaluable members of teams bringing a more experienced and structured approach to the assessment of problems associated with daily living skills and organizing meaningful activity. We have found them to be particularly adept at constructing rehabilitation programmes to help patients to return to some form of work. Their training in the 'use of the self' in mental health work provides a framework for many of the inevitable discussions around personal/ professional boundaries that arise in assertive outreach.

Few teams have succeeded in the UK in recruiting clinical psychologists. In part this reflects the job market but it may also derive from some resistance by psychologists to the more generic aspects of the role. This is a particular pity as many of the psychosocial skills appropriate for this form of work are highly developed within clinical psychology. International literature tends to be misleading as the term 'psychologist' is often applied to non-clinical graduates.

The issues surrounding the 'team approach' versus a key working role are dealt with in more detail in Chapter 5 and those concerning extended hours and 24-hour availability in Chapter 6.

Medical involvement

Psychiatrists have been integral members of outreach teams (whether they be more traditional CMHTs or ACT teams) from their inception. The DACT scale (Teague *et al.* 1998) rates the level of provision of an integrated psychiatrist as a core measure of model fidelity, suggesting up to one full-time psychiatrist for teams of 100 patients. Stein and Test's original study involved a team with a dedicated psychiatrist who was responsible for maintaining a focus on adequate medication. A recent systematic review of all forms of home-based care (Burns *et al.* 2001*a*) clearly indicates the significance of integrated medical input.

Support workers

Most US teams employ non-professional 'aides' who carry out both skilled and less skilled tasks in direct patient care. In the UK, support workers are involved in the whole team's case load; they do not have their own case load or care programme approach (CPA) key worker responsibility. Nethertheless, support workers will have clients that they see regularly and with whom they establish excellent therapeutic relationships. Their ability to engage with clients who may distrust the professionals (who carry more statutory responsibilities or have less 'street credibility') is invaluable. In our team the support worker is involved in supervising patients' self-medication, assessing mental state, practical assistance with shopping or transportation, and even venepuncture for clozapine blood monitoring.

Voluntary sector teams

Although the literature on assertive outreach is unambiguous about the need for medical involvement, and indeed the need for persistent and vigorous treatment, more recent developments have introduced doubts about it. In particular, the UK policy emphasis on assertive outreach as a service targeted on 'hard to engage' individuals (NSF 1999) has led to the development of such teams with a significantly reduced medical focus. These teams may be run by social services or the voluntary sector and prioritize non-threatening and long-term efforts at engagement. They will often see their role as encouraging disaffected and marginalized individuals to re-establish contact with health services, but not provide direct care themselves. They may not take formal responsibility for the patient (e.g. not take CPA responsibility) and often have a high proportion of non-professional staff. Many will have a significant input from user staff.

Such teams often have specific target groups—ethnic minority patients (in particular black African and African–Caribbean psychotic individuals) or homeless individuals. They clearly do play an important role in large anonymous cities, but their very individuality and variation makes detailed consideration outside the scope of this book. Many, though not all, of the approaches outlined here will be appropriate to most of them. Without a medical member there is no scope for initiating and effectively monitoring drug treatments or using hospital care routinely.

Such approaches are clearly exciting developments from which there will be much to learn; they cannot, however, be considered evidence-based. Assertive outreach teams established without medical involvement can not yet be recommended as a core component of a comprehensive mental health policy.

Alternative methods

Assertive community treatment is at the intensive and more medical end of a spectrum of models of case management for the severely mentally ill. ACT has, because of its medical and scientific bias, been subject to the most research. It has clearly become the dominant model and the one largely envisaged by the UK Government when it published *A National Service Framework for Mental Health* (Department of Health 1999a), *The NHS Plan* (Department of Health 2000), and *The Mental Health Policy Implementation Guide* (Department of Health 2001). Nevertheless, other articulated models do exist.

Brokerage case management (Intagliata 1982) is at the opposite end of the spectrum. It is neither intensive nor does it involve *in vivo* direct care provision. Brokerage links

Table 4.1   Elements of case management

	ACT	Brokerage	Strengths	Rehabilitation
Direct service provisions	Yes	No	Yes	Yes
Location	*In vivo*	Office-based	*In vivo*	*In vivo* or clinic/hostel/ hospital setting
Case load size	10–15	Up to 50	20–30	20–30
Frequency of contact	High	Low	Moderate	Moderate
Shared case loads/team approach	Yes	No	No	No
24-hour availability	Often	No	No	No

patients to appropriate services after assessment and care planning. Brokers are expected to monitor this care but not to provide it. Brokerage is therefore the only model that is not clinical case management.

The 'strengths model' (Rapp and Wintersteen 1989) has an articulated philosophy based on consumerism and engagement following the patient-led agenda. As the name suggests, the focus is on individual strengths rather than deficits or pathology. It stresses that people with severe and enduring mental illness can learn, grow, and change using the resources of their own communities, and aided by assertive outreach.

Rehabilitation-orientated case management draws on the principles of psychiatric rehabilitation such as working to reduce handicaps and disabilities. Put another way, the emphasis may be biased towards improving the patient's functioning rather than frequent and intensive efforts to manage symptomatology and community tenure.

Table 4.1 summarizes in broad terms the four commonly cited models of case management:

Conclusions

Assertive outreach benefits from having a clear model—or rather it did benefit. Starting with a rather charismatic service and strikingly successful evaluation, its configuration was accepted lock, stock, and barrel. Over the last 20 years confirmation of the value of the approach has accrued but also, perhaps, a realization that not all its components are equally important. There is an understandable tension between the desire to replicate a successful service and the desire to vary it somewhat so that the relative contributions of its components can be assessed. It is possible that not all were necessary anyway— the history of medicine is littered with unnecessary procedures being continued because they were originally associated with effective ones.

It is also likely that changes in the context in which the services are provided affect the importance of individual aspects. For instance, the brokerage emphasis (i.e. linking patients up with existing services) in early US case management (Holloway *et al.* 1995) faded rapidly as statutory services became better organized and more readily accessible. This emphasis is now being rediscovered in assertive outreach services in the voluntary sector for specially targeted groups such as the homeless.

The benefits of having a clear model with identifiable, essential components are enormous. There is, however, a risk of rigidity, of an ideology, arising around what is and is not 'real assertive outreach'. Such rigidity can be strengthened by the development of measures of model fidelity. Assertive outreach is probably the only mental health service structure to be subject to such measures. This, combined with the failure of later studies to totally confirm the magnitude of impact of earlier ones (a common finding in almost all health services' research), has led to heated debate. Key working versus the team approach and 24-hour availability versus extended hours are the two aspects of the original service description which give rise to most controversy. Because of their importance they are each given their own chapters.

Chapter 5

Key working versus the 'team approach'

In England and Wales, the care programme approach (CPA) (Department of Health 1990) requires that all individuals with mental health problems who are being cared for by specialist services should be registered on the CPA and that each should have a designated 'key worker'. There have been various changes to this legislation and changes of terms (Department of Health 1990). What was originally called 'higher level' CPA metamorphosed through 'levels 2 and 3' to 'enhanced'. 'Key worker' has sadly been renamed 'care co-ordinator', thereby perpetuating the confusion between broker-age and clinical case management (and possibly CPA and social services care management) (Burns 1997b).

Key workers are responsible for ensuring that their patient's care programme is kept up to date, carried out, and properly co-ordinated. While they may not be responsible for all aspects of care patients receive they are usually responsible for the major part of it. This is a model of care that is well established and fits well with traditions of multidis-ciplinary working. Trained professionals work together but shoulder appropriate individual responsibility.

The team approach is often proposed in stark contrast to the individual case manager or key worker required by the CPA. It is seen as a profoundly different approach. When some European studies have failed to find the same advantages for assertive outreach, the absence of a 'team approach' has been cited as a cause (Marshall 1996; Marshall et al. 1999).

Pathological dependency

In the original Madison team Stein was particularly exercised to reduce or prevent 'pathological dependency'. He had worked for a considerable period in a state mental hospital and was vividly aware of the risks of institutionalization (Barton 1959). The long-term mentally ill were often demoralized and anxious and, in such settings, read-ily lost initiative and self-confidence. The more the institution automatically met their needs the more dependent they became on it and, over time, less able to organize their own lives. Stein and his colleagues saw this lack of self-determination and competence as probably the major barrier for such patients in re-establishing an independent life outside hospital. The thinking behind the original team was very much along these lines—hence it was first called 'training in community living' (TCL), not 'assertive community treatment' (ACT).

Stein and his colleagues were also well versed in the psychodynamic theories that were current at that time. They knew that long-term relationships, when there is a significant imbalance in power (real or perceived) between those involved, can inhibit personal growth and self-determination. This concept of 'pathological dependency' is dealt with in detail in psychodynamic literature. Essentially, it is based in the observations that individuals with mental health problems often come to therapy with very low self-esteem. The very act of asking for help can be quite humiliating for adults who generally expect to be able to sort out their own problems. The experiences which have led them to seek help have often involved quite vivid and public confirmation that they are 'failing' in some way. This could be a demotion at work, a marital breakdown, or (as with many of our patients) failing globally at studies and employment because of their breakdowns, compounded by traumatic and disruptive hospital admissions.

Starting from this low ebb, the therapist's competence at helping the patient feel better can, paradoxically, reinforce their sense of inadequacy and personal failure. Each step forward confirms the gap between the patient's and therapist's personal competence. It underlines how much the patient needs the therapist and, therefore, how inadequate they are. Obviously, most therapy does not go this way, but some can. It was in order to reduce the risk of such pathological dependency that Stein advocated the team approach.

What is the 'team approach?

The team approach is based on the need for the patient to relate to all members of the team, not just their own special worker. If one case manager was responsible for too much of the patient's care then that relationship could become very unbalanced. The patient could view the case manager as supremely competent, in stark contrast to how they felt about themselves. They might attribute too much authority to that individual just as they had done to the hospital before them, and fail to develop confidence in their own autonomy. To counteract this, the team organized its work so that no patient could become over-dependent on any one staff member.

Similarly, a team approach lifts some of the burden from the staff member—it is not all their fault if things go wrong. Sharing the load across the whole team can prevent therapeutic pessimism. It avoids resentments building up between a key worker and a patient. It would be naïve to believe that such tensions do not occur—or that they are only one way. A well-managed team needs to be able to accept honestly that staff members can become exasperated and fed up with patients as well as vice versa. Being professional does not mean being a robot. Intensive, long-term work engages the case manager as a whole person and that inevitably brings stresses into the therapeutic relationship that need to be acknowledged.

The development of any special or exclusive relationship is prevented by actively ensuring that different parts of the care package are delivered by different team members.

In a very pure form, the same intervention is deliberately rotated between different team members (Bond *et al.* 1990). Sometimes the patient does not know the name of who is coming to visit them, just the agreed time and purpose and that it will be someone from the team. Although the DACT does quantify 'teamness' by asking how many patients have contact with more than one case manager in a given month, no published studies give any such data. Despite this absence of explicit knowledge of how it works in practice (or perhaps because of such an absence!) there are intensely held views in assertive outreach about the importance of the team approach.

The US emphasis on the team approach also needs to be understood in the context of their mental health practice of 20 years ago. This was then very individualistic, with a significant culture of isolated, office-based psychiatrists and little, if any, team work outside institutions. The situation in the UK was quite the reverse, with no tradition of individual psychiatrists working with the severely mentally ill. Teamwork has been the norm, spearheaded by social workers and CPNs in the community. The risks of unsupervised pathological relationships have always been less.

Current position

We have rejected the orthodoxy of the team approach for a number of reasons. Firstly, it simply does not square up with our experience of how individuals with long-term severe mental illness function. As a group they tend to be shy and have difficulty forming relationships. Certainly those hard-to-engage individuals targeted by assertive outreach teams have profound difficulties in establishing a relationship of trust. It takes time, commitment, and consistency to do it. Our clinical experience is that for anxious, suspicious individuals it is best to start with building up one relationship and then, gradually, extend the network. Some patients may never accept contact with more than one or two staff.

Secondly, we are also sceptical of the approach because our experience teaches us that the road to independence is through a period of healthy and supportive dependence. After all, we all became adults by slowly gaining our independence from our parents. We are convinced that well-trained staff can manage the therapeutic relationship (with adequate supervision) so that it meets legitimate dependency needs but supports healthy growth and avoids an inward-looking and claustrophobic bond.

Thirdly, there are also practical drawbacks with the team approach. Such a 'task-centred' approach has been superseded within in-patient nursing teams by the 'named nurse' system. The hospital setting is much more suitable to such a team approach—regular face-to-face contact of the team, continuous awareness and monitoring of a limited group of patients. Despite this, the task-centred approach is inefficient. It takes too much time and energy to administer and supervise—the continual allocation of tasks which have to be reported back on, the large amount of time needed to impart and share information and check that everything has been done. Also, patients do not like it. They want the security of knowing that some recognizable individual has an overview of their needs and brings continuity to ensuring their welfare. They also want an identified individual to turn to when they are worried and who they know will take a prolonged and proactive interest in their care and progress.

Mostly, we are sceptical because the reality and the rhetoric do not match up. During a study trip to many of the demonstration ACT teams in the US, one of us (TB) checked it out. While out on visits with case managers he routinely asked them who else was working with the patient they had just visited. Nearly always the answer was 'nobody— that's my patient'. This despite usually being told by the team leader during the visit induction that the service operated a fully developed 'team approach'. Key working seemed to survive the theory!

One report from a US team clearly states the potential drawbacks of the team approach:

> The team method of case management is time consuming and manpower intensive. Staff over-saturation with frequently changing information often results in long or incessant meetings, or communication attempts that are sometimes spurious. Staff have a tendency to 'tune out' because of over-arousal or overflow. Additionally, another problem with team case management is accountability in a system where there is no primary care manager except for charting, with resultant ambiguity about who will do the follow-up after treatment planning.

> (Degen *et al.* 1990)

How great is the difference?

In reality, the distinction between the two approaches is less than is portrayed. UK assertive outreach teams invariably offer a small network of carers within the team for most patients. At its very least there needs to be an identified secondary key worker to ensure that leave and sudden sickness are covered. We have found it valuable to ensure that joint working between the key worker and the secondary key worker is a reality— not just an administrative safety net. Patients requiring high levels of visiting, especially daily supervised medication, soon become used to most of the team. Often, certain team members will have special skills which involve them in the treatment of another key worker's patient (e.g. a nurse has to give the depot injection to an OT's patient, an OT has special expertise in finding employment and helps a social worker's patient with this). This is, however, very different from deliberately avoiding special relationships and spreading tasks around the team.

In a team that has run for several years it is quite possible for all staff to have had direct care experience with all the patients. It is virtually true for our service to 100 patients and should certainly be the case in smaller teams. Having direct contact makes handovers more meaningful and also improves the quality of contributions that the team members can make to routine and emergency reviews. This team-level discussion and monitoring of progress can also guard against introverted, pathological relation-ships. The team can comment when they see the key worker becoming over-concerned and preoccupied with detail. They also note when clinical goals have become restricted because of over-familiarity or staleness in the relationship.

Case study

A case manager reported at the second routine six-monthly review in a row that his patient had remained gratifyingly stable; there had been no crises. His colleagues congratulated him on how well things had settled (this had been a very volatile patient). However, they reminded him that a goal of pushing for structured daytime activitiy had been considered at the last presentation but rejected as premature. Now it should be the goal. The key worker had, understandably, focused on stabilizing the patient's medication compliance, almost to the exclusion of all else. His team-mates helped him raise his sights.

Not only that but the team can, and often does, offer to take over the load for a period if a relationship is particularly trying. By direct familiarity with the patient they can give advice and help without having to rely on the key worker volunteering the concern.

Case study

The team had been shaken by an unexpected suicide when a young man, who had been doing well, had committed suicided by jumping from a balcony. He had recently got a part-time voluntary job after years of a chaotic and semi-vagrant life. He had also, thanks to dogged detective work by his key worker, re-established contact with his mother, apparently to both their delight. The suicide was debriefed in the usual manner (see Chapter 26).

Over the next few months it became clear that the key worker had upped his level of monitoring across all his patients, especially one who had attempted suicided by jumping in the past. The level of close monitoring seemed to be raising, rather than reducing, his level of anxiety.

The team was able to discuss how most found themselves worrying when patients became stable after long periods of psychosis and when they started to talk about their 'wasted years'. We all recognized this as a risky period. As well as pursuing this, both in the team and in the individual key worker's supervision, one case manager simply said that he would give the key worker a 'break' and do alternate visits for the next month. In the event he did most. The key worker commented afterwards that being 'told' by a colleague what to do had been a great relief—there was no way he was going to ask for such an intervention.

Conclusions

Most patients cared for by assertive outreach teams are likely to have a wide range of needs and will benefit from contact with several of the team members. Consistency and reliability of care is of paramount importance with highly vulnerable and anxious individuals; it is important that they should not suddenly receive a visit from a complete stranger if their key worker is not available. Similarly, if joint visits (key worker and secondary key worker) are needed at times of increased stress it is preferable if both faces are familiar. Patients need to have relationships with more members of the team than just their key worker. The key worker relationship was never meant to be exclusive.

Some might consider this networking and multiple inputs to be a form of 'team approach', but we think this is confusing. What distinguishes the two approaches is the clear lodging of responsibility, across time and across functions, in the key worker. An orthodox 'team approach' deliberately avoids this for well worked-out (though we think, misguided) reasons.

While we clearly prefer the key worker approach there are important areas still to be explored and resolved about the degree of sharing of tasks within assertive outreach teams. For example, how should the balance between generic and specialist working be set? What is the role of the secondary key worker? Currently, these decisions have to be based on clinical judgement. Hopefully, over the next few years, carefully conducted studies might shed some light on these issues.

Chapter 6

24-hour availability and extended services

Availability seven days a week, round the clock ('24/7'), is one of the rallying cries of assertive outreach purists (Hoult 1986; Marshall and Lockwood 1998; Smyth and Hoult 2000). Like the team approach it is a central tenet of the assertive outreach ideology and was heavily stressed in early studies. Hoult's service in Sydney is the one where such crisis intervention, round the clock, is promoted in most detail. Interestingly, it is not known how often the original Madison service, while stressing the importance of 24-hour availability, actually made contact out of hours. Careful reading of the service details (Stein and Test 1978) indicates that this was on-call availability from home and very much a safety net rather than an active provision.

Mature ACT services rarely offer a full service at night. They rely on on-call staff from home who deal with problems predominantly by phone, by the use of an answerphone in some services, and by various methods of shared duty rotas and integration with the local emergency services (Stein and Santos 1998; UK700 Group: Burns *et al.* 1999a). As with the team approach, the gap between rhetoric and reality is wide for 24-hour services.

Crisis intervention

Crisis intervention has a long history in mental health writing. Caplan (1964) was the first to highlight its potential benefits. Responding to the psychological consequences of a major tragedy (a fire at a dance hall that killed many young people in a small town) he demonstrated the benefits of prompt action in dealing with what nowadays would probably be called post-traumatic stress disorder. Caplan was struck by how easy it was to access painful and traumatic experiences immediately after a crisis—in contrast to the slow, laborious process of overcoming defences and resistance in traditional psychoanalysis. He stressed how crises represented both 'a threat and an opportunity' and saw them as real opportunities for personal growth.

The approach derives from normal, not abnormal, psychology, and not with any understanding of psychopathology as we experience it. It was developed for essentially 'healthy' individuals, not those with a mental illness. Crisis intervention services grew from his work, although increasingly the emphasis moved from promoting personal growth to intervening quickly to avoid deterioration and damage in a target group with established mental health problems.

The crisis intervention literature demonstrates both a rapid growth of publications and services in the 1960s and 70s, following Caplan's book (Johnson and Thornicroft 1995) and also evidence of such services being short-lived (Cooper 1979). Despite this, the ability to respond to crises, 24 hours a day, seven days a week, was considered to be an essential component of assertive outreach teams (Hoult 1986; Stein and Test 1980).

As the concept of assertive outreach has broadened, the 'mobile support team', which has become the widespread model of acute care in Australia and in parts of Canada, has crisis intervention at its centre. Terms have become confusing and the divisions between 'home treatment' teams, 'crisis resolution' teams, and assertive outreach teams have been eroded. The ability to respond within hours at any time of the day or night to a crisis is central to the remit of home treatment teams (Smyth and Hoult 2000) and the crisis resolution teams that are mandated in the National Service Framework (Minghella *et al.* 1998; NSF 1999; Sainsbury Centre for Mental Health 1998). Although crisis response continues to be an essential component of an assertive outreach team, it is now rarely proposed as a defining characteristic.

24-hour crisis services

The need

Crises and out-of-hours contacts rapidly diminish as patients get to know their teams and teams get to know their patients. Deterioration is anticipated at times of stress and early signs are observed. Training for patients in the recognition of relapse signatures if they have them (Chapter 15) is a core skill in assertive outreach teams (Perry *et al.* 1999). With contact every day or so, it is likely that relapse can be spotted and predicted. That does not mean it can always be prevented and presentation to the emergency services in the middle of the night will inevitably happen occasionally.

The two questions to be answered are: would a case manager be able to do anything about it and are the opportunity costs of tying up so much staff time worth it overall? We audited out-of-hours on-call availability for three months in a well-established team and found only seven contacts for 100 patients. Two of these were about the same patient whom we wanted to admit but who had been avoiding us. Eventually, we were able to ensure that the duty psychiatrist admitted him. The other five were fairly trivial and would have been easily dealt with by an accident and emergency department.

The cost/benefits

The need for 24-hour services will, obviously, depend to some extent on the nature of the local mental health provision. The question is not just one of the possible benefits of a 24-hour service but the cost/benefits of such an investment. All mental health services operate from fixed budgets and decisions have to be made about best value for patients and families within limited resources. Outside office hours there are severe limitations on what can be done. Direct patient and carer contact is possible but there is little opportunity for any of the complex care planning and liaison which is a crucial part of the job. Nobody else is available at night—social services are closed, GPs are only available for emergencies, etc. In early US studies, where the cost of an in-patient day was so much more than that of a professional salary (Weisbrod *et al.* 1980) and where admission gatekeeping was otherwise absent, then 24-hour cover could pay for itself.

In a more co-ordinated local service, however, such as found in most of Europe and much of the US now, 24-hour availability for small groups of designated patients is disproportionately expensive and can also deter good staff. The Nacka project in Sweden was one of the earliest comprehensive outreach services in Europe (Stefansson and Cullberg 1986). This service found itself significantly compromised by its early commitment to a 24-hour service that was written into the service specification. Initially, this 24-hour service was busy and effective. As patients and other services learnt better how to access care, however, out-of-hours crises became fewer. The 24-hour commitment became effectively redundant and undermined the capacity and effectiveness of the whole service as so much resource remained tied up in non-productive availability.

Sustaining the service

In the successful replication of ACT by Hoult *et al.* (1984) in Sydney, Australia, they used an on-call system of one person on call between 11 p.m. and 8 a.m. On-call staff had very little to do between these hours during the 12-month study. Evaluation showed that patients and carers valued the potential availability of staff but seldom used it. In this country there is evidence of assertive outreach services having established 24-hour cover only to discontinue it after evaluation. One team in the north of England suspended 24-hour cover due to infrequent utilization, inappropriate use by a small number of clients (whose main problem was poor sleep), and the impact on staff morale of maintaining cover. Another assertive outreach team, comprising only five staff, abandoned the 24-hour on-call service as they were unable to sustain it with so few staff.

One high-profile voluntary sector assertive outreach team initially found that on-call staff were being woken in the early hours by non-crisis calls. The team used this experience to provide an educational approach to help develop coping strategies in the small number of patients making these calls. The number of inappropriate calls consequently diminished, leaving a very low volume of calls. No carers have used the on-call service. Staff morale is maintained by an on-call allowance which staff describe as a 'perk' of the job, given the low call rate. Staff still need to be available and sober when on call, however, and these requirements can be problematic in relation to childcare and social commitments.

One rehabilitation assertive outreach team has well-established arrangements with their in-patient ward, which acts as a filter of 'inappropriate' calls, but can 'bleep' the on-call outreach worker when needed. More recently, with the growth of inner-city crime, staff are increasingly unwilling to go into deprived and potentially dangerous neighbourhoods at night.

Contingency planning with the whole system

In the UK, where there is generally both approved social work and psychiatric availability round the clock and an overall shortage of trained staff, there is little gained by insisting on discrete 24-hour services for individual patient groups. Indeed, it could be argued that this insistence reflects an overly medical view of crisis which simply does not apply to mental health. There is no mental health equivalent of a heart attack or a perforated ulcer—breakdowns occur over weeks and even months, not hours or days (Burns 2000*b*, 2001).

For the 100 patients in our assertive outreach service, we prefer to work with the wider mental health and social care system in providing effective 24-hour access to provide services in a crisis. Providing existing 24-hour services with a contingency plan for each patient of the team is one way of helping the assessor make more informed decisions. In our locality, folders of ACT team contingency plans are held on the admission ward and the psychiatric intensive care unit, and with the duty senior nurse, the local A&E department, and duty social workers. These are all places and people to which our patients might present or be taken to in the middle of the night.

Peter's contingency plan (see Example 6.1) demonstrates how, for a particularly anxious patient who frequently presents, unnecessary admission to hospital can be reduced. Of course it works the other way and other patients' contingency plans can advise immediate admission by citing previous risks.

For the assessor to have confidence in such contingency plans, it is critical that they are updated regularly. We read out the contingency plan at each main review and send out updates when amendments are made. It is also vital that contingency plans make clear the availability of the team for follow-up the next day.

Extended hours

In contrast to 24-hour services, extended hours are almost universally endorsed by assertive outreach teams and in an expert consensus panel in the UK (Catty *et al.* 2001). Early studies in the US and Australia were based on a two-shift system providing services for about 12 hours per day. The shifts overlap in the afternoon. This approach is also being used in the UK in some settings (Smyth and Hoult 2000). Few teams favour restricting their services to office hours.

As an alternative to using a shift system some teams emphasize flexible working so that activities can take place in the evenings. These are usually activities centred around encouraging patient leisure (e.g. going to the cinema with a patient, helping them enrol in evening classes) or opportunities to meet with carers who may be at work during the day. In our team we specify a willingness to work up to one evening a week as flexi-time as a requirement of the job. Too much evening work in lieu of daytime work, however, is generally found to be disruptive. Staff miss out on too many meetings or are unavailable for joint working during the day. A careful eye has to be kept on this approach to extended hours if the smooth running of the team is not to be compromised.

Example 6.1

ACT TEAM CONTINGENCY PLAN	7.9.99

This patient has a clinical case manager (CCM) allocated to him/her. This CCM has only 12 patients and can offer rapid and comprehensive support. In your assessment of the patient's presenting problem please bear in mind the availability of contact which can be guaranteed the next working day. We are keen to help these patients learn to survive in the community with unnecessary hospital admissions. Advice on client management is given below.

Name: PETER Male/Female: MALE D.O.B.: 1.8.59 Address: Tel: GP: DR SMITH Address: Tel: 0208 788 xxxx	Hospital number: Next of kin: Address: Tel: Home: Work: Consultant psychiatrist: PROF. BURNS Diagnosis: GENERALIZED ANXIETY DISORDER / PARANOID SCHIZOPHRENIA Supervision register: NO Section 117: YES

Crisis management:
Avoid admission

Peter frequently seeks admission and presents to the ward invariably stating:

1. That he feels 'suicidal'. On assessment this is often non-specific and there is no intent.
2. That he has 'lost his medication'. He is currently on a Lorazepam withdrawal pro-gramme and is supplied the Lorazepam by the ACT Team. He can collect one day's supply only from his GP in an emergency. His medication at present is Olanzapine 10 mg bd, Lorazepam 1 mg bd.

Please send home and leave a message for his key worker.

KNOWN OTHER CONTACTS:
Roger – MIND – Tel No.
Ethel – Friend, Launderette – Tel No.

Contact arrangements for advice, help, or to leave a message: Bill – clinical case manager **During working hours: 9 am–5 pm, 7 days a week**	**Tel: 020 8877 xxxx**

Seven-day working

Working seven days a week has proved immensely rewarding. In our team we moved to seven days a week as we began to rely more on supervised daily medication (Chapter 11). We had found that patients were more likely to break down or get into trouble at the weekend (and particularly over weekends extended by national holidays). Medication compliance often faltered or alcohol consumption increased when there was nowhere to go and no visit expected. We had anticipated that the extended service would be most used for dealing with such crises, but have found quite the contrary—weekend working is almost exclusively planned visits and phone calls.

On the Friday handover, the weekend visits are agreed. These include a significant proportion of patients who are receiving daily supervised medication (planned routine visits). The next main group are those whose mental state has been unstable recently and who are reassured (as are we) by the regular contact (planned crisis visits). In the past, if we had felt that the risk of breakdown in such fragile patients was great, they might easily have been admitted as a preventative measure. Being able to see them every day often contains this anxiety. For many patients, a phone call to prompt the taking of medicine or to reduce isolation and anxiety is enough.

Weekend work is not rostered but paid for out of an identified overtime budget. This prevents staff feeling obliged to work weekends when they do not want to and also avoids too many absences in the week. Staff readily volunteer for weekend work and each weekend is split between two. The rate of visits is higher than during the week (an average of eight visits compared to five on a weekday) and the traffic is mercifully lighter. The visits are generally shorter, with predetermined functions. Any free time can be used to catch up with notes and paperwork.

Evaluation after six months of weekend and bank holiday working showed that 88% of all contacts in this period were planned routine visits; 10% related to planned crisis work; and only 2%, urgent situations or calls. Only one emergency contact involved a patient relapsing who needed admission. We regarded the absence of crisis and emergency activity as a positive outcome measure for the effectiveness of the service during core hours.

With only one staff member on duty, judgement is needed about how to respond to emergencies at the weekend. Many unplanned visits are fine—a patient rings up because they have run out of medicine, or they have a burst pipe and need help in organizing a plumber, etc. If, however, there is a rapid deterioration in mental state and it sounds like there could be safety issues, then the patient is encouraged to come to the ward or to A&E where the case manager can meet with him or her and assess the situation. Unscheduled visits to a day centre open at weekends would also be undertaken if staff or the patient contacted us. In truth, such unscheduled visits remain rare (due, in part, to the fact that just the knowledge of availability of the service reduces anxiety). Safety remains a vital issue to be considered when deciding on 24-hour service or extended hours.

Conclusions

Flexibility and access are key features of good assertive outreach working. A balance needs to be struck between total access and acceptable and rewarding work patterns for staff. Being regularly on call, with little productive work to do, is demoralizing for good staff who want to know that what they do makes a real difference. Well-established teams, in regular contact with their patients, find that what was previously described as a crisis, has, in reality, built up over days or weeks. Early intervention is rarely a crisis response.

Context is important and a 24-hour rapid response service is rarely needed if local services are good. The cost–benefit of such a discrete service for a small, well-engaged group of patients is hard to justify clinically. However, that does not mean that governments and commissioners will not demand it!

Chapter 7

The role of medication

Assertive outreach has developed, whether as a discrete service or as an aspect of generic CMHTs, mainly for the care of individuals with severe mental illness. The majority of such people suffer from schizophrenia, bipolar affective disorder, or a delusional psychosis. Altogether they constitute about 2% of the adult population. Patients suffering from these disorders nearly all benefit from medication over long periods. There are, undoubtedly, severe and persistent neurotic disorders (e.g. obsessive—compulsive disorder, eating disorders, a range of anxiety disorders) which also require intensive treatment and support without medication, but they represent only a small proportion of the case load of most services. So effective outreach services will need to clarify their attitude towards medications.

This chapter will deal with the place of medication in the overall work and practice of the team. Chapter 11 deals specifically with medication compliance enhancement and the chapters devoted to individual disorders pick up the specifics of the relevant medications. There are, however, more general issues that need to be addressed.

It is often forgotten that, in their original paper, Stein and Test recognized the importance of ensuring that their patients received their medicines. This received little attention in that paper, or in many of the subsequent high-profile assertive outreach studies, probably because most of the practitioners took it for granted. What they thought was innovative and characteristic of their new services was the broad, flexible, and responsive roles of their case managers. Regular prescription and provision of medication had been assumed as a core feature. One consequence of this is that assertive outreach staff may be attracted to the work because it has something of an 'anti-drug' or 'anti-medical' aura to it. In many ways this is entirely appropriate and understandable. This is a job with an explicitly holistic approach to patient care, valuing a willingness to move out beyond traditional professional boundaries.

Effective treatment and rehabilitation of individuals with severe psychotic illnesses, however, requires careful attention to optimal medication. Successful teams have to evolve an approach which recognizes the importance of medication and ensures that it is reliably and appropriately delivered, but does not let it erode or dominate their broader, more personalized service model. A realistic understanding of what medications can achieve, and what they cannot, is probably a good place to start. Equally, a recognition of the very real problems that their side-effects pose for patients enables the case manager to engage in an informed discussion of the pros and cons.

The role of maintenance medication in psychoses

Antipsychotic drugs helped drive the revolution in psychiatric care when they were introduced in the treatment of acute psychoses from the mid-1950s. How long to continue with the medicines was a pragmatic, clinical decision. Initially, they were viewed as treatments for acute episodes. Psychiatrists quickly learnt that stopping the medication as soon as the florid symptoms disappeared was often followed promptly by relapse. For some psychiatrists this confirmed a belief in a biological lifelong disorder, where the drugs were simply suppressing the acute manifestations. Many more kept their patients on drugs simply 'for safety's sake' and were reluctant to stop them, encouraging patients to put up with side-effects to lessen the risk of relapse.

Maintenance antipsychotics

Over the years, custom and practice has established that patients with schizophrenia are encouraged to remain on maintenance antipsychotics as prophhylaxis against relapse. This is particularly the case in Anglophone (UK and US) psychiatry and in Scandinavia, although much less widespread in other parts of Europe and the world. It is not entirely a culturally led decision, however, and there is good evidence for the protective benefits of maintenance medication. Some of the strongest evidence is from a series of random controlled trials using depot medication (Curson *et al.* 1985; Hirsch *et al.* 1973). (Depots were particularly useful because you could be certain whether the patient did or did not receive the medicine.) These studies demonstrated unequivocally that patients receiving the medicines stayed well longer and remained out of hospital longer. The picture is not entirely one of benefits to the patient, however. A study of a first onset cohort of patients with schizophrenia (Crow *et al.* 1986) found that although those receiving maintenance medication relapsed less and came into hospital less, they also did slightly less well in their vocational and social recovery than those without medication.

The early studies of Hirsch and colleagues (1973) confirmed that the proportion of patients getting antipsychotic medicines who relapsed was much lower than those who did not. But not all patients getting the medicines stayed well, and not all those without it relapsed. These studies initiated the search for the social stressors which precipitated relapse and the resultant identification of the role of high expressed emotion (Leff and Vaughn 1981).

The weight of evidence in favour of maintenance antipsychotics is now so overwhelming that few European ethics committees will permit placebo control trials in this area (i.e. they will not expose patients with schizophrenia, even if they give fully informed consent, to be without cover). Unfortunately, this evidence derives almost entirely from studies of a year's duration or less. We have no firm scientific evidence on which to base judgements of how long we should persist with maintenance medication. A European consensus statement suggested a minimum of two years after a first episode and five years after a repeat (Kissling *et al.* 1991). In practice, most services encourage patients to continue with their antipsychotics as long as they are prepared to, and most continue even after discharge back to their GP (Burns and Kendrick 1997; Kendrick *et al.* 1998).

It is highly likely that mental health teams overestimate the duration of continued maintenance medication required because we see the patients who relapse when they stop, while those who do not relapse, stay with their GP and get on with their lives.

Atypical antipsychotics and clozaril

The reintroduction of clozaril for the treatment of resistant schizophrenia (Kane *et al.* 1988; Kane and McGlashan 1995) and, more recently, the development of a range of new 'atypical' antipsychotics has significantly changed prescribing for schizophrenia. This will be dealt with in more detail in Chapter 15. It has, however, had more than pharmacological effects. Simply having a range of possible treatments, with different profiles of effects and side-effects, means that negotiation is not simply a token but a meaningful and concrete component in the therapeutic relationship. It is no longer simply a matter of taking the medicine or not taking the medicine but choosing *which medicine.*

Apart from clozaril, the evidence for significant therapeutic superiority of the atypicals is absent. Even evidence for drop-out and side-effect levels, when compared against more appropriate doses of older antipsychotics, is thin (Geddes *et al.* 2000). However, they 'feel' different and both patients and relatives seem to prefer the newer drugs. It would be easy to underestimate the importance of this element of choice and the empowerment that it can bring to individuals who have often felt themselves passive victims of their disease and powerless recipients of care.

Currently, none of the atypicals is available in depot preparation, but this is likely to change soon. Paradoxically, we have found their unavailability in this format to be sometimes an advantage. It can be used to structure discussions about compliance— talking through the potential advantages in terms of less motor side-effects and clearer thinking, and weighing them up with the need to take more personal responsibility for the treatment regimen. Rather than the limited discussions that centre round 'depot versus oral' older drugs (where the side-effects are essentially the same), there is a potential benefit to the patient of coming to terms with their illness and the need for prolonged oral treatment. Collaboration brings hope of less side-effects, rather than the simple avoidance of an injection.

Anticholinergics and monitoring of side-effects

When prescribing drugs over long periods for people with severe mental illnesses it is essential to monitor them carefully for side-effects. No effective drugs are entirely free of side-effects or of the risk of adverse events. With antipsychotic drugs some of the early side-effects are sudden and dramatic (e.g. dystonias, akathisia), while others may be insidious, developing over months or years (e.g. tardive dyskinesia, sluggishness, weight gain). Careful adjustment of dosage is essential to reduce the risk of side-effects and regular reviews (see Chapter 15) are essential.

Appropriate prescribing of anticholinergics for Parkinsonian side-effects will enhance compliance with treatment, but there is evidence that these are often continued unnecessarily (and the 'buzz' they give can lead to their misuse and street trading). They are often necessary at the start of treatment (when acute dystonias can also be a real risk), but the need for them reduces over time and greater efforts should be made to find an antipsychotic dose level that is therapeutic without requiring long-term concurrent anticholinergics.

Anticholinergics are often prescribed incorrectly for akithisia. This condition does not respond to them and is better treated with either benzodiazepines (Cunningham–Owens 1999) or beta-blockers (Fleischhacker *et al.* 1990), or with atypicals, including clozapine (Owens 1996). Akathisia is even more distressing for patients on older antipsychotics and is particularly noticed with flupenthixol and trifluoperazine. It is a sense of persistent restlessness, usually in the legs, but it can affect the trunk. The patient may inhibit movement but still experience the distress, or they may move around or fidget in a attempt to relieve it. Simply encouraging patients to 'put up with it' is hardly adequate. Attempts need to be made with benzodiazepines and beta-blockers, but in many cases the drug has to be changed. While patients are often remarkably tolerant of other side-effects, akathisia is rarely bearable over long periods.

Paying close attention to drugs to reduce side-effects is an important contribution to patient welfare. It is all too easy in our jobs to become blasé about the burden they impose (perhaps because in the past we have felt we had no choice). Patients appreciate the efforts made, even if they are not totally successful. In the most practical way it demonstrates real concern.

It is not the place in a book like this to give detailed advice about medication—relevant knowledge evolves far too rapidly. What is important is that outreach workers continually update their knowledge of psychopharmacology and ensure that they obtain regular reviews for their patients. We generally support the need for reviews to be structured both in time and in content. Nowhere is this more important than in the use of long-term antipsychotics and anticholinergics where the evidence is that patients are often left on excessively high doses of both for years on end (Holloway 1988).

The role of mood stabilizers

The last 30 years has also seen the accumulation of a body of evidence that the frequency of relapses in bipolar affective disorders can be lowered by taking regular lithium. In ten studies, 34% of those on lithium relapsed, as against 81% on placebo (Goodwin and Jamison 1990). This evidence is slightly more controversial (Cookson 1997;

Moncrieff 1997) than with antipsychotics. The studies were often older, the certainty about compliance less, and the natural lengths between relapses are so much longer which makes their interpretation more difficult. However, most clinicians consider that the weight of evidence is in favour of lithium prophylaxis despite the considerable range of side-effects and long-term physical damage associated with it.

More recently, other mood stabilizers have been introduced (carbamazepine, sodium valproate) whose relative benefits are, as yet, still being determined but are beginning to be as widely used as lithium (Khan *et al.* 1996).

Usually, the choice of mood stabilizer is determined by patient preference, as there is no clear indication of subtypes of mood disorder responding differently. More recently, there has been a growing impression that combining mood stabilizers can improve outcome (Freeman and Stoll 1998). With the growing interest in drugs such as lamotrigine (Fatemi *et al.* 1997) and depakote (Bowden *et al.* 1994) there are likely to be major shifts in practice in maintenance of bipolar patients. Because of their toxicity, maintaining patients on these compounds requires vigilance from the team. This will be dealt with in more detail in Chapter 16.

Antidepressants

Depression in the long-term severely mentally ill is often overlooked. Feeling low, tired, and hopeless can easily be attributed either to negative symptoms, to side-effects of the drugs, or to an empty and unstimulating life situation. There is evidence, however, that depression is common in schizophrenia and other delusional psychoses (Siris 2000; Zisook *et al.* 1999). It is common in the wake of an acute relapse when there can often be obvious causes of remorse and disappointment. Nonetheless, symptoms can be alleviated and functioning improved by antidepressants as well as increased support and encouragement.

As with any depressed patient, tablets alone are rarely enough and attention to problem solving and support is essential. Visits need to be increased and the very real risk of suicide considered. It is important not to overlook the potential benefit of antidepressants for our patients. They need to be chosen with care, prescribed at therapeutic levels, and continued long after symptom resolution. The choice of antidepressant is outside the scope of this volume and will, obviously, change with new developments. Whichever is prescribed, however, needs to be monitored for side-effects and also to ensure that it is not continued unnecessarily.

Benzodiazepines

A striking feature of the Italian community mental health services which have attracted such acclaim, is that Italian psychiatrists are much more generous with psychotropic drugs than their UK counterparts. In particular, they prescribe more benzodiazepines, both for sleeping and for the control of daytime anxiety. UK psychiatrists tend to be very puritanical about the use of benzodiazepines in the wake of evidence of their addictive potential. With the advent of atypical antipsychotics (which often are non-sedating) we have become increasingly aware of the sedative and anxiolytic properties of the drugs we prescribe. It is fairly obvious, in retrospect, that phenothiazines were often used in high doses in acute relapses as much for their sedative as their anti-psychotic effects. Now that sedation is a separate element in the management of acute psychosis, we have rediscovered its value in the periods of stress in the long-term management of psychotic patients.

We have increasingly found moderate doses of benzodiazepines (e.g. diazepam 5 mg tds) to be extraordinarily helpful in periods of agitation and stress with psychotic patients in the community. Treatment usually is only for between a few days and a couple of weeks. We have found no evidence of dependency or of a demand for continuation of the medicines in this group. Similarly, we have found prompt prescribing of adequate sleeping tablets to make survival outside hospital feasible. Psychotic patients with troubling delusions and hallucinations need a decent night's sleep to cope. It is also during the night that the support and distraction that much treatment can provide is absent. Prompt hypnotics are also a common feature in self-medication contingency plans for our bipolar patients.

Periodic, structured reviews

Patients with long-term problems may change very slowly over long periods and there is plenty of evidence that familiarity with them can lead to our missing these changes (Wooff *et al.* 1986, 1988). In Chapter 27 we highlight the importance of not simply relying on routine clinical practice but of using regular, structured assessments of clinical functioning. There are a range of such assessments for antipsychotic side-effects and the value of regular, structured screening for side-effects (Chaplin *et al.* 1999) is as important (if not more important) as that for clinical and social functioning. The patient's clinical and social functioning are likely to be uppermost in the mind of the key worker when they meet; drug side-effects can be easily overlooked.

Conclusions

The management of medications for specific problems will be dealt with more in the relevant following chapters. The thorny problem of how to improve compliance with medicines (or 'adherence' or 'concordance' as it is often called) will be picked up in more detail in Chapter 11. For the severely mentally ill patient, who needs a flexible outreach service, medication is likely to play a significant role in their management for many years. The last thing these patients need is mixed messages about the value of drugs in their treatment. The purpose of this chapter is to highlight their importance and to stress the need to devote time and energy to adjusting and monitoring their administration.

The message is not that correct medication is the only thing that matters. Far from it. Simply that medication is an equally important strand in a complex provision. For some patients it is uncontroversial and remains in the background, for some it is a source of continuous conflict within a broader treatment package, and, for very few, it may be the only currency of contact. It is focused on here separately because it is easily forgotten, perhaps either because it is thought of as simply the doctor's responsibility or because it draws less on the whole personality of the case manager.

Detailed advice on individual medicines (doses, interactions, etc.) is not appropriate in a book like this. Similarly, the exact arrangements for ensuring regular medical oversight will vary from team to team (e.g. between rural and urban settings). What does not vary is the need to take medication seriously as a strand in our patients' management—one that deserves respect and skilled attention.

Chapter 8

Compulsion and freedom

Issues of free will and personal autonomy are at the heart of all mental health practice. Although there are overwhelming similarities between psychiatry and the rest of medicine, there are some fundamental differences. Those of us who work in this field are aware that some sense of 'alienation' (either from the normal self or from those around us) is central to the experience of mental illness. In neurotic and depressive disorders, the primary complaint is often of 'not being my usual self', of being 'anxious, worried, pessimistic, preoccupied' and so on. In psychotic disorders, the perception of the world we live in is changed—the familiar becomes threatening, neutral acquaintances become persecutory and random, irrelevant events become charged with personal meanings.

Of course, people with all sorts of physical illnesses also experience themselves 'changed' and may find their environment unbearable. However, they link this to the illness and rarely feel for any length of time that they as individuals have irrevocably changed, or that the environment itself has changed. They recognise that it is their lowered resources or heightened sensitivity that accounts for the altered experiences. In mental illnesses, the patient has the challenge to try to restore their normal self image, to re-establish a normal relationship with themselves. In more severe psychotic illnesses, the challenge to the patient is to restore his or her usual perception of the surrounding world and relationships with individuals in it. Heuristically, we can capture this by saying that mental illnesses manifest themselves in relationships—either relationships with the self or with those around them.

Assessing insight

In the most extreme forms, the patient is described as 'lacking insight'. Insight is hard to define but remains an essential term that we keep returning to. The more closely one examines it, however, the slippier it gets. There is no one point of disjuncture—the range of individual world views is enormous. When does one decide that a strange view becomes 'a delusion', a period of pessimism becomes a 'depressive distortion'? These are, inevitably, complex individual judgements. Sometimes it is obvious: out of the blue, an accountant, father of two and a pillar of the local scouting movement, tells everyone that his body has been substituted by aliens. We have little doubt that he is unwell and that his ability to interpret his experiences is flawed. What, however, of the legions of people who are convinced that alien abduction is rife and that they know individuals who have been taken away and fundamentally altered before being returned to earth? Few of us would confidently call this a delusion.

Clinically, however, insight is an essential day-to-day concept in mental health work and degress of insight have long been acknowledged—'he's completely devoid of insight', 'she has some insight'. In an attempt to bring greater rigour to this, scales are being developed to measure levels of insight (Birchwood *et al.* 1994; David *et al.* 1992). These are used mainly in research studies to link functioning with neuropsychosocial tests. Valuable though these scales are in research and conceptual development, we have not found them routinely useful in our clinical work.

Birchwood (1994) has suggested three components of insight:

Components of insight

♦ Awareness of illness

♦ Need for treatment

♦ Attribution of symptoms

Birchwood *et al.* 1994

We usually judge impairment of insight by assessing the strength and pervasiveness of hallucinations and delusions. The assessment requires due attention to cultural norms and the context. The experience of cosmic influences and force fields running through a room has a totally different significance when recounted by a young New Age traveller than by an isolated 60-year-old widow. Similarly, the evolution of the ideas and experiences will influence our judgement. 'Bizarre' ideas which come out of the blue are much more suggestive of illness than preoccupations and convictions that have evolved over many years. What both of these contextual issues contain is some form of judgement about how much the person is 'his normal self'. It is not the normality of the idea generally (i.e. within the general population) that we are judging but its *normality for that individual*—how much he or she is 'alienated' from their normal view of themselves and the world. In many ways it is this very specificity to the individual that can make our judgements seem arbitrary and subjective to outsiders.

Disorder of the brain or disorder of the mind?

Whenever societies are sufficiently wealthy and settled they distinguish mental health care from general physical care. Psychiatry is seen as an established medical discipline but it *is* different from dermatology, neurology, etc. Although some European countries still insist on joint neurology and psychiatry training for psychiatrists, the practice is invariably different. An eminent neurologist, Henry Miller in Newcastle, began an influential article on psychiatry with the sentence 'Don't get me wrong, many of my best friends are psychiatrists' and then went on to describe psychiatry as '*Neurology without signs*'. Several equally eminent academic psychiatrists have also insisted that mental illnesses are just brain illnesses and that it is simply a matter of time before our discipline disappears. The facts speak against this, and the obituary may be premature. The difference reflects the clinical manifestations and how we manage mental illness, not whether it is located in the brain or not. We know that multiple sclerosis and Parkinson's disease are brain disorders, but there is no expectation that psychiatrists should take responsibility for them.

What separates mental illnesses and their management from general disorders is the 'alienation' described above, and the centrality of the therapeutic relationship as a tool in treatment (and not just a vehicle for it). The other profound difference is the need, at times, to override the patient's wishes and impose treatment even when that patient is fully alert. Issues of compulsion and personal freedom lie at the heart of the practice of mental health care and cannot be avoided in any system.

Compulsion in assertive outreach

All the same issues about how to balance individual liberty with the need for treatment in the absence of insight affect assertive outreach teams as they do any other form of mental health care—indeed more so. As we have improved continuity of care with our patients we now make decisions about when to intervene at much earlier stages in deterioration. This greater knowledge about their condition does not make our job easier—quite the reverse, it makes it harder.

When mental health services waited for patients to be brought to them the degree of disturbance was often very marked before opinions were sought. Patients were often suffering profound delusions and hallucinations and in conditions of severe distress and self-neglect. The conclusion that they were not in a fit state to decide for themselves was fairly obvious. Now, we often have to make decisions confronted with deterioration that, in itself, is not life-threatening or dramatic but which we know is the start of an inevitable decline that may result in such consequences. How justified are we in intervening early to prevent such distress and damage?

Early intervention

Some argue that the early use of compulsion by assertive outreach teams means that patients are disadvantaged. In effect, our contact with them may lower the threshold for overriding their self-determination and so, it is argued, assertive outreach diminishes, rather than increases, patients' autonomy. Others argue that waiting until the indications for admission are obvious and unequivocal only serves the needs of staff rather than patients. It makes the decision easy but the patient and their family pay the price, both psychological and social, of more severe relapses. Whether or not early intervention reduces or increases the amount of time in hospital cannot be answered with any certainty: there have been no specific trials.

The clinical view of many assertive outreach staff (including us) is that early intervention may reduce both the severity and duration of the relapse—'nip it in the bud'. This is not, however, self-evident and it can be legitimately argued that treatment reduces the severity of a relapse but that its time course is less affected. What evidence there is, is confusing. Overall, assertive outreach seems to reduce the duration of hospital stays but not the number of admissions (Mueser *etal.* 1998). The data reported do not, however, distinguish voluntary from compulsory admissions. In some studies, more intensive follow-up has been associated with increased admission rates (Curtis *etal.* 1992; Franklin *etal.* 1987; Tyrer *etal.* 1995) which have been attributed to better identification of clinical need. Again, one cannot draw any firm conclusions about the impact on compulsory admissions.

Knowing 'too much'

Another problem with assertive outreach is that decisions can be more difficult when one 'knows too much' about the patient and their circumstances. Assertive outreach workers are likely to have a very holistic understanding of their patients. The content of delusions and hallucinations may make a lot of sense to the case manager and their symbolism be all too obvious when you know the patient's history and what he or she is struggling with. How does one respond to a young schizophrenic man who becomes preoccupied with delusions of changes in his abdomen when you know it reflects his anxiety about his mother's recently diagnosed cancer of the uterus? Being too close can mean missing the wood for the trees (Wooff *etal.* 1988). Identification with a patient you have worked with for a long time can delay accepting the inevitable—hope can cloud judgement.

Compulsory admissions

Mental health legislation varies markedly between countries (and even between regions within some countries). Scotland has different legislation from England and Wales; each state in Australia or the US has its own statutes. The current legislation in the UK is under review and likely to change radically in the next few years. The final format of such changes is unclear but it is likely that compulsory treatment will be disentangled from the need for hospital admission. How personality disorder is dealt with will become more prescribed and, with that, assessment of capacity and of treatability as grounds for compulsion will be reviewed. Probably the only thing that is currently certain is that the review process and bureaucracy will increase. There is no point in recounting the details of practice here. Rather, the general issues impinging on assertive outreach practice will be addressed with some thought about the impact of community treatment orders. This latter is of particular importance to assertive outreach staff as we are the ones who will be asked to use them.

Protecting the therapeutic relationship

We have made clear above that we consider some use of compulsion to be an inevitable and justifiable component of good comprehensive mental health care. It is not something to be ashamed of or something from which we should distance ourselves. Nor is it something to be too worried about. With eight years of experience of managing 100 patients (of whom the majority have been admitted compulsorily at some time by us), we have found that they do forgive us. It is a remarkable fact, but one that we need to remind ourselves of regularly, that very few patients harbour a grudge for any length of time about compulsory admissions. Many remain convinced that we should not have done it, but they are still happy to see us and treat us decently. They often recognize that we have our job to do and that this is part of it. Assertive outreach teaches us that honest disagreement is perfectly compatible with a respectful and even warm relationship.

Importance of honesty

We would go further and propose that honesty is the most fundamental component of an ethical and successful long-term relationship. Deception should be avoided unless there is real risk of danger. The practice of getting someone else to effect the admission ('to protect the relationship') is short-sighted. Patients will have to be told that we endorsed or even initiated it. They will, quite correctly, interpret our leaving someone else to 'do the dirty work' as weakness and lack of commitment to them.

Just because a compulsory admission is unavoidable does not mean that how it is done will not make a difference. Having a familiar face around during a frightening and distressing experience (as it is highly likely to be, especially if the police have to be involved) makes it more bearable for both patient and family members (see Chapters 5 and 10). The value of some comforting words should not be underestimated:

> Don't worry Alice, I'm here, and will make sure that nobody hurts you. The police are just here to make sure nothing goes wrong. I'll come to the ward with you and I'll make it my job to see that you're back home as soon as possible. You know I wouldn't agree to you going in unless I thought you really needed it. Yes, I'll make sure the cat is fed.

Knowledge of the patient's anxieties and vulnerabilities can ease the process. You know their delusions and fears, so only you can attempt to reassure them. At the simplest level, it helps to know the layout of the flat and the identities of the people involved.

In several instances, case managers have found their involvement in these dramatic periods (when the patient is often at their lowest ebb) can serve as an important shared experience. Later it can be worked through to strengthen the alliance. One of the strengths of mental health nurses as case managers is that their involvement in such emotionally charged encounters, and their ease with direct physical contact, makes the relationship more vivid. The patient experiences it as a 'real relationship', not simply a contract with a disinterested, albeit conscientious, professional.

We find it best to acknowledge the disagreement openly and in as matter-of-fact a manner as possible. We explain why we are arranging a compulsory admission, listen whilst the patient 'takes it on board', and explore where we differ. In the end we aim for the patient to understand our actions, not necessarily to agree. We often 'agree to disagree'.

Although we strongly advocate honesty and transparency in the process of compulsion, commonsense and judgement must prevail. There are occasions where avoiding direct confrontation is prudent. Alone at home with an aroused and hostile patient who asks directly 'Well, are you going to section me?' it may be best to say 'I've got to think about it, but obviously it's possible if things go on like this', even if the real answer is 'yes'. This fuller answer may have to be given when you have support and are in a position to achieve it safely. Similarly, there have been times, usually at the start of trying to engage with a new patient with a long history of hostility to case managers, when other members of the team take the responsibility. It should be a rare occurrence and, if it has to be repeated with the same patient, it is probably worth radically rethinking their management.

Balancing the risks and benefits

As mentioned above, decisions on compulsory admission are often made more difficult, rather than less, when one knows the patient well. Assertive outreach staff need to pay more attention to the balance involved in assessments, and decisions should always involve consultation with the team, unless it is a very extreme emergency. Even then, doctors, social workers, and case managers need time to discuss. Four common issues complicate the decision in assertive outreach teams and should always be considered:

- Familiarity with the patient, fondness for them, or a sense of being their 'advocate' can mean that painful decisions are delayed too long.
- Admission can mistakenly be considered a 'failure'.
- There is a greater ability to sustain ill people out of hospital (even if it is not in their interests).
- There is also, however, greater understanding of the risks of deterioration and of the potential benefits of treatment.

Compulsion in the community

Much of the current debate about compulsion in the community oversimplifies both the nature of decisions and the nature of human relationships. Most of the important decisions we make as adults involve elements of both free will and elements of compulsion. Usually, the compulsion is experienced as a limit on the alternatives we can contemplate because of the impact on those we care about or love. Is the decision by an alcoholic to come in for drying out because his wife has threatened to leave him a free choice? Clearly not, although he would be a voluntary patient. When a young anorexic woman accepts admission, how do we disentangle the contributions of her mounting fear of dying (free will) from her respect for her parents' distress (compulsion)? There are limitless shades of grey in how free and voluntary decisions to accept treatment are—only in the most extreme cases is mental health law involved.

Power relationships

Few significant relationships are absolutely equal or single stranded. To the extent that any relationship is important to us it will, inevitably, compromise freedom. We will conduct ourselves to protect that relationship. We do not want to lose it and therefore it exerts a form of power over us—'I can't do that. What would she think?' Indeed, one explicit purpose of establishing a supportive and trusting relationship with a patient (developing effective engagement) is to be able to influence decisions later. While the relationship may be open and respectful there is a hope that, at least in some aspects, it will contain the power to influence.

We need to recognize that when we exert such influence we may often restrict an individual's personal freedom. Of course, they are ultimately at liberty to break the relationship, but that is easier said than done. Such a liberty may be more symbolic than real if the patient feels very dependent on us. For example, our recommendation may be seen as the only means of getting a change of accommodation or a welfare grant. We may even have articulated this:

> I can only really recommend you for the mental health quota flats if I'm able to say that you're better now and accepting treatment. Otherwise they won't consider you able to manage a tenancy.

While the 'blame' is placed with the housing department, we should acknowledge that we are using an element of compulsion here. American case managers refer to this as 'leverage' and consider it an essential component of effective outreach. They argue that developing engagement is one means of developing 'leverage'.

It is important to be honest in confronting the power relationships that do exist within mental health practice. We would reject the cynical view that engagement and therapeutic alliances are simply about getting power. They will not work unless they are driven by, and contain, a genuine wish to support the patient's own desires. On the other hand, we delude ourselves if we deny that there is authority and power in the relationship and pretend that everything apart from compulsory admissions are entirely free and consensual. Nowhere is this self awareness more important than in working with isolated and vulnerable individuals who may feel they have no options.

The risks of abuse

If we do not consciously monitor the power within these relationships it is easy to over-look abuses. Just because we would say 'no' to someone who tried to encourage (make) us, against our inclination, to go to a day centre, does not mean that our patient feels they can say 'no'. If you are the only person they regularly see they may be very frightened of losing your support and, consequently, prepared to go along with things you suggest that may be deeply unrewarding for them.

The Milgram experiments (Milgram 1963) of the 1960s remind us how powerful hierarchy is in human relationships. In these psychology studies, ostensibly self-confident subjects administered what they were led to believe were high-voltage shocks simply because they were told to do so by someone authoritative. Most of us are blind to the power we exert while being exquisitely sensitive to the power that others exert upon us!

Ethically, it is important to recognize the power we have if we are to avoid abusing it. Would it be ethical to withhold a tenancy as an incentive to improve compliance? How ethical is it to provide lunch at a depot clinic? This has been described as one way of improving uptake. But are we sure that it is a fair trade off when the patients may not want the injection but have no other source of cooked food? Perhaps the most stark examples are when patients (usually very poor patients) are paid to take treatment. It has been shown to improve care in areas as diverse as dentistry, tuberculosis, and cocaine addiction (Giuffrida and Torgerson 1997). Is this really ethical? How infinitely more complex the moral question when the illness may subtly impair capacity.

There are no simple, once-and-for-all answers to such questions. We raise them here to highlight the complexity of even the most benign and empowering therapeutic relationship. We certainly do use leverage and even gentle blackmail when we view the alternative consequences as serious. The purpose of this discussion is to remind ourselves of our need to constantly consider the ethical dimensions of our work, particularly the balance between individual liberty and the potential therapeutic benefits of treatment. Power and compulsion are part and parcel of our relationships with our patients—they are not simply the concerns of the approved social worker and the consultant when they arrange an involuntary admission.

Supervised discharge and community treatment orders

Many countries now allow for compulsory treatment of severely mentally ill individuals outside of hospitals. The current law in England and Wales (the 1983 Mental Health Act) is simply an updating of the 1959 Act, and reflects the thinking current in the 1950s. At that time it was inconceivable that severely ill individuals would be outside hospital and so the wording of the Act equates compulsion with admission. Times have changed but the wording of the act has not. 'Liable to be detained' is still the benchmark for compulsion.

Leave on Section

In truth, however, practice has changed considerably. Patients admitted for compulsory treatment could be allowed home on leave (Section 17 leave as it is called) while officially not being discharged. This leave is recognized as an essential part of an extended assessment and also of rehabilitation. After all, how could one be sure that the patient had fully recovered when assessed only in the controlled environment of the ward? Similarly, the patient needs the chance of regaining confidence in handling the stresses of every-day life while still arguably benefiting from the support and structure of the Section.

The status of leave on Section has been the focus of considerable controversy. In the 1980s, a small group of patients were maintained on repeated periods of Section 17 leave. This was rather unfortunately called 'long-leash' management and involved recalling the patient to hospital for a night to renew the treatment order for a year (Sensky *et al.* 1980). The practice was subject to judicial review (Hallström 1985) and deemed illegal, although it continued in Scotland. Extending the Section in order to continue Section 17 leave is illegal in England and Wales, although it is legal during the natural full length of the Section (either 6 or 12 months).

Some teams consider the use of extended leave to be an abuse of the legislation. Our reading of the code of practice and the 1994 'ten point plan' (Burns 1994) leads us to accept it as being in the spirit of the law and good practice. We have certainly used it extensively in assertive outreach and find it works essentially in the same way as supervised discharge (aftercare under supervision).

In the wake of the Ritchie report into the care of Christopher Clunis (Ritchie 1994), the debate about compulsory treatment in the community was renewed. The Royal College of Psychiatrists put forward a proposal for a community supervision order (CSO) (Royal College of Psychiatrists 1993) but this was not accepted by the government. Major concerns at the time were the public belief that force would be used to administer treatment against a patient's will, in their own homes, and that the proposals would conflict with European human rights legislation. In truth, the proposal explicitly dismissed any idea of forcible treatment in the home and it also did not have powers for automatic readmission if the patient refused treatment. It proposed that if the patient refused to take treatment they had to come to the clinic for assessment and that that assessment would follow the same standards as those currently in place for compulsory admission. In effect, if the patient was not severely ill at the time they refused the treatment then they were free to do so.

Supervised discharge

The newly passed supervised discharge legislation is, in practice, virtually the same as the 1993 proposal. It requires the patient to live at an agreed address (just like guardianship) and to allow access to the key worker. If the patient refuses to take the treatment they can be obliged to come to the clinic for assessment. That's all. There is no power to force treatment nor any sanction (such as automatic admission) that follows from refusal. Like extended Section 17 leave it ensures regular contact and the power to recall for assessment. Yet, despite these limited powers, we have found it very useful in assertive outreach and use it and Section 17 leave regularly.

Not a substitute for engagement

The power is about persuading the persuadable. We have the same experience as those who use compulsory treatment orders (CTOs) in Australia (Vaughan 2000)—it is valuable for a small group of patients with whom one has some relationship and who can agree to it. It is of no value whatsoever in the absence of a basic therapeutic relationship. It is not a *substitute for engagement* but a *tool in engagement*. The patient who flatly says 'no' will still say 'no' even if on an order. There are many patients, however, who although lacking insight into their illness retain a respect for law and can understand the mutual obligation imposed by such legislation. We always present it as a mutual obligation—they are obliged to see us regularly and we are obliged to come regularly to them and see how best we can help.

Case study

Jane had suffered from a florid paranoid delusional disorder for nearly two decades. She was convinced that her son, in long-term fostering, was the offspring of a prince and that she was weak because she was being poisoned via the drains under her flat. She attributed this to a plot to kidnap her son. She is a talented musician and lives a lonely life, with several cats, and apart from fortnightly visits to her son, has no regular contact apart from us. When untreated she neglects herself to dangerous degrees, living in squalor and not eating, increasingly preoccupied with poison from the drains.

With regular depot medication she remains concerned about a possible plot to kidnap her son, still occasionally complains about strange emanations from the drains, but is able to look after herself and her cats, play her music, and get out shopping. She enjoys the contact with her key worker. She adamantly denies that she is ill and is opposed to all medicines because of delusional convictions about numbers and influence. She does, however, accept that her supervised discharge is legal and (although she knows that it does not oblige her to take medicine) welcomes our contact and readily takes the injection. She has recently discussed a willingness to take oral medicines but we are taking it slowly.

In a team supporting just over 100 patients we usually have up to 10 on supervised discharge or Section 17 leave at any given time. One or two have been on these orders for well over a year, but most stay on them for 6–9 months. We feel that, in their own environment, patients can consolidate the clinical gains that can be made with consistent treatment in hospital. Like our colleagues in Australia, we have found it important to restrict the focus of the compulsion as much as possible—to regular contacts when we can encourage (though not force) medication. We do not impose day-centre attendance or psychological treatments. They would not work and we think go beyond what is ethical.

Advantages of a community treatment order

Our use of compulsion in the community is controversial, and we present our thinking and experience for what it is—not as a definitive solution. Whether or not a compulsory treatment order will be an advance on compulsory supervision is an open question. On the one hand it is honest—the main reason psychiatrists put patients on supervised discharge is to get them to take medicines (Bindman *et al*. 2000). Patients clearly know this even when we are absolutely explicit about the limits of the powers. On the other hand we know from experience that the powers are only of any value if they build upon some level of trust and engagement.

One powerful argument against CTOs is that if the law were to make the treatment rather than the contact obligatory, then staff would not work so hard on engagement. We wonder how it would work in practice. Already we have patients who, despite supervised discharge, have failed to co-operate with treatment. None of us feel that we would be willing to simply 'threaten' them. There might be, however, a small number at the threshold where being told that the medication is obligatory would make a difference.

The Royal College of Psychiatrists' CSO proposal included a time limit (3 years) beyond which the order could not be renewed. This was thought essential to avoid the 'catch-22' of patients being kept on the order on the grounds that it had kept them well or, conversely, on the grounds that they remained ill and in need of treatment. Predicting the long-term course of psychotic illnesses is not an exact science. It was foreseen that the situation could arise where a patient had recovered well enough to come off the order but it could be argued that this improvement was *because* he or she remained on it. How could one resolve this? The College felt that it should be assumed in the patient's favour both to avoid unnecessarily restrictive care and also to reassure the public (and potential patients).

Current thinking does not seem to have a time limit. We would anticipate that clinicians would exercise judgement and that review tribunals would need some convincing that an order should be extended when someone has been well for several years.

Conclusions

This has been a long chapter with few firm conclusions. Debates about balancing effective treatments against personal rights will continue to be at the centre of assertive outreach. There is no definitive answer as the balance point is determined as much by factors beyond the illness as by aspects of the illness. Just as society changes, the context changes and the threshold for compulsion is altered. The social acceptability of disorganized behaviour (and hence the stigma and discrimination stemming from such behaviour) depends on the tolerance and expectations of the local community. Risks also depend on where you are. Wandering off the ward is no big deal in a large mental hospital with extensive grounds but can be disastrous in a small district general hospital unit on a busy dual carriageway. Even climate makes a difference! Simply wandering in the winter in Canada or Scandinavia can result in exposure, frostbite, and even death.

Having a caring and involved family and some social stability radically alters the need for compulsion, which may account for much of the cultural variations. Their erosion is likely to explain at least some of the recent remarkable increase in compulsion in the UK (Wall *et al.* 1999).

The debate about compulsion in each individual case needs to be given space in team discussions, and the unique circumstances around each case should be acknowledged.

No team member has a monopoly on the thinking. Although it is codified in law, it is first and foremost an ethical decision, and ethical codes derive from all of us.

Team discussions about compulsion are often good starting points to remind us of the power issues in our relationships with our patients (and perhaps with each other!). There is no place in assertive outreach with severely mentally ill people for a naïve denial of dependency and power. Psychotherapists have a long tradition of exploring these relationships (in particular understanding how transference distortions introduce dependency and power). These are no less relevant because we are dealing with more severe disorders. We have not found having external facilitators to explore such issues helpful, although we know other teams do. Our observation is that such facilitated groups often focus excessively on team issues rather than patient issues. We feel that boundaries and autonomy are core issues for routine team meetings and supervision and that they should not be ignored. The scandals of abuse in the old mental hospitals arose because good staff forgot to question their practice with very dependent and difficult patients. It behoves us to make sure that it does not develop in assertive outreach.

Chapter 9

Cultural sensitivity

It would be true to say that we approached this chapter with more foreboding than any other in this book. Nowhere is there such fierce controversy in modern mental health services than that raging around the care of ethnic minority groups. In many ways it mirrors the sound and fury that emanated from the 'nature versus nurture' battles about families and schizophrenia in the 60s and 70s (see Chapter 15). It is an intensely politicized area. The very strength of feeling on the various sides of the argument (and the passion with which they continue to be advanced) indicates the absence of convincing or conclusive evidence for how to proceed. This is no simple 'either/or' issue—there are almost as many conflicts as there are protagonists!

We do not wish to take sides, but suggest that oversimplifying the difficulties of providing mental health care in a multi-racial and multicultural society (particularly casting the debate in terms of exploitation and racism) can alienate both staff and potential patients. It inhibits the trust and openness necessary for mental health care, and it severely constrains dialogue. Following our clinical habit we consider it more productive to give all the protagonists in any conflict the benefit of the doubt. We assume that both sides have patients' and families' welfare at heart and aim to relieve distress and safeguard dignity. Conflicts are best understood in terms of differing perceptions and perhaps incomplete information. It rarely helps to write off an opponent's viewpoint as simply mischievous or deliberately malicious. The aim should be to achieve a 'good enough' consensus from which to work.

Individuals from black and ethnic minority communities undoubtedly have specific mental health needs that are poorly served in most industrialized countries (Audit Commission 1994). There is also overwhelming evidence that rates of mental health problems are raised in some of these groups, such as schizophrenia in African and Afro-Caribbean men (especially second generation) (Harrison *et al.* 1997). Suicide rates have been found to be higher in the UK for young Asian women and young black men (Soni–Raleigh and Balarajan 1992; Bhugra *et al.* 1999). Conversely, there is concern that rates for take up of treatment is worryingly low in some ethnic minority groups such as the Asian population generally and Chinese and far-Eastern immigrants in particular. Take up of psychological therapies is low in all ethnic minority groups. These findings are not restricted to the UK.

Given the powerful social determination of help-seeking behaviour in all illnesses it should come as no surprise that there is variation in the perception and acceptance of what mental health services have to offer. Far from it. Deciding when unusual behaviour is 'illness' is a social process. Social groups will decide what is acceptable and what is unacceptable behaviour—it is a major component in how any group defines itself. When someone's behaviour is thought to be unusual or abnormal there may then be a whole range of ways of perceiving it. Is it creativity, eccentricity, religious possession, evil, or illness? Transcultural psychiatry reminds us that there can be an equally broad range of responses to a judgement of illness dependent on theories of causation and beliefs about treatment.

Learned sociological texts have been written about the way different societies respond to 'deviant' behaviour and about models of 'illness attribution' (Kleinman 1980). It is not necessary in a book like this to outline these various theories and how they relate to severe mental illness. Nor is it possible to discuss the power relations that lead to racism of both personal and institutional forms. We must, however, remind ourselves of individual and organizational responsibilities to tackle racism and ethnocentrism. It is vital that practitioners are aware that there is more than one way of understanding what is going on. Such an understanding is needed to make sense of patients', and their families', responses to their illnesses (as seen from essentially a Western, rationalist medical perspective) and how they perceive the treatments offered. It also reminds us that our understandings of these disorders are simply 'good enough' theories—none of us has ultimate truth.

Assessing the local situation

Effective community services must know the community that they serve. One of the great strengths of a locality-based service is that it can be tailored to specific needs. To do so requires knowing about them. Although much of this knowledge will be available informally, built up over time, it is worth making the effort to collect it formally, either by the team or by the larger service, and writing it down. Collective knowledge is not always available knowledge.

Case study

We had struggled for some time to maintain contact with a particularly elusive patient who we knew attended a Pentecostal church just a couple of miles outside our area. Only during his second systematic review did one of the team members identify the particular church and confirm that they would be willing to help us maintain contact. When we tried to work out why we had not known this before, it became clear that that team member had been on holiday for the previous review. As a member of the West African community she was an invaluable resource about these Pentecostal groups and their varying attitudes towards services like ours.

The NHS *Mental Health Policy Implementation Guide* (Department of Health 2001) gives a brief overview of the types of information that a service needs, and which should be written down and easily available.

- Ethnic breakdown of general population
- Community languages spoken
- Religious diversity
- Housing types (including homelessness)
- Unemployment
- Any vulnerable groups

Department of Health 2001

A local resource file should be kept covering all these areas. Having a resource file is not much use of course unless people get into the habit of using it. We would suggest that the resource file is reviewed at least annually by the team—probably best on a team 'away day' when the operational policy is being reviewed (Chapter 26). Otherwise, individual team members may continuously update the file when they come across valuable information but nobody else becomes aware of it. Similarly, obsolete information must be removed. If the file gets too bulky it will not be much use either. Information needs to be well edited and targeted; it also needs to be practical. For each of the headings above we would note the contact details and procedures for accessing the various groups and organizations.

The provision and access to interpreters for patients for whom English is a second or third language is an indication of good organizational practice. The use of trained interpreters rather than friends or family is preferable for a full assessment. How many of us would disclose our thoughts, fears, and beliefs via our parents or partners? Concerns about sexuality, religion, persecution, or passivity are most likely to be withheld if mediated through the patient's associate.

Cultural awareness training

Most employing authorities provide cultural awareness training for staff. Our own Trust requires a minimum of one day a year for all clinical staff and two days a year for clinical managers. Cultural awareness training has matured over the last decade and shed its rather confrontational and punitive reputation from the early 1990s. It is now usually externally facilitated and needs sensitivity to ensure that it does not become a vehicle for airing grievances and prejudices. Its purpose is to help us learn more about diverse cultural attitudes, expectations, and assumptions and to allow us to explore any prejudices, misunderstandings, or blocks that we may have. White, middle-aged men often approach them with real anxiety, fearing that they will be blamed for everything! Increasingly, however, these training days are now enjoyable experiences drawing on role play, anecdote, and a modicum of self-disclosure. Participants *learn about* themselves and their cultural assumptions rather than being *told about* them.

Staff backgrounds

In a team composed of staff from a wide range of backgrounds (see 'ethnic matching' below), increased cultural awareness is needed so that we can work well together, not just with our patients. We do not consider that a 'colour blind' approach is to be striven for. Quite the contrary. Services should be 'colour sensitive' (La Grenade 1999). Just as our patients are unique individuals with their personal and cultural backgrounds, so our staff also bring the richness of their varied cultures to our day-to-day work. This is a strength which can be utilized in ethnic and cultural matching. It also places an obligation on us to realize that the same event is not always the same experience for each of us involved. Teams need to be able to talk frankly about their experiences, including racism, both from their work and their social lives, so that they can support each other properly.

Case study

Al had been key working John for over two years. It had been demanding but productive work. Both Al and John are Afro-Caribbean. John has a substantial forensic history, including dangerous violence when psychotic. After over 18 months of stability John had begun to deteriorate, refusing medicines, smoking cannabis excesssively, and avoiding contact. Eventually Al made contact and ascertained that John was seriously unwell and would need asssment, probably for compulsory admission. Because of John's previous violence, the police insisted on the tactical support squad. Along with the consultant and social worker from the team, an extremely unpleasant (but brief and ultimately safe) assessment and transfer to hospital was effected. None of the team thought that anything else would have been possible and we were unanimous that this was the right thing to do. It was John's first admission without injury.

Although we all agreed on it being the right thing and were relieved that it had been achieved, the experience had been different for Al than for the consultant. Both had found it distasteful and menacing. But for Al, the sight of a young black man being subdued by an all-white group of police officers in full riot gear was hard to bear. He talked after of his sense of 'betrayal' of John, mixed with a feeling that the police felt the same way about him. He wanted to demonstrate his solidarity with John (remembering times when he had been stopped and searched by the police) yet equally strongly assert his difference as the responsible professional who had instigated the whole process.

In team feedback there was relief and praise that Al had organized the admission, but also a recognition that it was not easy for him to do it and no embarrassment in talking about these issues. Luckily, John did well.

Ethnic representation/matching

Population matching

Much has been written about the pros and cons of ethnic matching. We do not subscribe to a rigid dictate that black patients need black key workers, or that women patients need women key workers, and so on. Such a dictate would, anyway, sit poorly with the notion of shared responsibility or 'team approach'. On the other hand, it is essential that the overall configuration of the team should roughly represent the population it serves. In inner London, a multi-racial team is clearly essential. The same may not be true of, say, rural Ireland.

We subscribe fully to the concept of ethnic representation—both so that the team can be taken seriously by its clientele and (more importantly) so that it can understand the experiences of its clientele (patients and families and many of the support agencies). At a purely practical level, some gender and ethnic matching is essential. Many Asian families will not contemplate female members being treated by male staff—most of our female patients who need depot medication have this administered by female nurses. Some Asian patients have only poor command of English and it would be perverse not to provide them with an Urdu- or Hindi-speaking key worker if one is available.

Specialist teams

In London, there are teams with specific remits to work and engage with black patients. Often this arises from local pressure to improve access and cultural acceptibility where this has been thought lacking. This approach often favours commissioning services from the independent sector. Non-statutory, black mental health services (with ethnically matched professional and non-professional staff) avoid the stigma of statutory psychiatry. Some commentators go as far as to say that:

> Black communities have an inherent mistrust of the formal mental health care system.
>
> (La Grenade 1999)

One such black service is Antenna in North London:

Antenna is a pioneering initiative in London set up jointly by the local statutory mental health service and groups representing black African and Afro-Caribbean communities. The aim of this assertive outreach service is specifically to engage a target group of 16–25-year-olds from these communities who are experiencing mental health problems. The whole team is drawn from this cultural background and includes a consultant psychiatrist. Feedback from stakeholders identified the need for a service that confidently addressed the cultural and socio-economic issues as they relate to the black community. The service is proactive.

Black men in some localities in London experience 40% unemployment and may have been disadvantaged by the education system. The assertive outreach service may seek to engage patients by helping them back into education and work. Where a team is based in the voluntary sector the interface with statutory services is critical for patients with more severe disorders who inevitably require support in the form of prescribing, costed services such as housing, home care, or meals on wheels, and compulsory admission or treatment.

Patient matching

Patients who have experienced considerable racial harassment (in the UK this particularly affects young black men) may have difficulty trusting white staff. They may find it easier to relate to black staff who they know will understand what they have been through. If patients make it clear that they feel this way it makes sense to try and achieve it. On the other hand, one must be realistic. As the above example of John's compulsory admission demonstrates, this shared sense of solidarity will be sorely tested. Bitter recriminations will result if too much is made of it. The temptation to over-identify with the patient, against authority, must be carefully balanced with a recognition that *the key worker is part of the establishment* and, as such, is able to mobilize a full range of care and support for their patient.

Where we do have ethnically matched key workers we are careful to ensure that the secondary key worker is of a different cultural background. Also, the involvement of other team members will lead to a balanced exposure for the patient. Trust established with the key worker can then (we hope) spread to other staff members as the patient and family experience them working together and see how they treat each other with respect. Too total a dependence on an ethnically closely identified key worker can lead to problems when that key worker is absent unexpectedly.

Problems with matching

Sometimes, ethnic closeness can be a problem and one needs to recognize this. Patients (though more often families) who have felt discriminated against in the past may also feel discriminated against in this situation. Though very uncommon, we have, on a couple occasions, come across families who have talked of 'health care apartheid'. In both instances things improved when feelings were aired and issues discussed, and in neither case was a change of key worker pursued.

Below are some pitfalls in the key worker/patient relationship from a cultural and psycho-dynamic perspective.

Assumptions and responses by key workers

- **Colour blindness:** assumption that the minority patient is the same as the majority patient.
- **Colour consciousness:** all problems result from the minority status.
- **Cultural transference:** patient's feelings result from the key worker's race.
- **Cultural counter-transference:** key worker's feelings towards the patient result from their own race.
- **Cultural identification:** the key worker from a minority background defines all problems as racially based.
- **Identification with the disadvantaged:** the key worker from a minority background denies their status and power.

From Bhugra and Bhui (2001)

The benefits of improved alliance through identification can be at a price. Many patients (and families) understandably project the restrictions on achievement imposed by the illness on other, more common causes. We see in Chapter 19 how young men may prefer to attribute their symptoms to alcohol or drugs rather than schizophrenia—it seems somehow more acceptable. Most ethnic minority groups have common experiences of racial discrimination which lend solidarity and social cohesion. For a young black patient, unable to get a job because of his psychotic illness, it can be reassuring to blame racism. It is no longer simply '*his problem*' but '*society's unfairness*'. Working closely with a key worker from a similar background, who has faced similar obstacles, can rob the patient of that defence or, conversely, the key worker can identify too closely with this perspective.

Case study

Anne, a female Afro-Caribbean patient, formed a good relationship with her female African key worker. This was a considerable achievement as she had always been difficult to engage (particularly because of her complex and stormy relationship with her father who had significant mental health problems to contend with himself). The father initially welcomed the new key worker and supported all her recommendations. He emphasized how much she was on Anne's side and how skilled and conscientious she was. Over time, however, the father's support for the key worker became increasingly idealized. It was clear that he saw her as the daughter he had never had and was holding her up as an example for Anne, undermining her slowly growing self-confidence.

Despite quite intensive work with the pair, nothing seemed to reduce this demoralizing idealization. In the end, Anne herself asked for a change of key worker and has begun to work well with a white female nurse. Her father occasionally comments that it is easier for white people to get good jobs than for him and his daughter. He is less involved in her care (which has some downsides) but Anne is clearly enormously relieved not to be continually contrasted with her previous key worker.

Racial harassment and abuse

Zero tolerance

Zero tolerance towards racial or sexual harassment or physical threat is a welcome addition to the policies of most health and social care organizations. Clear statements to this effect are posted prominently in A&E departments and throughout hospitals. Our local Trust policy on this is stated in a notice at the entrance to all wards and in all out-patient departments. Making a reality of such a policy is not, however, that easy.

It is a good first step that the policy is unequivocal. It is no longer assumed that 'good' or 'experienced' staff will simply take such harassment in their stride as part of the job. This was certainly the attitude twenty or so years ago, when staff were expected to 'toughen up'. Being tolerant to such abuse was considered a professional virtue, almost part of the Hippocratic oath. A commitment to equal treatment for everyone, whatever their political or personal views (which we would agree is a core professional value for health and social care staff), was often confused with a personal tolerance of quite unacceptable behaviour.

It is not by chance that health and social care staff are generally more tolerant of abusive behaviour in patients and clients. We are used to dealing with individuals in crisis. People who are confused or in great pain and distress may say and do things they would never do otherwise, and for which afterwards they are often embarrassed and remorseful. Few of us would hold against them offensive remarks or a glancing blow from an acutely paranoid and scared individual. Being able to rise above unkind remarks is essential when dealing with acutely psychotic individuals. In hypomania particularly (Chapter 16), it is essential not to take to heart what is said (which can often be very accurately personal and pointed). These are symptoms of the illness and to be discounted. Subsequently, one may need to acknowledge and work through their impact when the patient is more recovered.

The central issues relate to dealing with established attitudes and behaviours. It is for managing racial harassment within the day-to-day behaviours of individuals that zero tolerance is needed. Mental health care is much less paternalistic in its practice than before. The benefit for the patient is that the relationship is more respectful and equal. The cost of this equality is that the patient has responsibilities. One of those responsibilities is to treat staff with respect and decency and to act as much as possible as a responsible citizen.

Words and deeds

People can and do, think what they like. Our legitimate concern with racial harassment and abuse is what people do, *not* what they think. As children grow up in a more multicultural and varied society, with schools that address issues of racial and cultural tolerance, we can hope over time for more inclusive, less prejudiced attitudes. Working in the community with mentally ill individuals (already the object of stigma and discrimination), however, the immediate effects of racial harassment and abuse have to be addressed.

When racial harassment and abuse is discussed it is often assumed that it is always abuse of the (usually ethnic minority) patient by white members of staff or the public. This is, undoubtedly, the most recognized, but not the only, form in which it occurs. Society is highly sensitive to these manifestations and there is a growing consensus about not tolerating them. As suggested in the discussion of zero tolerance, ethnic minority staff must be accorded the same rights as any other in this matter.

There are three forms of racial harassment which are of specific importance in outreach work:

1. Harassment of the patient or family by neighbours and the general public
2. Harassment of neighbours and public by the patient
3. Harassment of staff by patients or their families

Harassment of the patient or family by neighbours and the general public

Protecting patients and their families from racial abuse is clearly one of the roles of an outreach worker. As an advocate for their rights this means making sure not only that they are not discriminated against either because of their mental illness but also on the grounds of their ethnicity. The two are often intertwined, sometimes deliberately. Racial intolerance can be dressed up as a fear of psychotic behaviour when neighbours request an eviction. Resentment against immigrants and asylum seekers can make the position of patients and their families intolerable, with mounting tension leading to relapse. Dealing with these situations requires tact and careful judgement. Simply acceding to hostility and organizing a move may involve enormous upheaval for the family. It can also reveal a loss of vital supports whose existence and importance had been masked by the conflict.

Legal procedures

At its most extreme it is possible, with the help of the local authority, to instigate proceedings against harassing neighbours which can result in *them* being evicted and even prosecuted. We have never done this and would be concerned about the degree of risk it would carry for our patients in terms of reprisals and added stress. We have tried to talk to neighbours when patients and families give us permission. Sometimes it has been possible to increase tolerance when neighbours have had a clearer understanding of the situation—why the family has had to flee persecution, why the patient is unable to work, how hard they are trying to get better with treatment.

It is not, however, easy to change attitudes and our success with such interventions has been minimal. The grim reality is that many severely mentally ill patients in the community will live in fairly deprived areas and be subject, daily, to levels of harassment that most of us would find very difficult to accept. Where such harassment clearly breaks the law, when there are threats or open hostility, then it is our duty to support patients and their families in obtaining justice. Often this means supporting them in contacting the police and keeping up the pressure to get charges pressed.

Harassment of neighbours and public by the patient

It is all too easy to forget that our patients can also harbour and express racist or sexist attitudes. These can be intensified during acute relapses—it is not at all uncommon for paranoid delusions to involve specific cultural and ethnic groups (black patients feeling persecuted by whites, white patients by the IRA, or by Asian groups). On the whole, this is not so difficult to deal with. Both staff and neighbours are able to write off what is said (or sometimes written) in acute episodes. The risk is greater when the patient is not known locally. We have had hypomanic patients assaulted because of uninhibited racist remarks they have made in pubs or in the street.

What to do if the patient or family have racist attitudes that are not related to the illness? We still have a duty to care and cannot simply write off patients because, for example, they come from a far right nationalist family and are derogatory and insulting about black people, or are from an extremist Hindu family and make disparaging remarks about Muslims. In such circumstances it is important to maximize the chances of successful engagement. This involves not allocating a key worker who will excite such prejudices. Many of us feel uncomfortable doing this—it is as if we are colluding with the racism. Our approach, however, should be to strengthen the positive rather than focus too much on the negative. Avoiding a match which is likely to be unsuccessful is not essentially that different to meeting a preference for a specific type of key worker (e.g. if a patient specifically asks for a female key worker).

We have found a softening of attitudes over time with some of our very prejudiced patients. As they get to accept their key worker they become more positive to the team and its members, irrespective of their individual ethnicity. They can form warm relationships with team members and look forward to their visits while we know, from conversations with their key worker, that they still have strong prejudices against that individual's background. We have no hard evidence that this experience of working with a multi-racial team does generalize for bigoted patients but our experience is generally positive.

Distinguishing thoughts from behaviours

At a more practical level, patients and their families may need help in learning not to antagonise their neighbours by racist behaviour. Just as we often work hard to encourage patients not to share their delusional beliefs too widely, we can use the same procedures to help them inhibit racist remarks and behaviour. A pragmatic approach is more likely to succeed than a moral one. The style emphasizes the risks and consequences of such behaviour. Just as cognitive behavioural therapy for hallucinations (Chapter 25) aims to modify the response to them rather than their occurrence, the aim is to help patients keep their racist views to themselves rather than attempt to stop them having them.

This approach makes a very firm distinction between thought and action. We make clear to the patient that, although we do not share his or her beliefs, and indeed disapprove of them, it does not stop us wanting to help. However, we are not going to collude with expressions of such ideas. It is rather like the clergy's obligation to 'love the sinner but hate the sin'. Firm but non- confrontational responses to racist remarks should be used: 'I don't want to hear about that', or even 'I'm not going to listen to any more of this. I'll come back tomorrow when you're able to focus on the task in hand.' Refusing to listen to racist remarks about ethnic minority staff is a very concrete way of demonstrating what is and what is not acceptable: 'Okay, I understand you're upset about Krishna's last visit. I'm happy to hear about what he did that upset you—but not about who he is.'

No matter how hard one tries, patients and their families may persist in racist behaviour towards neighbours or other patients. They will have to suffer the consequences. Day centres and hostels increasingly ban patients who persist in racist behaviour. Even in-patient wards may discharge patients for such behaviour if their condition allows it. Housing associations and local authorities will evict persistently racist tenants, though obviously only as a last resort when they are mentally ill. We have on several occasions had to rehouse patients because of racist behaviour. Most often this has been to protect them from retaliatory violence from other tenants, but on more than one occasion is was to pre-empt an eviction.

Harassment of staff by patients or their families

Most of us have been roundly abused in times of crisis (e.g. during a compulsory admission, when patients have to be restrained). It is unpleasant, but not a big deal. It is much more wearing when it is persistent and in cold blood. Usually such abuse is directed at in-patient staff when patients are compulsorily detained. In this situation there is little alternative but to tolerate it.

We can rationalize that the anger stems from the compulsion and the racist content is probably an expression of their sense of helplessness. Staff are well able to distinguish racist abuse that is driven by psychotic experiences from that which is an expression of anger or long-held racial beliefs. Motive clearly does make a difference. The former is strikingly unhurtful whereas remarks that are meant to hurt, usually do. Rapid control of the psychosis is probably the only solution in either situation. Where the abusive remarks arise from the psychosis they will recede; where they are anger at detention, then detention can be lifted as the psychosis is controlled.

Staff need to be protected from racist remarks and, within the ward, reorganizing shifts and nursing patterns may be necessary. Racist abuse of white and Asian staff is no less common than that of black staff. Black and Asian patients can be equally guilty of such behaviour. White on black racist remarks may be getting less, reflecting society's increasing intolerance of them. It may be that zero tolerance policies are often interpreted rather simplistically in terms of old patterns of racism. We need to treat racism equally firmly irrespective of its direction.

Racist remarks by families also need to be treated firmly (after allowing for initial distress). Most services make it explicit that they will not deal with family members who behave in a persistently racist manner. Logical though this is, it is far from easy or simple. Do we withhold family work to reduce Expressed Emotion for a patient who (though not actively racist himself) lives with bigoted and insulting parents?

In all aspects of managing racism within mental health, judgement has to be exercised. This is very much an area where the focus must remain on the patient's welfare. In each individual case the pros and cons of confronting racism have to be weighed up against damage to the therapeutic alliance and the potential of the treatments to make a significant difference over time. A clear and unequivocal policy (such as that of zero tolerance) has benefits but it should be interpreted with clinical judgement in each individual case.

User and carer involvement

Active involvement of user and carer groups from the various ethnic minority popula-tions served is one of the most effective ways of improving local cultural sensitivity and acceptability. Such involvement should be encouraged not just on an individual case basis but at all phases of developing and monitoring services. Open days, when teams invite the local population to hear about their work, are invaluable. Specific invitations to local religious and ethnic leaders and representatives are never wasted. Often staff are anxious about this, fearing that they will be criticized for failings, and are reluctant to engage in this public dialogue. In truth, it is rarely confrontational. Least of all because there are likely to be several groups present, each with a different agenda. They learn about each other as well as about us, and we about them.

Engaging such groups early and often means that they can give invaluable advice about how best to provide care and support for their members. They can often clarify simple misunderstandings. For instance, when Asian patients in South London requested traditional healing (prayer or dietary advice from a mosque) this did not in fact imply a criticism of our medical approach (Greenwood *et al.* 2000). We had assumed that requests to take a patient away to a mosque to attend a series of rituals suggested that the family had little faith in Western medicine. Not so, we were informed. They clearly appreciated and wanted the benefits of medication, but they also wanted the added benefits of their familiar interventions. We also learnt from them how hopelessly inadequate terms like 'Asian' are. Increasingly, we use the country of origin, not the region, in our discussions (e.g. 'this Somali man', 'this Bangladeshi family').

The other advantage of close involvement with user and carer groups from ethnic minorities is their spontaneous willingness to help and the offers of support they bring. It is probably not a cliché to propose that many immigrant groups still have stronger and wider support networks than the white British. The variety of such groups makes it difficult to predict where their strengths will lie—hence the simple approach of making sure that they understand as fully as possible exactly what we do so that they can tell us directly how they can contribute.

Political correctness

Concerns about political correctness are particularly acute in the area of ethnic minorities and in mental health generally. It is good that we have realized that casual generalizations can be demeaning to individuals with an experience (whether personal or cultural) of being treated as second-class citizens. Observing that patients in mental hospitals were always referred to by their first names by staff (to whom they replied using staff titles), Maxwell Jones insisted on mutual first names in his therapeutic communities (Jones 1952). He realized the asymmetry of hierarchical relationships. What seems like a friendly familiarity from above may be felt as humiliation from below when you have no choice about it. Long-term unequal relationships are really only acceptable if they are entered into freely. Language should be used carefully so that it does not hide unacceptable power relationships.

What was central to much of the understanding of the complexity of relationships in therapeutic communities 30 years ago has become commonplace. We are sensitive to how language (often with the appearance of friendliness and humour) can gloss over, or even strengthen, prejudices and practices that if examined carefully we could not defend. The success of the women's movement and the fight for genuine equal rights for all members of society has rightly obliged us to examine language more closely and to be careful how we use it.

This has undoubtedly benefited former vulnerable and marginalized members of society. Witness the unacceptability of previously common words (e.g. idiot, spastic), along with a heightened awareness that individuals are more than their labels. Changing terms can reduce stigma, though it is naïve to assume it abolishes it. In the field of mental handicap there has been a deliberate practice of changing the terms for individuals with limited intellectual capacity. This policy is aimed at improving the understanding of the limitation while continually stressing that this is just one aspect of the individual. In exactly the same way we use the term 'person with schizophrenia' or 'schizophrenia patient' rather than 'schizophrenic patient' or 'schizophrenic' because individuals with this disorder say they feel written off by terms like 'schizophrenic'. There is no absolute logic to this—most people with asthma do not mind being referred to as 'asthmatics' (there is no social stigma attached to that term, and neither does it imply a complete identity).

There are very real advantages of such careful use of language (avoiding stigmatizing terms and using inclusive terms whenever possible) for individuals with severe mental illnesses. They find themselves stigmatized and undermined routinely in the mass media. It is an aspect of our advocacy role for them that we scrupulously avoid such practices and foster the use of more neutral and accurate language.

Stereotypes

Recognizing a person's individuality means avoiding the shorthand assumptions of stereotypes. Not all young black men will want to attend a community music group; not all white men will be interested in football; nor do all Asian women want to socialize with other Asian women. Racial stereotypes are a form of prejudice. They need not even be negative to be prejudicial—why assume a Jamaican will be a good dancer?

Mental health work can be fun!

The price sometimes paid for such political correctness is that professionals can come to believe that any levity or humour in their work is a sign of disrespect for their patients. This is to throw the baby out with the bath water. Mental health work is based in honest relationships and these are complex, shifting, and often unequal. When Maxwell Jones insisted on greater equality of relationships in his therapeutic community it was not to abolish status and interpersonal differences, but to help examine them and understand them better. Paradoxically, this approach made members more self-conscious about hierarchy and status. It is self-deluding to work with severely mentally ill individuals and pretend that the relationship is an entirely free and equal one. It is not and cannot be. That does not mean that it cannot be respectful and honest.

An honest relationship between individuals will allow for humour (as well as for impatience, annoyance, and frustration). As a team we have learnt to be more free with each other as we have learnt to be more supportive and understanding. When we appointed our first user worker we were anxious that we would have to stop expressing our frustration with patients in team meetings or making jokes about what we do. She soon disabused us of these anxieties. The last thing that she wanted, she said, was for us to be 'walking on egg shells' around her. She knew that we respected her and her work. She could tolerate and join in the banter but, if it went too far, then she, like any of us, could say so.

We need to complain about patients when things are difficult, just as members of a family complain about each other but remain committed. If the relationship slides into dislike or fear, then we are not able to do a useful job. Being able to let off steam prevents, rather than promotes, relationships deteriorating.

A multidisciplinary and multicultural team will also have endless opportunities to find the funny side in difficult situations. There are realistic and healthy tensions between doctors, nurses, social workers, occupational therapists, and psychologists which can be a source of pleasure and enrichment in the work, as well as of conflict. Being able to talk openly about differences is more likely to lead to effective joint working. Similarly with ethnic differences. Pretending these do not exist can only lead to misunderstanding. Being able to enjoy the differences and to gently tease one another seems to promote respect and support. Taking pleasure in the humorous aspects of what at times can be grim work is essential for survival.

Case study

Ed (an Afro-Caribbean case manager) was reporting back on an incident when he had been assaulted by one of his patients. He had gone to give the patient her routine depot injection and found her in the kitchen baking. Baking was one of the activities that we had been able to interest her in. Unfortunately, on this day she had also been drinking and was very irritable. She shouted at Ed saying that she did not want his injection. She pushed him backwards covering him with flour and breaking his new expensive glasses. Ed withdrew immediately, althought the patient had begun already to apologize.

At feedback Ed was more upset about his new glasses (of which he had been very proud) than of any real worry about being hurt. He was also annoyed that he had flour spilled all over his jacket and face. Andy (a West African case manager) replied that he should not complain that much about his glasses: 'It's not that bad Ed. After all, you went in black and you came out white. Michael Jackson would have paid a fortune for that.'

The above anecdote may seem tasteless or politically incorrect in some situations. It certainly did not feel that way to those involved. Humour provides a safe area in which differences of experience and expectations can be acknowledged and explored. It allows us to get to know more about each other without being intrusive or pompous.

Apart from explicitly abusive or offensive language there are no easily imported absolute rules about what can, and what cannot, be said between team members. How it feels will often be the best guide. It will only be a good guide, however, if the team has an open culture where less confident members *really* can indicate if they feel put down or embarrassed by comments. Senior team members must ensure such a culture is sustained (e.g. by ensuring expression from all in team reviews, by putting time aside in team days to allow reflection and criticism, and by being open to criticism themselves). However, being at the top of the pyramid they are the least well placed to judge the tone. This is not easy to do and there will undoubtedly be mistakes and times when individuals overstep the mark. However, in the long run this is surely better than safety at the cost of rendering the team mechanical and unsupportive.

Conclusions

Cultural sensitivity generally mirrors the core tasks of mental health workers. Our job is to understand each unique individual with whom we work. This involves understanding their history and how they see the world around them. We need to recognize that the same event will be experienced differently by those involved and that sensitivity and respect must always be used to avoid giving unnecessary offence. Differences may arise because of mental illness or because of a different cultural expectation or because of the personal history of that individual.

For example, a political street demonstration could be a frightening experience for a number of reasons. For one individual it is so because they are paranoid and refer the events to themselves; for another individual it is because of traumatic experiences in their war-torn homeland; or perhaps it is a reminder of a drunken and out-of-control father. And to yet another, it is because they are excessively anxious and controlled, taught from childhood to keep their emotions to themselves.

Cultural diversity is a great strength in mental health teams because it deepens our understanding of human experiences by illuminating them from different perspectives. It makes the job more difficult, however, because we need to be aware of a greater range of needs and responses and, perhaps, because consensus is less easy to achieve. It requires us to be more sensitive to how we behave, to be aware that what we do may not be interpreted in the way we mean it. It needs us to be more careful and thoughtful about how we use language, and it runs the risk that, scared of offending others, we become 'wooden' and less accessible as humans. It reminds us, however, that there is no unassailable primacy for any one world view.

Racism has to be confronted in this, as in any other profession. A balance needs to be struck between carefully monitoring our behaviour to identify prejudices and allowing ourselves to relate as whole individuals. The very complexities of the situations confronting mental health workers in the community prevent any oversimplified and sloganized approach to social inclusion. These situations will continue to present us with incredibly complex ethical challenges where there is no single right answer—another reason why the job is never boring.

Part II

Health and social care practice

Chapter 10

Engagement

Introduction

Engagement is the most overused and under-defined term in the assertive outreach vocabulary. Definitions range from the ability of teams to retain patients in the service, to attempts to describe the qualities required of the patient/worker relationship. Table 10.1 classifies the varied activities and strategies that together can help build regular contact, promote a therapeutic alliance, and maximize our ability to provide long-term continuity of care to those patients who have come to be known as 'hard to engage'. The selected vignettes and discussion of the strategies in this chapter should equip the reader with a working definition and a toolbox for practice.

Table 10.1 Classification of engagement-related activity and intent

Constructive approach	Informative approach	Restrictive approach
◆ Befriending	◆ Assertive outreach; frequent and persistent contact— direct or indirect	◆ Use of statutory powers under 1983 Mental Health Act: — Section 25 after care under supervision —Guardianship — Section 17 long leave
◆ Collaborative or patient-led agenda	◆ Regular contact with patient's family and carers where no direct contact with patient	◆ Appointeeship
◆ Strengths-focused interventions	◆ 'Doorstepping'; regular attempts at contact despite refusal of access	◆ No 'drop out' policy
◆ Non-judgemental, nurturing approach	◆ Observation of patient's home environment when access denied	
◆ Advocacy and empowering approach	◆ Contact and information gathering through third parties (e.g. neighbours and local community) where necessary	

Table 10.1 (*Continued*)

Constructive approach	Informative approach	Restrictive approach
◆ Home or community-based interventions	◆ Contact with housing and benefits office	
◆ Preference for 'mainstream' activities	◆ Contact with GP	
◆ Practical assistance and problem solving		
◆ Social and recreational activity		
◆ Assistance with financial and welfare benefits		
◆ Employment assistance and support		
◆ Support and problem solving for family and carers		
◆ Obtaining or preserving accommodation		

This classification describes the spectrum of activity from those interventions aimed at building a genuine therapeutic alliance, through monitoring strategies, to the ultimate legal sanctions when all else fails and the clinical picture dictates. These three strands will be described in more detail in this chapter. It is very often the *intention* of the activity that classifies it as 'engagement'. For example, home-based services and interventions are not necessarily related to engagement, but where they are driven by a desire to make services more acceptable to patients' needs and circumstances then home-based services do enhance the process of engaging. We often focus on why patients fail to engage with services and less about why services fail to engage with patients (Sainsbury Centre for Mental Health 1998).

Housing, benefits, and employment activity are all social care interventions in themselves. They appear in our classification because where they are clearly the patient's priority their fulfilment will foster a positive attitude towards services. This may then help create the conditions necessary to initiate or change treatment.

Engagement should not be seen only as a means to an end; social and recreational activities can have direct positive effects on quality of life and mood. Most patients referred to assertive outreach, however, will have a compelling need for treatment with medication and enhanced compliance. As outlined in Chapter 4, we see people frequently in order to monitor their mental state. We monitor their mental state in order to offer treatment. Successful engagement with a key worker or services will facilitate work with a patient on other difficult issues such as personal hygiene, money, aspirations, relationships, and sexuality. How many of us would discuss these topics with a stranger?

Constructive approach

Two quotes encapsulate this concept:

> Very few people seek help from mental health services with enthusiasm.
>
> (Onyett 1992)

> The foundation for effective assertive outreach services will be 'engagement' and 'persistence' with a constructive rather than restrictive approach to keeping track of people.
>
> (Sainsbury Centre for Mental Health 1998).

With any new referral it is important to spend time explaining to the patient why they have been referred, how assertive outreach may differ from their previous experience of mental health services, and what the opportunities and benefits are for them. This information should be backed up with written material and the patient's views should be sought. This in itself demonstrates a collaborative and negotiated approach which may feel different and new to the patient. Often, patients may be reluctant to change from their existing key worker or to receive any form of service. Individualized reasons for assertive outreach, stressing how the new team will provide extra resources to enable the patient to survive outside hospital, avoiding readmission and relapse, helps ensure that the transfer is not seen as any form of criticism of the previous team or key worker. In this way constructive attempts at engagement start from the very beginning.

Many patients will be able to provide their own agenda, given some support and non-judgemental prompts. Where engagement is difficult, these patient-led 'wants' should be the starting point, unless the need for clinical treatment is critical.

The Sainsbury Centre for Mental Health commissioned 'user-led' research into patients' views on assertive outreach (Beeforth *et al.* 1994). Patients described assertive outreach as generally preferable to standard psychiatric care for a number of reasons. Firstly, many valued the relationship with staff, which became more 'authentic' (closer to a normal friendship). Patients appreciated the availability, reliability, and ability of their key worker to offer practical help. The availability of interventions and support for carers was recognized as desirable, as was the emphasis on empowering patients and promoting mainstream activities. In general, patients preferred the strengths' model (Prance 1993; Rapp and Wintersteen 1989), with its focus on strengths, interests, and abilities. This model views the 'consumer' as the director of the helping process and emphasizes that even those most severely mentally ill can grow and change. While the strengths' model has its limitations as the foundation for a whole service, its concepts (and particularly its emphasis on the patient's agenda) provide an excellent philosophy for engaging constructively.

Case study

Arthur lost his cleaning job 10 years previously due to developing paranoid beliefs and increasingly derogatory and disabling auditory hallucinations. Always a loner, he had become extremely withdrawn and neglected. He believed everyone could read his mind as he heard people castigating him for his heretical or treasonable 'compulsive thoughts'. He had no insight into the psychiatric nature of his condition. He was distressed by his experiences and had a history of barricading himself in his flat for fear of being thrown into prison. As a result, access to his flat was extremely difficult.

On referall, his flat was spartan and neglected. He had worn the same trousers for three years—they were stiff with grime. Arthur stated that he did not wish to be visited regularly at home and if it was more than once a month he would have nothing to say or report since his life was so limited. His only activity was a weekly visit to the local post office, which he described as an ordeal.

The first task was to describe to Arthur how our approach might differ from what he had experienced previously. He would not have to 'report', nor would he be questioned. He was encouraged to think of his key worker's visits more as befriending and supportive. He might, in time, want his key worker to accompany him on his weekly shopping trip, to make it less of an ordeal. Arthur was not much impressed by these proposals and access remained difficult.

On a subsequent visit, his key worker needed to use the toilet and discovered it did not flush. Lifting the cistern, he saw that a piece of plastic had broken in the flush linkage. Arthur had been tipping bowls of water in the bowl to flush it for about five years. A twenty-minute trip to the ironmongers, fifty pence, and some rather unpleasant handiwork secured a working flush. This proved to be the defining moment in the engagement process. His key worker had proved himself useful and perhaps trustworthy. From this small foundation, other interventions were possible over the years, perhaps the most satisfying being an outing to buy some new trousers.

An almost universally powerful engagement tool is knowledge of the state welfare benefit system and related sources of extra finance. Since the majority of our clients are wholly dependent on welfare, an ability to obtain disability living allowance, a community care grant, or a holiday grant, increase our acceptability in the patient's eyes.

Informative approach

The term 'informative approach' has been used to describe monitoring and observation. The team may be required to undertake this for a patient who has disengaged or is at risk of doing so. It may not always be seen as constructive by the patient but it is not restrictive.

Tensions often exist between the team's duty of care and the patient's desire for self-determination, their privacy, or reluctance to be viewed as mentally ill. Assertive outreach involves taking responsibility for care. Persistent contact, direct or indirect, provides an early warning system for social or clinical crises. This is only if the right enquiries are made and the worker is alert to the signs. We aim for each patient to be seen on average twice a week. However, contact ranges from seven days a week for some patients to only once a fortnight or so for some 'graduating' patients. Obviously these contacts are mainly to deliver interventions and services but we should always be monitoring and observing. Each visit permits informal assessment of appearance, sleep patterns, mood, irritability, hostility, compliance with medication, red utility bills, eviction notices, damaged furniture, street drugs' equipment, alcohol, etc.

Ford and Repper (1994) interviewed 20 case managers working in assertive outreach and 10 CPNs. None of the CPNs would have accepted a new referral's refusal to see them after the first attempt; all, however, would have passed them back to the referring agency within six attempts. In contrast, 19 of the case managers said that they would continue indefinitely to attempt to engage and make contact.

If direct contact is refused then indirect monitoring and information gathering can become a substitute. In the current climate, failure to monitor (and document!) can lead to criticism if an inquiry follows an untoward incident involving that patient. The first step is usually to seek the family's views on their relative's health and need for services. Families may be reluctant to help directly, by giving access, if this risks conflict with the patient. By maintaining contact with the family, feedback on mental state and compliance can be obtained. Third-party sources of information can also provide knowledge of the patient's routine, places frequented, and friends. Likewise, home visits when the patient is not at home can be a useful opportunity to look through the window, check for piles of unopened mail, and bump into neighbours. Indicators of relapse vary from patient to patient and dirty dishes or mouldy take-away cartons cannot always be reliable evidence. Smashed windows, burn marks, and insecure premises are more worrying. Where the patient has a history of hostility it is generally not advisable to peer through the letterbox since stories (probably apocryphal) do abound of workers being attacked through letterboxes. Entering premises on your own when the door has been left open by a chaotic or preoccupied patient, in order to have a look around, is also hazardous.

Neighbours will often volunteer information, especially when they are involved. It is rarely necessary to outline your professional relationship when making basic enquiries with neighbours. In many cases a simple 'have you seen the gentleman downstairs recently?' elicits a history of nocturnal shouting and screaming, or other problems only too apparent to the neighbours.

Enquiries with the council can produce other possible indicators of relapse, such as complaints by neighbours or recent arrears. Housing and benefits departments will usually take your name and telephone number as a contact and inform you when problems arise to enlist your help in resolving them. If the weight of evidence becomes overwhelming, then a medical or Mental Health Act assessment is worth trying. Such information gathering can inform risk assessment:

Case study

Olu is a 38-year-old man with a long history of paranoid schizophrenia. Numerous admissions over 25 years, often via the police on Section 136, prompted his referral to assertive outreach. His experiences led to mistrust of services and avoidance of follow-up and treatment.

Case study (*Continued*)

Olu was withdrawn and always a loner who had no contact with his parents. He had long been labelled 'hard to engage'. He had told social services that his parents had moved back to Nigeria and attempts to contact them for Section 3 consultation proved fruitless. Attempts at contact with Olu were met with either his empty council flat or, if he was at home, expletives and the door remaining closed. Even following treatment in hospital, when he became more open, he would barely tolerate a five-minute interaction. Alternative approaches were needed to break this cycle of repeated 136 and 135 admissions, together with the associated risks of rent arrears and distress.

Information on Olu's mental health status could be ascertained indirectly from the reaction to your knock when he was home. He was rarely home during the day, requiring persistent, early morning visits. The ferocity of expletives when grossly unwell would prompt joint visits. With mounting concerns, we eventually decided to talk with immediate neighbours. We had to overcome major doubts, balancing confidentiality with risk. In the end, there were three main reasons for this course of action:

1. Olu's appearance and behaviour were such that the neighbours could be in no doubt about his mental health and social needs.

2. Previous risks existed, both generally and to the neighbours.

3. No relatives were in contact.

Restrictive approach

Restrictive approaches come last, after a long period of attempts at engagement and information gathering. Not all patients who refuse contact will justify this. If someone appears to be coping reasonably well and no risks other than future relapse are apparent, the team may have to accept minimal direct and indirect contact until such a time as the situation deteriorates. Difficult ethical issues arise in cases where compulsion is prolonged or repeated, and these require team discussion.

Case study

Whilst a Section 135 warrant was being arranged, Olu was picked up on a Section 136 by the police, some distance away, and brought to our local hospital. It was agreed that we would use a restrictive approach.

He was converted to a Section 3 with treatment consisting of depot medication, as all previous attempts with oral medication complicance had failed. 'Intensive inreach' of three or more visits to the ward weekly, by his key worker, continued and Olu's mental state improved quickly, as always. After three depots he was given extended leave with the proviso that he attend the ward for his depot every two weeks and meet his key worker in the alternate week. These arrangements were transferred to supervised discharge, requiring him to attend the ward twice weekly for the purpose of offering treatment and allowing access to his 'supervisor' (see Chapter 8, 'Compulsion and freedom'). He had a good relationship with the ward staff and chose to have his depot from them. He also often got breakfast.

At the time of writing Olu has been out of hospital for two years and his supervised discharge has been renewed twice. He defaulted on his depot after six months and, when seen at home, complained of side-effects. His depot was reduced and he restarted. The benefits of a protracted period of treatment and contact continue to accrue. He has taken himself for a haircut, removing many years of matted 'locks'. His neighbours are more supportive of him and greet him on passing. He is warmer and less guarded in relationships. He has not been in trouble with the police and has allowed his key worker to accompany him to the housing office to sort out his arrears.

Finally, out of the blue, his mother phoned the team base to enquire after him. Both parents had remained local residents, despite Olu's previous claim! We were able to give glowing feedback on progress to his mother and encourage direct contact. She allowed us to give Olu her phone number and said she would visit her son. They have yet to meet.

In the Ford and Repper (1994) interviews referred to earlier, it was clear that some people were more uncomfortable with this aspect of the work:

> Some case managers were concerned that they could be restricting clients' rights to refuse a service. In practice this issue had to be balanced against the case manager's responsibility to provide a service to clients who could be at risk of neglect, self-injury or of harming others.

Multidisciplinary team discussion and liaison with families provide ways of checking out our ethical judgements about whether, or when, to act restrictively.

Mental health legislation varies both within the UK and internationally, and is likely to change soon (see Chapter 8). The anachronistic wording of the Mental Health Act in the UK means that patients can effectively be discharged from hospital whilst still under some requirements of their compulsory admission. This is called 'being on leave'. Three aspects of 'leave' are particularly relevant to engagement—long leave, supervised discharge, and guardianship. These are discussed here, along with appointeeship.

Long leave

While the granting of leave should not be used as an alternative to discharge, we have found, for some hard-to-engage patients, that it enhances contact and compliance with medication and reduces the time spent in hospital.

Case study

Olu was given increasing periods of Section 17 leave to test out medication compliance and contact. The fact that he remained liable to be detained if he did not return or comply with the depot was discussed fully with him. He was pleased to be allowed home quickly and accepted the 'trade off' of still being on a section. He quickly earned long leave which carried on under Section 17 for several months until he was transferred to supervised discharge. Without this restrictive approach, previous experience had shown that he would drop out within two to three months.

We have experienced some local concern about the use of Section 17 long leave. Ward staff worry that they still have some responsibility to provide a leave bed. Our agreement is that once a patient has been on Section 17 long leave for a week, the assertive outreach team is fully responsible for them. They are reviewed along with community patients, and a bed does not need to be kept. Consultant responsibility across in-patient and community care helps. A separate in-patient consultant may feel uncomfortable giving several months' leave to a patient they are not following up themselves. Where further statutory restriction is needed, aftercare under supervision (supervised discharge) should be discussed well in advance of expiry.

Supervised discharge

Properly called 'aftercare under supervision', these new powers were introduced in April 1996 (Department of Health 1995) partly as a response to the moral and media panic surrounding well-publicized homicides by the severely mentally ill, such as the case highlighted by the Clunis Report (Ritchie 1994).

Powers of supervised discharge can be applied to any patient who has been detained in hospital and require the patient, once discharged, to co-operate with a treatment plan or face recall to hospital for assessment. They include the power to 'take and convey'. They are intended for patients who would present a substantial risk or who would be unlikely to receive aftercare services without these powers. The conditions of the treatment plan can be that:

- The patient resides at a specified place.
- The patient attends at a place and time specified for the *purpose* of medical treatment, occupation, education, or training.
- The patient allows access to their home to the supervisor, any registered medical practitioner, or approved social worker (ASW) and to any other person authorized by the supervisor.

For assertive outreach teams it makes sense for one of the team, the patient's key worker, to be the named supervisor. Supervised discharge can only *require* the patient's attendance for medical treatment; if the patient refuses the treatment, there are no more powers. The patient cannot be detained and an application for admission for treatment would need to be considered if the patient was currently unwell enough to satisfy the criteria. We have found that our local police will not assist in recall to hospital under supervised discharge.

Despite these drawbacks we have had surprisingly positive outcomes from a dozen or more uses of this legislation with our most intractable patients (Burns 2000c). We have rarely needed to invoke the powers of recall since most patients do recognize that they have entered into a legal contract.

Guardianship

Supervised discharge has largely replaced the little-used powers of guardianship.

> If a patient needs to receive after-care within a formal structure but he or she does not meet all the criteria for after-care under supervision, guardianship under Section 7 of the MHA 1983 may be used.
>
> (Department of Health 1999*b*)

Whereas supervised discharge aims to keep a formerly detained patient out of hospital after discharge, guardianship is seen as a possible alternative to admission or to continuing hospital care. Guardianship is applied for by a social worker, making application to the local authority, together with a comprehensive care plan. The guardian can require the patient to live at a specified place, attend for treatment and so on, and give access to their home to staff detailed in the Act. We have no experience of its use in our patient group.

Appointeeship

Where a person is in receipt of DSS benefits, arrangements can be made for payment to a person on behalf of a claimant unable to act. That person is appointed by the DSS. It can be anyone—a social worker, even a DSS employee. No medical evidence is required. No legal safeguards exist and no monitoring of the appointee's use of the money takes place. However this procedure is quick and easy compared to the Court of Protection.

(Brayne and Martin 1990)

This quote is from two solicitors demonstrating the contrast of appointeeship with the more rigorous Mental Health Act powers.

Appointeeship can be used as 'leverage' in the engagement process.

Case study

When Mark was referred to the assertive outreach team, he already had an appointee in the finance department of the local social services. The appointee was an administrator who transferred money weekly into an account that Mark could access, for his personal use, through a bank branch or cash card. The appointee took care of all bills and matters relating to housing and welfare benefits.

Mark suffers from schizophrenia and was particularly chaotic and 'hard to engage'. His mental state was worsened by non-compliance with prescribed medication and also regular 'crack' cocaine use. He required more and more money to maintain his habit and was involved in petty theft and even managed to defraud the bank. The bank decided not to prosecute but refused him as a customer, leaving the appointee with no means of giving Mark his money.

After discussion, the team decided to act as an intermediary between Mark and the appointee by agreeing to dispense his money. Three times a week we hand over £30, on condition that Mark attends the team base. This condition was initially because Mark was seldom at home, but it does bring the following advantages:

- Regular contact to monitor mental state, level of intoxication, level of neglect, etc.
- To offer treatment in the form of supervised medication administration.
- To offer social intervention in the form of drugs counselling, lifts to the supermarket, other practical help, and budgetary advice. Mark is encouraged and assisted to spend money on food to get him through the week, before he spends it on cocaine.

The leverage that appointeeship confers means that Mark is now receiving medication, supervised three days a week, plus other aftercare services. It is made clear to Mark that receipt of his allowance is not dependent on his acceptance of medication. His mental state has improved and he has fewer days without food in the house.

Failed engagement

Failure to engage constructively with a patient is stressful for assertive outreach workers since it frustrates our desire to succeed. In our experience, staff, particularly new members, find the patient's rejection of their considerable efforts and the high expectations of the model difficult. We have to remind ourselves that other teams have tried and failed and that is often why the patient has been referred. We have certain skills and smaller case loads, but a few patients will still evade all attempts at contact. Individual and team support systems, as described in Chapter 26, help staff to depersonalize the problems.

In our experience it is the more able patients who are most likely to drop out (McGrew *et al.* 1995). One patient used the complaints process eloquently, citing harassment. Another patient moves out of his flat as soon as he is discharged and even his family does not know where he goes until he appears in some distant hospital, mute and catatonic.

Measuring and defining engagement

Keys to engagement (Sainsbury Centre for Mental Health 1998) states that 'assertive outreach teams can achieve engagement for 95% of people with the greatest difficulty'. In common with others, it offers no clear definition of how this engagement is measured or teams evaluated.

The Dartmouth ACT scale (Teague *et al.* 1998) offers standards for model fidelity, and two of its components measure engagement. The first states that services have a 'no drop out' policy which is measured by whether the service engages and retains clients at a mutually satisfactory level. The team is scored with anchor points from an annual case-load retention of 50% moving up in scores to a maximum 100%. Secondly, the use of 'assertive engagement mechanisms' such as street outreach and legal powers are measured. The Dartmouth ACT scale recognizes that assertive outreach teams need to use both constructive and restrictive approaches to be effective.

Herinckx *et al.* (1997) cite the dearth of randomized trials of ACT which examine retention of patients in services as an outcome variable. Randomized studies will indicate attrition rates for dropping out of the research but not indicate if these patients also dropped out of clinical care. The Herinckx study randomly assigned patients in Portland, Oregon to one of two assertive community treatment teams ($n = 116$) or to standard community mental health centre care ($n = 58$). Interestingly, one of the ACT teams was staffed by 'self-identified mental heath consumers'. Patients from all three teams were followed up for up to two and a half years. At the end of this observation period the combined ACT teams were able to retain 68% of their patients, compared to 43% in standard care. There was no difference in drop-out rate between the ACT team staffed by consumers and the traditionally staffed team. Much of the drop out occurred in the first nine months. Nearly 20% of patients assigned to standard care never successfully connected with the service, compared to 2% of those assigned to ACT. In this study, analysis of patient characteristics such as age, highly symptomatic patients, diagnosis of schizophrenia, and presence of drug or alcohol abuse showed no association with engagement or retention.

In a meta-analysis by Bond *et al.* (1995) retention was defined as uninterrupted services over a twelve-month period. Nine studies of assertive community treatment were reviewed. Of the four with control groups, two demonstrated greater retention for ACT and two, no difference.

The UK700 study (Burns *et al.* 2000) defined engagement-related activity as any patient contact which fostered a positive client attitude to treatment and the service. Only constructive engagement was rated under engagement—appointeeship would be rated as 'finance' and Mental Health Act activity as 'mental health'. The proportion of face-to-face activity recorded as engagement (as defined above) was marginally greater in intensive case management (ICM) with case loads of 10–15 (at 16%) than in standard care with case loads of 30–35 (at 14%). A greater difference between the two groups was the fourfold increase in the rate of attempted (failed) contacts for ICM compared to standard care:

> Case managers with smaller caseloads did strive more vigorously to maintain contact (more telephone calls and failed visits).
>
> (Burns *et al.* 2000)

Conclusions

Engagement is a term used exclusively by professionals and regarded with suspicion by some patients. Patients may not share our positive associations with phrases such as 'preventing people falling through the net'. Is this the sort of net that fish are caught in or the one that saves the trapeze artist? It is important that we are sensitive to alternative perceptions—our 'conscientious persistence' may be our patients' 'harassment'.

We believe that for this group of patients engagement occurs between the patient and a key worker more effectively than between the patient and the team. The interpersonal skills of the individual worker (such as compassion, empathy, and a nurturing approach) cannot be easily described in writing. The team must foster this approach, having the flexibility to take a patient to the cinema or the swimming pool and valuing these most satisfying and enjoyable forms of engagement. Engagement is not a separate function in itself but permeates everything that we do in this work. It is also not restricted to the early part of treatment but persists throughout our contact with patients.

Chapter 11

Medication compliance

Compliance, concordance, or adherence?

When patients are admitted with another relapse of their psychotic illness there is often discussion about whether they have been taking their medicines regularly. It is common in mental health practice to find that they have either stopped taking their tablets altogether or have been irregular with them several weeks before admission. The debate then arises about whether they have broken down because they stopped taking the medicine or stopped taking the medicine because they were breaking down. Whichever it is, failure to take medicines as prescribed has been unequivocally demonstrated to increase the risk of relapse (Curson *et al.* 1985; Hirsch *et al.* 1973).

Traditionally, this has been referred to as compliance—the degree to which the patient *complies* with the prescribed treatment regimen. Although it is most often discussed in relationship to medicines, compliance or non-compliance issues can be crucial in all aspects of treatments. For instance, how well patients comply with prescribed diets or exercise regimes is likely to be a factor in outcome variations in some conditions. We will confine ourselves here to issues about medicines (and in particular psychotropic medications). Helping patients comply with the broader treatment package is addressed throughout this book and engagement (Chapter 10) is particularly relevant.

Non-compliance can be either covert or overt (Curson *et al.* 1985). Covert non-compliance is when the patient implies that they are co-operating with the prescribed treatment but, in reality, are doing so only partially or not at all. This is very common indeed. Overt non-compliance occurs when patients simply refuse to accept the proffered treatment. One of the advantages proposed for depot medication is that although it cannot guarantee 100% compliance it can ensure that there is no covert non-compliance. If the patient is not taking the medicines then it is clear to all involved.

Recently there has been something of a reaction against the term 'compliance' because it is taken to imply altogether too passive a role for the patient. In the spirit of greater emphasis on negotiated treatments and patient influence on choice, 'adherence' to the agreed regime has been proposed. Even more recently the term 'concordance' has been used to drive home the equality of the relationship. Only time will tell if either of these terms will supplant compliance, which is still the term most commonly used. We will stick with compliance here to avoid confusion but would underline that it should not be assumed to imply a passive or submissive role for the patient. Far from it. It is best practice to emphasize negotiation and encourage patients to take as much responsibility for the content and conduct of their treatment as possible.

The extent of non-compliance

There is nothing especially psychiatric about medication non-compliance. Hardly anyone seems able to take tablets regularly over long periods. A simple check of your bathroom cabinet will confirm this! It is especially so if the consequences of forgetting them are not immediate. Studies of patients taking antihypertensives indicate that just over half take them reliably (Johnson *et al.* 1999). The same finding emerges from studies of tuberculosis therapy (Menzies *et al.* 1993).

Mental health professionals often make the mistake of citing diabetes as a non-stigmatizing example of the need to take prolonged treatment, when encouraging their patients to persist with antipsychotics. This is probably a mistake. As with antihypertensives, the patient on antipsychotics will probably feel better, not worse, in the days immediately following non-compliance. The risks (whether of relapse or, for the patient with high blood pressure, a stroke) are in the future. For the diabetic, the importance of medication is immediately reinforced by the discomfort associated with missed doses. Yet even in diabetes, compliance is often poor.

Causes of non-compliance

The causes of non-compliance are varied and the situation for each individual will need to be assessed. Not only does it vary between individuals but it can also change over time in the same individual. Although we have listed 'causes of non-compliance' it is generally better to think positively in terms of strategies for improving and supporting compliance. This is not just playing with words. The starting point with our patients is the difficulty of sustaining long-term treatment, and when we explore the issues it is to make things easier, not to apportion blame.

Human nature/disorganization

As mentioned above, there are some general, non-specific factors which interfere with compliance. We are keen to help our patients live as normal a life as possible and minimize the impact of their illness on them. The more successful we are with that, paradoxically, the more the risk of forgetting to attend to their medicines. We refer to this as 'human nature'. Once there are more interesting things to concentrate on, it is not surprising that attention is directed to them and away from managing the illness.

Many of our patients lead fairly unstructured, indeed disorganized, lives. A lack of routine makes it even more likely that medicines will be forgotten. Successful regimes often necessitate that medicines are always taken at a regular point in the day (e.g. with breakfast or when returning from work in the evening). This relies on getting up at a regular time and having breakfast or having a job to go to. In the absence of such personal routines our interventions may be directed to introducing some structure.

Side-effects

Virtually all effective medicines have some side-effects. In the case of antipsychotics, mood stabilizers, and antidepressants these often include distressing motor effects such as stiffness and tremor, gastrointestinal and urinary tract problems such as constipation and dry mouth, and also general sedation. Weight gain is particularly distressing for many patients.

Undoubtedly, drop out from treatment and poor compliance can be a consequence of side-effects. Monitoring regularly for these and ensuring that they are minimized by optimal dosing and, if need be, with adjunct medication, is essential if patients are to persist (Chapter 7). Acknowledging the importance of side-effects and discussing them frankly can help in itself. The common fear that talking about them will scare patients off is not borne out by experience (Chaplin *et al.* 1999; Chaplin and Kent 1998). Sometimes patients interpret side-effects as a worsening of their condition and explanation and honest reassurance can go a long way to preventing discontinuation.

It has been the more benign side-effect profile, rather than increased effectiveness, that has been responsible for the rapid shift towards the newer antidepressants and the atypical antipsychotics in the last few years.

Insight/denial

So far we have been stressing problems with compliance that are common to all disorders. Lack of insight is often blamed for poor compliance in psychotic patients. Obviously this is important. A striking feature of psychoses is that the patients are often unaware of the extent of their illness or even deny it altogether, ascribing their discomforts to external agencies (persecutory individuals, direct interference with their thoughts, etc.).

Insight is, however, a complex concept—it is not simply a matter of having it or not. Both Birchwood (Birchwood *et al.* 1994) and David (David 1990; David *et al.* 1992) have proposed three components. Insight scales have been developed which recognize that there are degrees of insight (David *et al.* 1992) and even these have only demonstrated a weak association with compliance. All of us have worked with patients who are completely devoid of insight and yet happily accept treatment for an illness whose existence they deny. Similarly, most of us have had the frustrating experience of watching patients who have recovered well, acknowledge that they were ill and are now better, and yet refuse to take the treatment that will continue to help.

Increasingly, we conceptualize this area in terms of health belief systems. These vary enormously in our multicultural society. The simple scientific model of illness used by most health care staff is not necessarily shared by our patients, whether psychotic or not (Laugharne 1999). Patients' explanations for illness may even include New Age thinking about the influence of ley lines, a belief in voodoo, or the experience of demonic possession (in some Pentecostal Christian churches).

Different groups within society can have equal information about an illness and come to quite differing views about the relative importance of its consequences. A striking

Components of insight

David *et al.* (1992):
- Recognition that one has a mental illness
- Compliance with treatment
- Ability to relabel unusual mental events (delusions and hallucinations) as pathological

Birchwood *et al.* (1994):
- Awareness of illness
- Need for treatment
- Attribution of symptoms

example is how many young people continue to smoke despite the overwhelming evidence about the risks. It is not that they are unaware of the consequences. However, the balance between immediate gratification and long distant complications such as strokes and lung disease seems different to them compared to health care professionals (who are regularly confronted with these consequences). It can be difficult for us to fully comprehend this. A study of diabetic patients demonstrated that many of them assessed the relative importance of good blood-sugar control totally differently to their doctors (White *et al.* 1996). The patients were focused on the short-term problems (hypos) and the doctors, on the long-term risks (retinopathy and neuropathy). Each focus determines a different strategy for compliance.

For many of our patients the risk of a relapse may simply not seem that important compared to the inconvenience of side-effects. For the most disabled and socially marginalized there is simply not that much at stake. If you have a job, a family, and some social status you are likely to put up with almost anything to avoid an acute psychotic episode. If you are living on your own, ostracized by your neighbours and with low self-esteem, then intermittent periods in hospital are not that much of a price to pay to avoid feeling stiff and sluggish.

In summary, we find the shorthand term 'insight' of limited value in our work. It is almost invariably about constructing a space in which to negotiate a set of complex and, often, conflicting values.

Denial often contributes to poor compliance and may seem indistinguishable from poor insight. It is different, however, and needs to be worked with. Denial is normal and often very adaptive. Most of us use denial from time to time so that we can put aside difficult issues and get on with life. Usually, we then come back to them when things are less stressful. Denial protects us from painful emotions and preoccupations—it has been shown to be positively beneficial in some circumstances and may be one of the reasons why trauma counselling can be counterproductive (Mayou *et al.* 2000).

In a local, unpublished piece of work some years ago, young black men with poor compliance were asked why they did not take their medicines. We had anticipated that the answers would be entirely complaints about side-effects or a lack of belief that they were ill. Several did give these reasons but an equal number told us that they simply wanted to forget about their illness for a time and carry on like everyone else. They had not lost sight of their illness but actively chose to try and ignore it for a period. Denial in psychotic patients requires the same attention that it does in non-psychotic ones; they too need help in coming to terms with the pain of the illness.

Surrounding views

It is not just the patients' views about their illness and treatment that matter. Compliance with treatment is powerfully influenced by the opinions of those the patient depends on and relates to. Family attitudes matter enormously. Do the parents or spouse also accept that the patient is ill and benefits from the treatment? One meta-analysis of Expressed Emotion work with families has even suggested that the improvements found are accounted for by improved compliance with the medicines as the family is able to pull together better (Razali and Yahya 1995).

People that the patient meets socially are likely to be unsupportive, if not actively opposed, to their continuing medication. They will often only meet the patient when he or she is relatively well (since the patient will either be in hospital or more isolated when ill). Consequently, they will attribute any residual problems, along with side-effects, to the drugs and compare the patient to how they themselves are. This is dramatically demonstrated by a study of societal attitudes towards the treatments of mental illness (Jorm *et al.* 1997) where medications for schizophrenia came low on the list, long after the commonest suggestion, 'get out a bit more'. Some countries (notably Australia and Norway) have engaged in national programmes to improve public understanding of mental health and the WHO is leading an international drive to reduce stigma in schizophrenia.

At a more local level, community mental health workers will have to devote time to changing attitudes of those individuals that they identify as 'key' in improving compliance. There is evidence that educational initiatives for local neighbourhoods can help. A brief programme to help local acceptance of an aftercare hostel for mentally ill individuals demonstrated a clear link between rejecting and controlling attitudes towards them and poor knowledge about mental illness (Wolff *et al.* 1996). These authors found that inviting the neighbours in was successful in improving understanding and reducing rejection.

Improving compliance

Just as there are many contributing strands to poor compliance, so there are a number of approaches that can be used in trying to improve it. Where the emphasis lies will vary according to the assessment made of the particular circumstances of an individual patient. Similarly, the emphasis for an individual patient may also vary markedly over time—there is something of a hierarchy in the interventions with patients often 'graduating' from one to another. In the descriptions that follow we move from the more general approaches (we would use with all patients) through to more specific and targeted approaches (for patients with severe compliance problems). We would not like to give the impression, however, that there is a rigorous science here, nor an unvarying sequence. There is a range and it is vital that staff make sure they are familiar with it and can apply other strategies when the current one is not working well.

The therapeutic relationship

Probably the most important determinant of whether a patient takes their treatment is how well they get on with their case manager. Most of the research that has been done in this area has been on compliance with medicines and the relationship with the prescribing doctor, but it is illuminating. Patients who feel their doctors are competent, compassionate, and genuinely interested in them as individuals will take treatment, often despite troublesome side-effects (Frank and Gunderson 1990). This seems so central to assertive outreach that one can overlook it. The holistic approach to helping patients, that characterizes this work, is crucial to sustaining long-term compliance. Time and energy spent on engagement (Chapter 10) is not simply a luxury but a core contribution to both the patient's well being and their treatment. Nagging is no substitute for a thoroughly grounded relationship!

There is strong evidence that a good therapeutic relationship (sometimes called a 'working alliance') can predict outcome in the severely mentally ill (Priebe and Gruyters 1995). While this may in part be that those patients who can form warmer relationships are generally less ill, it is highly likely that the improved outcome also reflects their better compliance with the treatment from staff with whom they engage more and trust.

Education

It is vital to make sure that patients are well informed about the purpose of their drugs. This means a detailed (and often repeated) explanation of both their long-term benefits and also their more immediate effects on arousal and symptoms. It will often involve some simple explanation about the relationship between emotional arousal and psychological functioning.

Hogarty, who has worked for many years developing psychological strategies to improve outcome in schizophrenia, considers that the regulation of mounting anxiety is the key to remaining well (Hogarty *et al.* 1995). The Yerkes–Dodson curve (1908) (see Fig. 11.1) is helpful and convincing. It emphasizes how some level of stress and arousal is both normal and beneficial but how over-arousal reduces performance (and can lead to breakdown). The role of medicines to bring arousal back to within the normal range can then be explained.

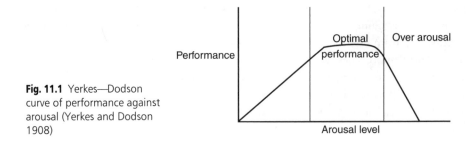

Fig. 11.1 Yerkes—Dodson curve of performance against arousal (Yerkes and Dodson 1908)

A full explanation of the therapeutic purpose and effects of the medicines will involve explaining about side-effects and risks. There is no evidence that an honest and frank description of the risks reduces compliance (Chaplin and Kent 1998). On the contrary, it reassures patients that you know what you are talking about—they will probably already have had experience of the side- effects.

There is a rapidly expanding library of professionally produced information on these drugs (leaflets and videos from pharmaceutical companies) which can be used to supplement personal explanations. It is rarely helpful to substitute an individualized explanation totally with such prepared material. The more targeted and personalized it can be, the more likely to be taken seriously. For instance, we have found that the video of the film starring Diana Ross, about the effects of clozapine on a woman with severe schizophrenia ('Out of Darkness', Odyssey Films, 1994), is particularly appreciated by our black patients who are more able to identify with her. We have also found that unless patients' particular questions can be honestly addressed, they lose interest in printed material.

Education also must include family members and those who have significant influence on the patient. This educational endeavour can go beyond simply outlining the rationale for the treatments and include a careful analysis of the stress points in a patient's life so that they can be anticipated or avoided. This approach is central to the 'psychoeducation' component of behavioural family management aimed at reducing high Expressed Emotion (Mari and Streiner 1994*a*) and is dealt with more in Chapter 25. Even with patients who live alone, a good understanding of what interferes with compliance can help improve it.

Case study

Barry had been settled on his oral trifluoperazine for some years and was happy with it. He had not been admitted for several years, lived with his parents, and had a part-time job in a warehouse with his dad.

Twice in the last year he had become tense and complained of poor sleep and admitted readily, to direct questioning, that he had stopped his medicine for a week on each occasion. We initially thought that he was experimenting with whether he still needed it, but this proved not to be the case. He explained that on both occasions he had been on a family holiday and, while away, had gone to the pub with his dad and his dad's footballing mates (who knew of his illness). One of them encouraged him to stop taking the medicine, saying that it was making him slow and sluggish and that doctors always played safe.

Although he reinstated his tablets on returning home, it was then that his destabilization manifested itself. He discussed this with his father who explained the importance of his medicine to his friend, and there have been no further such incidents.

Prompting and supporting

We have made clear that we consider most of the difficulties in compliance to be best understood as 'normal'—i.e. our aim is to help somebody with a difficult task rather than try and find out why they cannot cope with an easy task. In practice, this means that we must support and prompt them in their task. We regularly check with them how it is going (see the section below, 'Monitoring and structuring') and commiserate with them about the difficulties of complying. We congratulate and encourage them in their success. A positive, committed attitude really works. If the staff member does not really think that the medicines are important, then their support will be compromised. We have seen this very much in our team as we have gained experience with clozapine. It has become increasingly easier to start and maintain patients on clozapine as team members have seen other patients improve. There is no substitute for the genuine enthusiasm that then infuses the support and encouragement offered.

Support and encouragement can be powerfully enhanced by involving other patients, if they are willing. Patients will often listen more willingly to the case made by another patient who has experienced the same effects and side-effects and endorses that the medicines have made a real difference to their lives. We have gained immeasurably by having a user worker who often draws to great effect on her own experience of the benefits that maintenance medication has provided for her. Seeing her holding down a rewarding and important job despite (or because of?) her medicines encourages compliance both by demonstrating that they are tolerable and by giving a sense of hope and a goal to aim for.

Prompting and supporting are not passive procedures. Although they seem non-specific (as with the therapeutic relationship), they will only happen if they are taken seriously and kept high on the list of priorities. Medication has been overlooked some-what with the more exciting psychosocial developments within community psychiatry. As outlined in Chapter 7, teams need to explore any resistance to promoting appropriate medications and ensure that it is taken seriously by everyone—it is not just the doctor's job.

Monitoring and structuring

Simply focusing on the medicines (albeit briefly) at each visit strengthens compliance. Learning to ask the question 'have you taken all your tablets?' in a positive way is the first step. Having emphasized how difficult it is to remember to take medicines over long periods, and having stressed how normal that is, the concern can be expressed as a collaboration: 'OK, let's see how you've done with the medicines this week. How's it gone? Did you forget any days or have you remembered them all?'

Such a query can easily be accompanied by a pill count. If compliance is poor, then it is often best to prescribe on a weekly basis. This allows a rapid count of how many tablets are left over and hence how many doses have been missed. The problem can be quickly identified and quantified. It is crucial to be able to do this in a way that is not seen as persecutory or suggesting a lack of trust. Many staff we meet think this cannot be achieved and that the therapeutic relationship will be the first casualty of such a manoeuvre. Clumsily done, this may be the case, but our extensive experience is that it is eminently acceptable to most patients. Properly and positively presented, in the spirit of genuine collaboration, it is seen as evidence of conscientiousness and concern, not persecution. With any new technique, it is probably best to try it out several times with patients who are compliant. When you feel comfortable with it, extend it to more problematic patients.

As well as asking and checking, many patients can be considerably helped by aids such as dosette boxes. The case manager can fill these up with the help of the patient, as a joint task, in one of their visits. Alternatively, in some cases pharmacists will dispense into them. The advantages are obvious, especially for patients taking a range of medicines for their physical health. It is not unusual for a patient to have to take up to 20 tablets a day—we have one such patient who has a complex regime for his Parkinson's disease. With lots of tablets, it is very easy to forget or get confused ('Now did I just take that?').

If the patient wants to deceive us, then he can dispose of the pills. This happens sometimes—but simple forgetfulness is by far the commonest reason. Where the patient is thought to be deliberately deceiving, then daily supervised medicines or depot medication (see below) may be the only alternative.

Supervised medication

One of the major advantages of dedicated assertive outreach teams is that they can offer intensive supervision of oral medicines. This can involve regular visits, up to twice daily in extreme situations, to make absolutely sure that the prescribed medicines are being taken. In our team this can include treatments not only for mental health (antipsychotics, mood stabilizers, anticholinergics, antidepressants) but also for physical health (e.g. insulin, antihypertensives). 'Observed meds', as the Americans call it, is one of the hallmarks of ACT teams

Out of our current group of just over 100 patients we expect about 10–15 to be on 'observed meds' at any time. For just over half of these it will mean a daily visit, seven days a week, to deliver the medicine and stay with the patient while they take it. For the remainder, the visits can be between three and five times a week. The longest we have had a patient on daily supervised medication is now 18 months, and we do not anticipate stopping it. For most patients, daily visits are continued until it is judged that the medication routine is a fully accepted part of the patient's way of life. For this to be a viable proposition the medication needs to be effective as a single daily dose.

The most common single daily dose is of atypical antipsychotics (often clozapine). Because of its sedative side-effects, patients prefer to take it as late in the afternoon as possible. We have considered the possibility of a 'night run' for such medications but, on balance, have abandoned it because of concerns about safety and also because the late afternoon delivery seems to work. Some patients take the bulk of their dose at the delivery and are left to take a further dose themselves either in the morning or sometimes just before retiring. Though this may seem illogical—after all, if they are reliable about taking one dose, why not them all?—we have found it works. Firstly, patients with limited insight or commitment to the regime will often comply as long as they are kept well with the basic dose. This approach ensures that the bulk of the dose is taken regularly. Secondly, the daily visit keeps the drugs in the forefront of their mind, so that they do not forget the second dose. Thirdly, it is easy to check the intervening doses at the daily visit.

We emphasize the supportive function of daily supervised medication while also honestly acknowledging the supervisory component. Few patients have any illusions about the importance that we place on medication, so there is no catastrophic impact on the therapeutic relationship. For the process to succeed, the person delivering the medicines needs to believe in the importance of maintenance medication. Training in this is essential. Most of us feel uncomfortable with this 'controlling' aspect of the job and teams need time to talk through these issues. Even though experienced members may have been convinced of the value of the approach by previous successes, new members need to be able to express and explore their ambivalences. The 'user worker' in our team has taken on a substantial number of daily meds and her absolute endorsement of the approach ('I wish someone had offered me this years ago, it would have saved me a lot of hard lessons') speaks volumes.

The visits are often short and *the patient's case manager should not always conduct them*. This is important, because it is when the case manager is off that we need to be able to rely on regular medicines. A couple of times, early on, we found patients accepting regular supervised medicines from 'their' case manager without problem but adamantly refusing it from another team member (even when they knew that member) when their worker was suddenly absent. If the relationship is initially particularly fragile, the case manager may establish the routine, but second and third members should be introduced as soon as possible.

The delivery of daily medicines is co-ordinated for each week at the main review meeting and the names of those responsible written up on a notice board. This ensures that the whole team knows who is on supervised medicines so that if anyone is away sick, then their visits can be redistributed. To save on travelling time, geographical 'clusters' of patients on supervised medicines are often dealt with by one person.

The emphasis on supervised medicines and the change from a five-day to a seven-day service have been the two innovations in our team which have had the most obvious effect on readmission rates. We have to regularly remind ourselves of this when staff complain about the limited job satisfaction that comes from simply delivering medicines.

It may be dull for us but it makes a real difference to the stability of our patients' lives. With more stable patients, who are able to shoulder some responsibility themselves, we can move on to other strategies to improve compliance.

Depot medication

No matter how much work goes into developing a strong, supportive, therapeutic relationship (encouragement and monitoring of medication, etc.), there will remain some patients who simply will not take their medicines. For such patients, where the consequences of relapse warrant it, depot medication is the only feasible alternative. In the UK and Scandinavia there has been a tradition of quite heavy reliance on depots, with up to 50% of patients with schizophrenia maintained on them. This is less so now with the advent of the atypicals, but still accounts for a sizeable proportion of mainten- ance treatment. Even in our assertive outreach team, with the availability of seven-day supervised medication, about 15 of our 100 patients are on depots. Most of these have been tried, often repeatedly, on supervised atypicals, and failed. Several of them are subject to some forms of compulsion. Currently, there are no atypicals available as depots, but this is likely to change in the very near future with the possibility that the balance between daily supervised medicines and depots may change.

Usually, the case manager administers depots (if they are a nurse) on a visit to the patient's home. While this is the preferred method, there are some patients who are so hard to track down that we have found it more reliable to get them to come to a ward or day hospital to get it. Good, fail-safe communication between the ward and the team is essential if this is to work and missed doses spotted.

Compliance therapy

New evidence-based intervention packages aimed at improving compliance have been developed in recent years. Reliance on unstructured counselling, education, and 'nag- ging' of patients with psychosis has waned and the benefits of a structured programme of compliance therapy, conducted in formal therapy sessions, is recommended.

A randomized controlled trial compared a brief course of compliance therapy with non-specific counselling. The number of sessions was small (4–6) and their duration could be shortened if the patient was aroused or distracted. They rarely took more than 30 minutes and the whole course was spread over just 2–3 weeks. The authors concluded that it is both practical and highly effective in improving compliance with medication in psychotic in-patients (Kemp *et al.* 1996). Despite problems with attri- tion in the sample, those followed up at 6, 12, and 18 months maintained improved observer-rated compliance over the control group (Kemp *et al.* 1998).

Kemp, Hayward, and David have produced a manual and a video setting out their programme of compliance therapy for psychotic patients (Kemp *et al.* 1997). The approach is based on collaboration, cognitive behavioural approaches in psychosis (Kingdon and Turkington 1994), and motivational interviewing techniques used in substance abuse (Rollinick *et al.* 1992). Whilst the randomized controlled trial consisted of exposure to 4–6 sessions of compliance therapy, the manual sets out 12 sessions divided into three phases.

Content of the three phases of compliance therapy

Phase 1: reviewing illness and attitude towards therapy

- Review illness history and previous experience of medication.
- Concentrate on reflective listening and establishing rapport.
- Elicit the patient's stance towards treatment, culture, background.
- Avoid challenging directly denial of problems e.g. 'why does your family think there is a problem?'
- Acknowledge negative experiences.
- Link medication cessation with relapses.

Phase 2: exploring ambivalence to treatment

- Explore ambivalence towards medication treatment e.g. side-effects, misunderstandings, denial, stigma.
- Consider advantages and disadvantages e.g. 'what bothers you the most about the medication?'; 'how has it helped?'
- Identify target symptoms for treatment from patient's feedback.
- Explore cautiously psychotic symptoms and beliefs that limit compliance.
- Highlight benefits of treatment and use metaphors e.g. 'try to see your medicine as a protective layer or an insurance policy'.

Phase 3: reducing stigma

- Encourage self-sufficiency and recognition of early relapse signs.
- Establish normalizing rationales to deal with stigma e.g. prevalence, comparisons with physical illness, famous sufferers.
- Predict consequences of stopping medication.
- Encourage maintenance treatment as a freely chosen strategy to enhance long-term quality of life.

(adapted from Kemp *et al.* 1997)

The authors believe that compliance therapy can also be used effectively in the community by key workers. For assertive outreach, the intensity of contacts, relatively generous time resources, and long-term relationships with patients make this approach practical and desirable. The basic tenets of the approach are familiar to mental health professionals and training can be included in psychosocial intervention courses or in training and development activities within the team. Limitations to the approach stem from the intellectual and cognitive demands on the patient. Patients with severe cognitive deficits, negative symptoms, sedation, thought disorder, or poor concentration will struggle with the formalized approach.

Conclusions

Assertive outreach exists to deliver effective treatments. There is no point in engaging with patients and monitoring their well-being unless there is something to offer them. We have good treatments (pharmacological, psychological and social) but they do not work if they are not applied. With psychological and social treatments, we are often in the driving seat once engagement has been achieved. With drug treatments, we know that they are generally followed only roughly and inconsistently by most patients. It is a sobering thought that we could probably achieve almost all the added benefits (in terms of relapse prevention) that can be gained from our range of psychosocial interventions, simply if the medicines we prescribe were taken regularly.

We have emphasized in this chapter how vitally important improving compliance is. The paradox is that experience tells us that a narrow focus on compliance is likely to be counterproductive. If our patients think that we are only interested in them taking the tablets, we can be sure they will not do it. Improving compliance will only work in the long run if our efforts in that direction are part of a wider, genuinely patient-focused, approach. Similarly, we would caution against being too 'technical' about it. Our approach is to stress the normality of the problem and to search for long-term solutions. It is important to learn and provide the motivational interviewing approaches. But it is even more important to convey an understanding that living with a long-term, severe illness is a difficult and demanding exercise and 'to err is human'. There is no place for moralizing and criticism. The benefits of improved compliance are enormous and worth the effort.

Chapter 12

Hostility

Introduction

We use the term 'hostility' to encompass a range of behaviours that we might encounter whilst working in the community with people suffering severe mental illness. These behaviours are not exclusive to our patients; in daily life we might encounter passive aggression, intimidating behaviour, verbal aggression, and threats—especially whilst driving a car! Actual physical violence, however, remains rare both in our practice and in society. Homicides by people with mental illness are, mercifully, infrequent events and as such are statistically difficult to predict, despite increasingly sophisticated risk assessment procedures (Munro and Rumgay 2000).

This chapter will discuss the politics, incidence, assessment, and management of challenging, hostile, and violent behaviour from an assertive outreach perspective. We seek not to control patients but to work with them collaboratively and safely wherever possible. Patients and patient advocacy groups dislike the current preoccupation with risk, which can lead to more coercive legislation and practice. It also discourages positive risk taking where individuals may learn from their successes and failures. There is a danger that assertive outreach could become a system of policing and medicating patients to reduce a perceived risk to the public.

Incidence

Since the murder of Jonathan Zito by Christopher Clunis in 1992 (Ritchie 1994) there has been intense public concern in the UK about violence by the mentally ill. Reports of seemingly random homicides perpetrated by the severely mentally ill in the community, have created a public perception out of proportion to the evidence. A consequence of the Ritchie report is mandatory external inquiries into any such homicide. The result is media attention on three occasions for each tragedy—the event, the court sentence, and publication of the inquiry. Not surprisingly, the public's perception of the risk is exaggerated by such coverage. The current perception is one of a rapidly increasing risk (almost of epidemic proportions) of homicides by the mentally ill. This is in stark contrast to the facts which demonstrate a low and stable incidence of homicides by the mentally ill since the 1950s.

Community care policies have had no impact. An average of 40 homicides each year are committed by the mentally ill, of which only six involve strangers (Taylor and Gunn 1999). The rate of homicides within the whole population is 600–700. The proportion of all homicides committed by mentally ill people in the UK is therefore below 10%—a rate found in countries with similar overall rates of homicide. In countries with higher rates of homicide (e.g. the USA), the proportion attributable to mental illness is lower.

The relative risk of violence from the mentally ill is even less worrying against the background of a steadily rising rate of violent incidents in general over the same period. Violence by the severely mentally ill accounts for only a small proportion of violent acts (Coid 1996).

People with schizophrenia and severe bipolar affective disorder are, however, statistically more likely than others to commit a violent offence (Coid 1996). Patients suffering a major mental illness are more dangerous than the general public in terms of self-reported violence and official records of arrests and convictions. For male patients, the risk of violence increases fourfold and for women, the increased risk is less, but still considerable. Coid found that mentally ill patients shared the same risk factors for violence and criminality as the general public—being male, unemployed, younger, and from a lower social class. However, even controlling for these factors, the association between mental illness and increased violence remains.

Risk factors and risk assessment

Risk assessment should be an integral part of the care programme approach. A clinical risk assessment should take place as part of the referral process for any new patient to an assertive outreach team. An example of the risk assessment documentation we use is given in Example 12.3 and is presented in conjunction with a case study.

Risk assessment is, however, not an exact science — far from it. Munro and Rumgay's (2000) study of 40 homicide inquiry reports, concluded that in 29 the violence could not have been predicted. Twenty-four of the offenders did have a history of violence or high risk factors for violence, but only eight could have been assessed as high risk at the time of the homicide. In only three of the cases was the danger predictable, and in these only days prior to the homicide. For assertive outreach the lessons of frequent contact and rapid intervention are clear:

> These findings suggest that more homicides could be prevented by improving the response to patients who start to relapse, regardless of their assessed potential for violence, than by trying to identify high risk patients and targeting resources on them.
>
> (Munro and Rumgay 2000)

Table 12.1, from Coid (1996), outlines current knowledge of risk factors associated with increased violence.

The best predictor of future violence is previous violence. A risk history from patient and relatives, psychiatric notes, and, where available, criminal records, will provide most of this information. Most patients referred for assertive outreach will be well known to services. The referral process must include effective written and verbal handover of information on risk as well as clinical state.

Table 12.1 Patient risk factors for violence

History	Environment	Mental state
• Previous violence	• Lack of social supports	• Persecutory delusions
• Substance abuse	• Lack or loss of accommodation	• Delusions of passivity e.g. thought insertion
• Poor compliance with medication, especially recent discontinuation of medication		• Emotions related to violence e.g. anger, irritability, suspiciousness, hostility
• Poorly engaged with services		
• Social restlessness and rootlessness		
• Recent severe stress		
• Evidence of planning such as obtaining weapons		
• Specific threats made by patient		

(Adapted: Coid 1996)

Noffsinger and Resnick's review (Noffsinger and Resnick 1999) concluded that substance abuse is a greater risk factor for violence than is mental illness. Substance abuse significantly raises the rate of violence in both the psychiatric and general population (Steadman *et al.* 1998). In a longitudinal follow-up study, Swartz *et al.* (1998) concluded that substance abuse, combined with poor compliance with medication, is likely to predict a higher risk of violent behaviour among the severely mentally ill. Lack of contact with specialist mental health services and specific psychotic experiences (particularly paranoid beliefs about specific people) were also associated (Swanson *et al.* 1997).

Clearly, patients with dual diagnosis, with histories of previous violence, or who are poorly compliant with treatment and follow-up, will be of particular concern to assertive outreach teams and key workers.

Individual approaches

Risk management planning on an individual level is based on accurate risk histories and knowledge of the current risk and risk factors. This may in practice be very simple: 'If Jason is intoxicated when he answers the door, make your excuses and walk away.'

Some patients need two trigger factors. Beverley has assaulted two key workers and two doctors. On each occasion she has been high, or becoming high, plus she has been demanding antidepressants which the team has been anxious not to give her. Clearly for Beverley, her ability to accept refusal and her range of coping strategies are severely diminished when she is high. We know that elevated mood reduces most people's inhibitions. We also know that intoxication has the same effect.

These sorts of risk management plans can be easily incorporated into daily practice. Writing them down helps formalize our thinking and allows information to be shared across the team. Care plans, contingency plans, and risk management plans (see Examples 12.1 and 12.2) can contain simple statements and instructions and are often most effective when written as concisely as possible:

> Avoid conflict when high. May make demands that cannot be satisfied e.g. 'give me some prozac'. Refusal of demands leads to assault when high. Make excuses and leave; do not wait to rationalize, argue, or discuss.

De-escalation

The ideal is to talk down an aroused patient using psychological de-escalation and problem-solving techniques. This will only be possible and appropriate in the early stages of conflict before serious escalation occurs. The decision to attempt to resolve the situation through discussion will hinge on your knowledge of the patient, specifically their cognitive abilities and personality. Conflict caused by delusional beliefs about you, or feelings of persecution, are unlikely to respond well if the patient's mental state or level of intoxication are significantly impairing their ability to process information. Where psychology and problem solving are considered unlikely, retreat at this stage is preferable, as in the care of Beverley given above.

The decision to leave should not be presented as a punishment to the patient and can instead be presented in a neutral, matter-of-fact way: 'I'm sorry if I have upset you, maybe its better if I leave now and come back another time.' This is a 'face-saving' statement—you accept responsibility for what has happened so that the patient can feel that they have won the argument.

Anger may not lead to aggression in patients with strong internal inhibitions, or where there is no suitable target for the aggression. External inhibitions that help to prevent aggression include fear of consequences or retaliation, material losses, and embarrassment. As professionals we have a responsibility not to challenge patients inappropriately, hold overly negative views about their motives, or to engage in attempts to dominate. Such staff attitudes can be powerfully transmitted by demeanour and tone.

Where problem solving is possible, then psychological de-escalation techniques can often prevent aggression. We should listen and acknowledge the existence of the problems, show concern and understanding, and attempt to depersonalize the issue. Often disputes occur over medication, either when we withhold anticholinergics or sleeping tablets or attempt to improve compliance with the current prescription. Explaining to the patient that decisions are made by the team or by seniors can diffuse the personal focus of the grievance: 'I have nothing to gain personally from you taking medication. But with your history the team's opinion is that you will have more chance of staying well if you stay on the treatment.'

Problem solving in this instance might include making the treatment more tolerable by adjusting the dose and managing side-effects. By personalizing themselves, as distinct from an identity simply as a nurse or doctor, key workers can distance themselves from conflicts that arise from their role. Careful disclosure of personal information about your family, using first names and so on, is a recognized strategy in hostage situations.

Non-verbal techniques are familiar to most of us practicing in mental health. Intense eye contact and staring should be avoided as it is usually perceived as hostile. Intermittent 'normal' eye contact, maintaining a distance that does not threaten the individual's personal space, avoiding 'squaring up' by standing at a slight angle to the patient, and a relaxed posture all help (Davies and Frude 1993). People who are aroused, and those prone to paranoia, have enlarged areas of 'personal space' which, when encroached, make them feel uncomfortable and on edge. Kinzel (1970) demonstrated that violent prisoners identify larger personal spaces than those who are non-violent. Keeping a safe distance and towards the front feels safer for all of us. Similarly, touch may be reassuring for some more sympathetic patients but is generally intolerable for more aggressive and aroused patients.

Remaining calm is the stock response often used when dealing with an aroused person. However, if the patient has a grievance and wants you to sort it out, remaining calm and quiet may give the impression that you are not going to deal with their complaints or demands with the required urgency. 'Mood matching' recognizes this. Davies and Frude (1993) suggest that we match the patient's aggression with a similar degree of arousal directed into concern, involvement, and interest—but not with a similar degree of emotion. This can be difficult to achieve in practice and, together with the use of humour to diffuse situations, is a strategy that requires confidence.

Symptom management

In the community we use medicines to manage symptoms that persist for months and years. Only rarely are we required to administer medication for acute rapid tranquilization. In avoiding hospital admission and the risk of assault on carers and staff, medication can be successfully used to manage symptoms such as arousal, paranoia, and mania in the short term. Frequent contact and a flexible response according to agreed relapse plans can mean the early introduction of antipsychotics or benzodiazepines. Daily team discussion and the availability of medical staff can permit daily titration of medication, for example, with a patient who is becoming manic. Agreeing these responses, and the threshold at which they are introduced, with the patient, at a much earlier stage, will minimize conflict and help compliance.

Early attempts at the pharmacological management of a relapsing patient reduce the risk that they become aggressive and may help to avoid the hospital admission which may result from aggressive behaviour. The combination of medication with psychological techniques can help avoid adverse incidents, compulsory admission, and the stigmatizing involvement of the police for severely relapsing patients.

Responding to physical assaults

In the event of a physical assault, it is worth rehearsing a repertoire of responses to minimize injury and maximize the chance of escape. It is also worth realizing that, in the heat of the moment, basic survival instincts may overwhelm any preparation or training. The techniques of breakaway are routinely taught to community workers, and regular refresher courses are advised. Breakaway consists of movements and blocks designed to release or protect a worker from a number of grabbing or striking attacks including strangulation, grasping of hair or clothes, punching, kicking, or attempted sexual assault where the attacker is pressing someone to the ground. All the techniques operate on the principle of reasonable force and the prevention of injury to assailant and assailed. Breakaway movements need to be used in conjunction with techniques such as telling the attacker to stop, assertively and repeatedly if necessary, and shouting for help. Should your attacker have a weapon, rapid escape is preferable to attempts to defend yourself. The main defence would be to place something between you and your attacker (e.g. a door or a chair) and to keep at a distance until escape becomes possible.

Case study

Graham is a 42-year-old man with a diagnosis of paranoid schizophrenia, characterized by suspicion and passivity experiences. He does not drink but smokes cannabis regularly. He was referred because of poor compliance with medication. He was considered hard to engage and hostile, and had had frequent hospital admissions, on several occasions via the courts for violent offences. He lives alone in a block of flats, having recently moved following disputes with previous neighbours.

Graham has a history of a serious assault on a neighbour for which he was convicted. This is the clearest guide to his level of risk. The abuse of cannabis is a further risk factor because of the possibility of it exacerbating his paranoid illness and lowering his inhibitions. A further risk factor is his discontinuation of medication.

Graham is guarded but not yet refusing access to his home, so there is the possibility of early intervention and home-based care. His history and the fact that he is already paranoid about his neighbours would suggest that admission for treatment may be safest. He has not made any threats to the new neighbours and there may be scope to reinstate medication to which he is known to respond quickly.

Graham's risk assessment, risk history, and care plan are presented in Examples 12.1–12.3.

The documentation spells out accountability for interventions and decisions, but does not leave this solely with one person. It will be noted that although the plan is discussed with the patient and attempts made to agree a relapse plan, Graham is not given a copy of his care plan. This is because of the possibility, mentioned in the plan, of breach of confidentiality should the neighbours be considered at high risk. Legal precedent is well established that mental health professionals have a 'duty to warn' identifiable third parties and generalized victims, but that breach of this duty renders the professional liable to civil action. Public interest has been found to outweigh the patient's right to confidentiality in such cases where the risk is real and would involve physical harm (Noffsinger and Resnick 1999).

Example 12.1

ENHANCED CPA/SECTION 117(2)REVIEW (delete as applicable)	
Patient's name: Graham K. Address: Flat3, Ingle House, Archer Street Phone: none Date of birth: 09/09/59 GP: Norris Phone: 582 xxxx	CMHT: ACT TEAM Phone: 020 8877 xxxx New patient: No If No, date of review: 20/4/01.............. Diagnosis: 1. Paranoid Schizophrenia .... F 20.0 2. .... F — — ·—

Assessed needs or problem	Intervention	Resp. of
Frequent relapse of paranoid symptoms	◆ Re-establish Depixol 50mg. IM two weekly ◆ Psychoeducational and compliance therapy approaches to enhance compliance with medication ◆ Practical assistance to mediate with potential stressors e.g. housing, finance ◆ Continue to educate Graham regarding harmful use of cannabis and link with paranoid relapse ◆ Establish collaborative relapse plan to include relapse signature, action to be taken by Graham and the team, and rescue medicine to be used	JH JH/ Graham
Risk of assault when unwell (see risk history and risk management plan)	◆ Frequent contact, 3 to 7 times a week. Joint visits only, **not to be visited alone** ◆ Low threshold for admission or Mental Health Act assessment ◆ Risk assessment on each contact to establish immediacy of any risk e.g. verbal threats against neighbour ◆ Consider breach of confidentiality to inform and liase with neighbour if high assessed risk and delay in admission	JH JH/ Dr Evans JH Prof Burns

Involved in care: D̶r̶ Psychologist CPN OT SW Ward nurse C̶C̶M Support worker other
Present at
meeting: D̶r̶ Psychologist CPN OT S̶W̶ Ward nurse C̶C̶M Support worker other

Discussed
with the patient?   YES   Copy to patient?   NO   Copy to GP?   Yes
Care co-ordinator (print):   James Howard   Phone: 020 8877 xxxx
Care co-ordinator (signature): ....   Date of next review: 20/10/01..............
Job title: Clinical case
                              manager   Patient's signature: ....

Supervision register?	YES	Care management?	NO	Risk history completed?	YES
Supervised				Relapse + risk plan	
discharge?	NO	Section 117(2)?	YES	required?	YES

Example 12.2

CONFIDENTIAL: RELAPSE AND RISK MANAGEMENT PLAN

Name: Graham K.

Categories of risk identified:

Aggression and violence	YES	Severe self-neglect	NO
Exploitation (self or others)	NO	Risk to children & young adults	NO
Suicide and self-harm	NO	Other (please specify}	

Current factors which suggest there is significant apparent risk:
(For example: alcohol or substance misuse; specific threats; suicidal ideation; violent fantasies; anger; suspiciousness; persecutory beliefs; paranoid feelings or ideas about particular people)

History of violent offences (see risk history). Currently has paranoid beliefs about his neighbours who he believes are touching him in intimate places. Also believes that Princess Diana is touching him. Poorly compliant with medication. Regular consumption of cannabis.

Clear statement of anticipated risk(s):
(Who is at risk; how immediate is that risk; how severe; how ongoing)

Believes that his neighbours are touching him, difficult to assess as is guarded and suspicious. Has not made any specific threats against neighbours but has a history of assaulting neighbours at previous address. Previous assault was severe, with the neighbour suffering a broken jaw. Risk is driven by psychotic experiences.

Action plan:
(Including names of people responsible for each action and steps to be taken if plan breaks down)

Joint visit by key worker (James H) and another member of team, plus team doctor (Dr Evans). Aim to negotiate re-establishing antipsychotic medication immediately in form of depot or supervised daily medication. Aim to assess if immediate threat to neighbour or to team members. If immediate threat he may require hospital admission, with possible compulsory admission under the Mental Health Act. If a delay in admission occurs due to completion of the section discuss with team and consultant (Professor Burns) breaking confidentiality to inform neighbour of risk. If risk considered manageable at home, negotiate frequent joint visits (James H plus team approach), preferably daily at first. **Not to be visited alone.**
To use safety check system with office prior to visit and establish checking-in time.

Date completed: 20/04/01   Review date: 07/05/01

This risk assessment may contain confidential and/or sensitive information provided by third parties. Such information should not be disclosed to the patient without prior consultation with the informant

Example 12.3

RISK ASSESSMENT DOCUMENTATION
Client's name: Graham K.

RISK HISTORY

Give details of any risk behaviour shown by the patient (actual or threatened). Each entry must be signed and dated
(e.g. previous violence; weapons used; impulsivity; self-harm; non-compliance; disengagement from services; convictions; potentially seriously harmful acts)

Non-compliant with medication since January 2001.

Verbally abusive to key worker (James H) in October 2000. Complaints about side-effects of medication.

Conviction for ABH (actual bodily harm), July 1998, assault on neighbour at previous address, broke neighbour's jaw. Sentenced with hospital treatment order, 3-month admission, July to October 1998.

Prior to this had disengaged from services since previous admission in February 1995.

Assaulted in-patient nurse during admission in February 1995.

Conviction for taking and driving away a motor vehicle, 1992, 2-year suspended sentence.

Team approaches

Inquiries into serious untoward incidents such as homicides, by the mentally ill, usually highlight organizational failures (Ritchie 1994). Failures in the clinical management and supervision of patients often stem from poor co-ordination and poor liaison between different agencies.

Assertive outreach aims to minimize fragmentation of services and maximize co-ordination of care from the resources of a single team. Staff dealing with hostile patients must feel safe and supported within the team and have opportunities to express their anxieties and ask for help freely, such as in a daily handover. The focus should be on anticipation through assessment and frequent contact, and prevention through team and individual responses. Should a member of staff be threatened or assaulted, then debriefing and support should be available from the team and management to cope with psychological, physical, and legal consequences. Employers have a statutory duty of care for the health and safety of their employees, so far as is reasonably practical, even when their employees have a foreseeable risk of violence at work.

Organizational risk factors that relate to the functioning, policies, and training of the team are:

- Systematic assessment of risk not carried out.
- Risk indicators denied or minimized by responsible professionals.
- Information not passed from one professional, or team, to another.

- Clinical responsibility not clearly defined or transferred appropriately.
- Inadequate resources in specialist mental health services and in the community e.g. hospital beds, housing, forensic services.
- Management fails to establish, implement, and train staff regarding policies for risk assessment, critical incident analysis, clinical audit, breakaway, and control and restraint.

(Adapted Coid 1996)

The team leader has a responsibility to ensure that communication, accountability, and training are optimized within the team. We all have a responsibility to raise concerns about patients and systems at the appropriate team meeting. Above all, the team must not be allowed to drift into complacency.

The duty of the employer and management towards health and safety is partly realized through providing training in de-escalation and breakaway techniques for all staff who come into contact with patients. This should include receptionists and ward clerks. There are several techniques used to prevent, manage, or resolve hostile and potentially violent incidents on an individual basis with community patients. Psychological and pharmaceutical approaches may prevent or ameliorate difficult situations. Physical escape, in the form of breakaway, can minimize injury should an assault take place.

Peer review/support

One of the functions of a good multidisciplinary team is to guard against individual complacency towards risk. The daily handover, clinical supervision, and individual patient reviews are all opportunities to discuss and problem-solve risk as a team. We may feel that our own relationship with a patient will protect us from assault. However, a relapsing psychotic patient or an intoxicated patient is just as likely to assault a member of their family, so we are not in any way protected by our perceived closeness to them.

Our team operates a low threshold for joint visits and a high degree of flexibility, so that a joint visit can be organized quickly and easily at the daily handover. It is one of the rationales for assertive outreach teams to have daily contact with each other and enough team members to give backup.

Many people unfamiliar with community working ask us if we visit patients alone. This question betrays a lack of understanding of the patient group and of assertive outreach. Most patient contact is one-to-one, in the patient's home. Patients are referred to assertive outreach because of a complex pattern of needs, of which intermittent hostility may or may not be a component. Joint visiting has a clear role in periods of concern, but is rarely a prerequisite. At the other extreme, a home visit may not be advisable even with two or more members of staff. For patients showing current signs of hostility or violence, indirect approaches such as telephone contact or contact with carers may be all that is possible until a Mental Health Act assessment, with police in attendance, can be arranged. It is important, however, that such periods of indirect contact are not protracted. If the patient can be persuaded to meet members of the team in a relatively safer environment, such as the team base or ward, this can offer greater backup and protection than in the patient's home.

Safety systems

Whether using an assertive outreach approach or not, teams need to have a clear and reliable safety check system. This can involve both a system for checking in at the end of the day and for checking in before and after visits to individual patients. A safety check system allows the tracking of team members' movements through a daily diary left with the secretary at the team base. The secretary's role is to receive calls and tick off each member of staff reporting back safe after an individual visit or at the end of the day. The team member's responsibility is to complete the diary and reliably check in.

The secretary must be confident that if the team member does not check in, is not contactable on their mobile phone, or traceable from diary entries, that they are in trouble and must summon assistance according to agreed protocols. An inconsistent system is almost worse than no system. It must be reliable and continuously reinforced through peer pressure, management supervision, and audit.

The safety value of mobile phones is often exaggerated. They enable team members to check in with the team base and for the person responsible for the safety check to contact staff who have not checked in for whatever reason. They are not, however, effective for summoning assistance during an assault since you will rarely have the time and composure to dial, unless you have managed to escape or lock yourself in a room. Mobile phones also suffer from failed signals or batteries, and should not be thought of as giving protection. Similarly, personal alarms are questionable in their ability to prevent violence and summon assistance. Valuable though these are, they do provide perhaps a false sense of security.

Critical incident analysis

Important lessons can be learned from critical incident analysis. The aftermath of a violent incident has sometimes profound effects on individuals and teams alike. Guilt, loss of confidence, anger, and disillusionment are all common responses. Individual debriefing by the line manager should seek to obtain information, give support, and establish if treatment or time off is required and whether the police should be contacted. Critical incident analysis comes later and involves the whole team discussing, in a constructive way, the antecedents, predictability, procedures, and both immediate and follow-up responses. Changes to individual and organizational practice, care and contingency plans, resources, and training needs will often be recommended. It is important that these changes are considered carefully and implemented, and not just confined to the incident report.

Prosecuting patients for assault

Some organizations operate policies of zero tolerance for assaults on staff (see Chapter 9) and use posters on wards and in clinics to inform patients that prosecutions will be brought against offenders. In practice it can be difficult to prosecute a patient receiving treatment for severe mental illness and police responses vary. Often the police will be reluctant to charge a patient unless the assault is severe or involves a weapon, even when a formal request has been made. Some health care staff are also reluctant to press charges against patients, although this convention is changing.

Decision making needs to take into account the seriousness of the offence, the mental state of the patient at the time, and the effect of prosecution on deterring future violent behaviour towards staff or others. If a patient is regarded as having the capacity at the time of the assault to know the consequences and the morality of the act, then prosecution is usually correct. The formality of a criminal record may protect and alert others should the patient move around the country, and may strengthen the patient's inhibitions and deter a repeat occurrence.

The Crown Prosecution Service has to consider the impact of proceedings on the defendant's mental health as part of determining if it is in the public interest to prosecute. Should the interests of justice be outweighed by adverse effects on the defendant's health, then proceedings will be discontinued. If the mentally disordered offender is undergoing or about to undergo in-patient treatment, then the police are unlikely to recommend prosecution for minor offences.

Conclusion

For those of us who have worked in both in-patient and community settings, our experience suggests that confrontation and hostility are far less frequently encountered with community patients. Collaborative approaches, and the greater sense of personal control that patients feel in their own environments, avoid the situational irritants, constraints, and transgressions that cause frustration and anger in hospital. Of course, patients can still interpret even neutral situations in a paranoid or distorted way, giving rise to conflict, and we still inevitably encounter such conflict in our role as a mental health professional.

Whilst hostility in assertive outreach may be infrequent, the potential consequences of a violent incident occurring in the relative isolation of the patient's home without the support of colleagues are serious. Furthermore, we know that the reliability of risk assessment is low (Munro and Rumgay 2000). We have a responsibility to protect ourselves through training and understanding of risk factors, by our attitudes and behaviour towards patients, and through the application of risk management plans to everyday practice. The organization in which we work has a responsibility also to provide training, policies, procedures, support, and supervision.

We all have a duty to educate our patients, their carers, the public at large, and policy makers, disabusing them of the perceptions of a rising tide of violent assaults by mentally ill people. Equally importantly we must make clear that such violence, when it does occur, is no more likely in this era of care in the community. Pervasive misconceptions about the level of threat posed by our patients have, undoubtedly, been responsible for making our work more difficult and less rewarding and our patients' lives much more difficult.

Chapter 13

Suicidality

Introduction

In the previous chapter we considered the risk management of harm to others. This chapter will focus on a behaviour that generates risk to the patient. Suicidality encompasses all of the following behaviours:

Suicide: a deliberately initiated act of self-harm performed in the knowledge of its fatal outcome.

Parasuicide: a non-habitual act deliberately performed in the expectation of a non-fatal outcome but which causes harm or will do so without the intervention of others.

Attempted suicide: a non-fatal act in which a fatal outcome may be expected.

Suicidality may be a result of an individual's recognition of the realities of coping with a life of serious mental illnesses and grief for the losses incurred. It may be that the illness prevents them acquiring the skills needed to cope with such setbacks and disappointments. Poor coping skills and the social and economic marginalization that can accompany serious illness are a common double burden for our patients. For those with positive psychotic symptoms, suicidality can be driven by command hallucinations, acute paranoid delusions of impending doom, or by the dysphoria that accompanies many patients' illness.

This chapter will describe ways of understanding, predicting, and managing self-harm in psychotic patients living in their own homes.

Incidence

There are difficulties with official statistics of suicide, as anyone who has been to a Coroner's Court will know. Currently, the same legal criteria apply to verdicts of suicide as criminal cases—it must be proven 'beyond reasonable doubt'. Where a suicide note is not left and witnesses' evidence is unavailable or inconclusive, open verdicts or verdicts of accidental death are often passed, despite a high probability of suicide (O'Donnell and Farmer 1995). Thus, the true suicide rate is undoubtedly underestimated in official statistics.

Figure 13.1 summarizes the annual incidence of suicide and parasuicide in the UK from a review by Gunnell (1991) which drew together official sources and suicide studies.

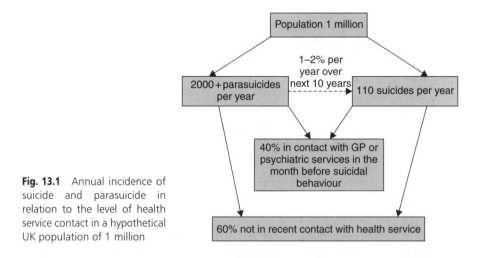

Fig. 13.1 Annual incidence of suicide and parasuicide in relation to the level of health service contact in a hypothetical UK population of 1 million

Male suicides outnumber female suicides by three to one. The trend over the last 30 years shows a rising rate of male suicides, especially in those under 45 years of age, and a falling rate for females. Parasuicide is more common in younger age groups and females (Gunnell 1991).

Suicidal thoughts are much more common than suicidal behaviour. Paykel *et al.* (1974) found 7.8% of the general population admitted having thought that life might not be worth living at some time. A further 1.5% had considered taking their own life. Gunnell (1991) estimated that 1% of those 1.5% experiencing serious suicidal thoughts go on to commit suicide.

Risk factors and risk assessment

The UK Government has set out ambitious targets for reducing suicide rates in both the general population (by 15%) and the severely mentally ill (by 33%) in England. *The Health Of The Nation* (Department of Health 1992) identifies the four diagnostic groups of mental illness which carry the greatest mortality from suicide:

Risk of suicide by psychiatric diagnosis	
Affective disorder	15%
Personality disorder	15%
Alcohol dependence	15%
Schizophrenia	10%

Community mental health teams have to provide outreach to individuals suffering from the whole range of these problems. For many assertive outreach teams, explicit criteria will exclude patients with sole diagnosis of unipolar depression, personality

Table 13.1 Risk factors for suicide

Illness	Personal factors	Life events	Culture and society
◆ Physical illness	◆ Single marital status	◆ History of parasuicide	◆ Economic depression
◆ Mental illness	◆ Unemployment	◆ Imprisonment	◆ Religious beliefs
◆ Drug or alcohol misuse	◆ Male	◆ Loss of job	◆ Poor social supports
◆ Non-compliance with medication	◆ Younger age	◆ Divorce	◆ Young Asian women
		◆ Family history of suicide	

disorder, or alcohol dependence (Chapter 3). This does not mean that we can dismiss the impact of these disorders, and subsequent risk factors, for severely mentally ill psychotic patients. Dual diagnosis patients (Chapter 19) and patients with secondary depression (Chapter 18) and personality disorder (Chapter 17) are covered in this book precisely because of their prevalence as concurrent problems for many patients referred for assertive outreach. Bipolar affective disorder patients are, of course, an integral focus of the work of such teams.

There are known complicating factors which raise the risk. Physical illnesses such as cancer and epilepsy, and, particularly, intrusive chronic pain and disability such as arthritis and even tinitus, are associated with increased rates of suicide. Young women in the UK from the Indian subcontinent are 2.7 times more likely to commit suicide between the ages of 15 and 24 (Soni–Raleigh and Balarajan 1992). Single men have suicide rates that are almost as high as for men who are divorced (Charlton *et al.* 1994). Widowed men have higher rates still. Men who are unemployed run between two and three times the risk of death by suicide than the average. One fifth of suicides were non-compliant with medication in the month before their death (Appleby *et al.* 2000).

Assessment

Assertive outreach targets patients with severe mental illness, who may be vulnerable to substance abuse, socially marginalized through unemployment, and with poor support networks. Most of the risk factors outlined above apply, so their simple application does not get us very far. Risk factors are derived from longitudinal analysis of large populations and may be of little specificity or sensitivity with regards to an individual patient (Morgan 1994). Individual clinical evaluation (which means routinely asking our patients difficult questions about the presence of suicidal thoughts, suicidal intent, evidence of planning, command hallucinations, and depression and hopelessness) is the best method of assessment. Recent changes in clinical features such as depression, hostility, distress, and anxiety indicate a higher risk of suicide than a patient who is consistently anxious or distressed.

Clinical evaluation is greatly aided by the use of structured assessment tools. The routine use of the Brief Psychiatric Rating Scale (BPRS) (Overall and Gorham 1962) will help pick up previously unreported depressed mood. Further assessment of depres-

orting Beck Depression Inventory (Beck
eel I would be better of dead' or 'I would
of hopelessness—'I feel that the future is
a particular warning sign for suicidality.
arly command hallucinations) we should
nd if they feel that they can resist them.
y have used the expression of suicidal
ing or controlling situations may require
of patients with personality disorder do

ide attempt or self-harm, and knowledge
uicide risk for each individual.
ot be predicted or prevented reliably, and
Suicide and Homicide (Appleby *et al.* 1999).
ors failed to predict any of the 46 suicides
al. 1991). The main problem is the large
application of statistical risk factors. Both
on is impractical as a goal for health care

n—concentrating scarce resources on identifying
.

(Wilkinson 1994)

omicide prevention measures, the activities that
of treatments, etc—are in fact aspects of high
quality care.

(Appleby *et al.* 1999)

Individual interventions

Risk management plans

The use of care plans and risk management plans to manage suicidality can be effective both in individual cases and at the team level. Increased contact with the patient is the most important immediate response in a crisis to reduce suicide risk. Many suicide attempts are predominantly impulsive—a response to an acute or transient stressful circumstance.

If the patient has communicated to you their suicidal thoughts you can assume that, on one level, they have a desire to stay alive and be helped. Delaying the suicidal impulse becomes the immediate goal together with practical assistance and problem solving where possible. To delay the impulse the patient must be able to exercise self-control, otherwise hospitalization is essential. An acutely psychotic patient, unable to deny command hallucinations, will benefit little from negotiation and counselling whereas, in depressive episodes, counselling techniques of restoring hope are very valuable. You can remind the bipolar patient that although they feel that nothing will ever improve they have a cyclical illness and peaks can replace troughs.

Remind the patient that as their key worker you will do whatever is necessary to help them through this situation, however complex. Finances, housing, relationships, and illnesses can all be tackled, probably one by one, and the patient can be helped to resist being overwhelmed by multiple problems.

Removing the means

Removing the obvious means of self-harm or suicide can reduce the likelihood of an impulsive suicidal act. In wards, great efforts are made to remove ligature points. In the community, these hazards cannot be controlled other than by admittting the patient to hospital. However, supplies of medication to the patient can be limited, hoarded tablets removed, and safe alternatives to more toxic medicines prescribed.

Many patients may be tempted to take an overdose given the opportunity but would not have the motivation or will power to take themselves to the railway line. Patients with a history of self-harm in the previous three months should not receive more than two weeks' supply of medication (Appleby *et al.* 1999). Be aware that illicit drugs and alcohol may be used to increase the effect of an overdose and to reduce inhibitions that would prevent someone from hanging themselves. Team members from different disciplines will need training on relative toxicity, signs of overdose, and the clinical management of overdose. *Do not wait for critical incident analysis to identify this need.* Team doctors can provide basic training in a team development session.

A patient's key worker, who happens to have occupational therapy or social work training, is informed by the patient that they have taken 20 lithium carbonate tablets, impulsively, half an hour ago. Clearly, the key worker will need advice, but the ability to recognize, assess, and relay information to the team doctor or to the ambulance service can aid intervention and indicate the level of urgency. The patient was able to tell of what they had done—so they are conscious. Are they unsteady on their feet? Have they vomited? Is there an empty bottle or packet to verify the amount taken? What strength tablets are they? Did the patient take anything else? Are there signs of other drugs or alcohol? Is lithium dangerous in overdose?

Patients should be encouraged to use the team, not just one individual, for support. If a patient phones feeling suicidal and his key worker is away, other team members must intervene and have access to relapse and contingency plans. Well-established arrangements for the team approach to working mean that patients who need intensive or crisis interventions are never denied them due to the absence of particular staff.

Restructuring social networks

As a longer-term strategy, patients need to be encouraged to use other supports in the community such as family, friends, drop-in centres, and the church. Helping isolated patients to restructure their social and occupational situation provides a long-term intervention for chronic low self-esteem, depression, and dissatisfaction. Many have lost their social status and supports through illness. Some who developed a psychotic illness early in life have never worked or formed relationships and social groups.

Coping strategy enhancement

Some patients have never learned the coping skills that help most of us deal with setbacks and failures. The teaching, and reinforcement through rehearsal, of simple strategies and courses of action to take when distressed can help patients avoid getting to the point of crisis and suicidal ideation.

Case study

Julie used to present herself at the A&E department saying she felt suicidal after arguments with her alcoholic partner. On two occasions she had taken a modest overdose of temazepam, believing that her partner would leave her.

Julie was encouraged not to argue with her partner when he was drunk, as this would never produce a satisfactory outcome. Instead, she should walk away to another room, have a cigarette, and listen to some relaxing music. She should remind herself that her partner was drunk, did not necessarily mean what he said, and had not walked out on her in the past ten years. If she was unable to contain her distress herself, she should call her mother. She could also contact the team.

What to do when a suicide occurs

One of the twelve points for safer services in the report of the National Confidential Inquiry into Suicide and Homicide (Appleby *et al*. 1999) is the establishment of assertive outreach teams to prevent loss of contact with vulnerable and high-risk patients.

In our experience, a typical CMHT or assertive outreach team can expect one or two suicides per year. Given the limitations of suicide prediction described above, it is important that suicides should not automatically be considered as a team failure. *We need a realistic recognition that suicide is part of the job.* We must not be complacent about it, but neither should we excoriate ourselves when it happens. The individual most closely involved with the victim is likely to feel crushed, saddened, and often guilty.

The team has two immediate obligations. Firstly, to support that individual, allowing them time to talk it through. They will often express exaggerated views of what they could have done but failed to do and sometimes an equally exaggerated judgement about the impact of things they have done. These concerns need to be heard and taken seriously, not dismissed. Only when they have been talked through in detail can they be weighed and placed in perspective. Assertive outreach workers' feelings may mirror those of the patient's friends and family. The team as a whole has an obligation to contact and offer support to the family and provide relevant information.

The second task facing the team is to conduct a review of the events preceding the suicide to identify anything that may have made it more likely or obscured the detection of warning signs. In England and Wales, the completion of the returns for the Confidential Inquiry into Homicide and Suicide (Appleby *et al.* 1999) is a useful framework for this process. Its very length and bureaucratic detail may help structure the process and reduce the sense of anger and defensiveness that can otherwise inhibit an honest enquiry. Lessons from critical incidents need to be incorporated into routine care. Involving the whole team in a critical incident analysis brings it together at difficult times and identifies strengths and weaknesses.

Gaps in documentation of risks are often identified after critical incidents. Clear team policies, team-based managers able to monitor the application of policy, and standardized documentation assist in consistent risk assessment. The examples presented of our documentation (Examples 13.1–13.3) indicate areas of risk and steps in formulating a clear response.

Assertive outreach teams are resourced and organized to respond as rapidly as possible to patients identified as at risk. Daily handover, availability of multidisciplinary team members, continuity of care, and regular review of patients all contribute to the safe management of suicidality. Our close knowledge of the patient may alert us to risks through clear contingency and relapse plans. Equally, there is a danger that familiarity leads to tolerance of ongoing risks such as suicidal thoughts and we fail to recognize when this may lead to suicidal behaviour. Clinical supervision and peer discussion of risky patients improves focus.

Case study

Richard is a 39-year-old man whose life has been devastated by psychotic illness. He finds the psychotic experiences (for example, believing that people are coming into his flat and putting pins into his body) extremely distressing. He also shows depressed mood and isolates himself from his family, friends, and services. He does not believe he is ill and does not believe the medicine helps the way he feels. He is also sensitive to the side-effects of medication.

He has had several long admissions to hospital and his symptoms have not reduced significantly with antipsychotic medication. The medication does, however, reduce his arousal and his accusations of others sticking pins into his body.

Several years ago, Richard attempted to hang himself on the ward. He has taken two overdoses of medication. Whilst reluctant to talk about these events, he indicates that they were a response to distressing and painful symptoms at the time, rather than a planned and thought-out assessment of his life.

Example 13.1

ENHANCED CPA/SECTION 117(2) REVIEW (delete as applicable)	
Patient's name: Richard G. Address: 112 Holden House, Winstanley Estate, Battersea. Phone: 0208 987 xxxx Date of birth: 21/08/62 GP: Jackson Phone: 0208 987 xxxx	CMHT: ACT TEAM Phone: 020 8877 xxxx New patient: No If No, date of review: 01/10/01 Diagnosis: 1. Paranoid Schizophrenia.　　F20.0 2. .... F —— —˙—

Assessed needs or problem	Intervention	Resp . of
Engagement, Isolates himself from services, family and friends.	♦ Aim to establish face-to-face contact twice per week. Use of telephone contact as required. ♦ Richard does not tolerate long visits. Explore Richard's wishes e.g. Company, leisure activities. ♦ Liaise with family. Improving level of contact. ♦ Explore local facilities e.g. library, drop-in-club. Help restructure social network.	BW
Long-term low risk of suicide in response to acute distress driven by psychotic symptoms.	♦ Maintain regular contact. ♦ Increase contact when acutely distressed. ♦ Assess for level of suicide ideation, command hallucinations, paranoia, suicidal intent, depressed mood, and hopelessness. Use team doctor for full mental state assessment.	BW
	♦ Consider admission if extremely distressed ± Mental Health Act if refuses informal admission. ♦ Offer medications for symptom relief and arousal. Risperidone long term. Diazepam short term. ♦ Limit supplies of medication to one week. ♦ Try to establish on Risperidone. ♦ Psychoeducation on illness and origin of distress. ♦ Explore the use of CBT when better.	BW

Involved in care:	Dr✓ Psychologist CPN OT SW Ward nurse CCM✓ Support Worker✓ Other			
Present at meeting	Dr✓ Psychologist CPN OT SW✓ Ward nurse CCM✓ Support Worker Other			
Discussed with the patient?	YES	Copy to patient?	YES	Copy to GP?	YES
Care co-ordinator (print):	Bob Walker		Phone: 020 8877 xxxx	
Care co-ordinator (signature):	....		Date of next review: 1/04/02	
Job title:	Clinical case manager		Patient's signature:...........................	

On supervision register?	NO	Care management?	NO	Risk history completed?	YES
On supervised discharge?	NO	Section 117(2)?	YES	Relapse + risk plan required?	YES

Example 13.2

CONFIDENTIAL: RELAPSE AND RISK MANAGEMENT PLAN

Name: Richard G.

Categories of Risk Identified:

Aggression and violence	NO	Severe self-neglect	NO
Exploitation (self or others)	NO	Risk to children & young adults	NO
Suicide and self-harm	YES	Other (please specify}	

Current factors which suggest there is significant apparent risk:
(For example: alcohol or substance misuse; specific threats; suicidal ideation; violent fantasies; anger; suspiciousness; persecutory beliefs; paranoid feelings or ideas about particular people)

Non-compliant with medication. Depressed mood. Social isolation. Says he will take the medication when he feels distressed. Current persecutory beliefs around people coming into his flat at night to interfere with his body. Denies suicidal intent.

Clear statement of anticipated risk(s):
(Who is at risk; how immediate is that risk; how severe; how ongoing)
Ongoing low risk of suicide. Risk increased during acute distress driven by psychotic experiences.
Action plan:
(Including names of people responsible for each action and steps to be taken if plan breaks down)

See care plan: Maintain regular contact. Bob Walker and team to increase contact when Richard more acutely distressed.

Assess for level of suicidal ideation, command hallucinations, paranoia, suicidal intent, depressed mood, and hopelessness. Use team doctor for full mental state assessment as level of distress or psychosis increases. Consider admission if Richard extremely distressed and multiple risk factors as above evident. Consider use of Mental Health Act if refuses informal admission.
Offer medication for symptom relief and to reduce arousal and distress. Risperidone moderately effective if taken long term. Diazepam effective short term to reduce arousal.
Limit supplies of medication to one week to ensure regular contact and reduce risk of overdose.

Date completed: 01/10/01	Review date: 01/04/02

This risk assessment may contain confidential and/or sensitive information provided by third parties. Such information should not be disclosed to the patient without prior consultation with the informant

Example 13.3

RISK ASSESSMENT DOCUMENTATION

Client's Name: Richard G.

RISK HISTORY
Give details of any risk behaviour shown by the patient (actual or threatened). Each entry must be signed and dated
(E.g. previous violence; weapons used; impulsivity; self-harm; non-compliance; disengagement from services; convictions; potentially seriously harmful acts)

1995: Overdose of antidepressant medication
1997: Attempted to hang himself on the ward
1999: Overdose of Temazepam

Conclusions

In brutal epidemiological terms:

There is little research evidence linking any health service intervention with a fall in suicide rates.

(Appleby *et al.* 2000)

We are not good at predicting suicide; nobody is yet. We must hope that establishing meaningful relationships with our patients, conducting assessments, and our clinical judgement will help identify suicidal intent so that early intervention can follow. A realistic approach to the inevitability of suicide when working with often damaged and distressed individuals is needed. We must learn lessons from such tragic events and avoid complacency while rejecting the pervasive 'blame' culture that equates suicide with a 'sense of failure'. Good mental health practice is based on establishing real relationships between patients and staff, so sadness after suicide is inevitable. It should not, however, develop into persecution or pathological self-doubt.

Assertive outreach can vary the level of support between several visits a day to once every other week or so, depending on the assessed vulnerabilities of our patients. Providing high-quality care and support, together with modern treatments and interventions to all our patients is the most effective way of serving and protecting them in the long term.

Chapter 14

Self-neglect

Introduction

Self-neglect often results from the demotivating, negative symptoms of schizophrenia together with the cognitive deficits that strip some patients of their ability to manage themselves and the outside world in a normal way. Social factors such as limited social networks, unemployment, and poverty may contribute to a sense of hopelessness or apathy towards self-care and care of the immediate environment. Reed and Leonard (1989) describe self-neglect as:

> A pattern of intentionally neglecting prescribed self-care activities despite access to available resources and knowledge.

This chapter will describe ways of managing self-neglect in psychotic patients living in their own homes.

Incidence

Little is published about self-neglect or its incidence in the general and mentally ill populations. The closest that we can come to an estimate of the incidence of serious self-neglect is through examining the numbers of people put on the supervision register for this category in England. Unfortunately, the supervision register is notorious for inconsistencies in its application by different clinicians. The risk to others is over-represented and the risk to self is under-represented.

> The Supervision Register policy has not resulted in the identification of a well-defined group. Its effectiveness is hindered by the lack of operationalised measures of risk.

> (Bindman *et al.* 2000)

Bindman sampled a group of 133 patients on the supervision register across England. Only 45 were registered as at risk of self-neglect. Of these, 16 had at some time suffered from weight loss as a result of self-neglect, and 7 had neglected themselves to a life-threatening extent.

Risk factors and risk assessment

Self-neglect has a low profile as an area of concern for mental health services. As a result, there is no standard measure or method of categorizing self-neglect (Bindman *et al.* 2000). Those whose relapse signature includes social withdrawal and psychomotor retardation, to the extent that they fail to eat and drink adequately, must be the main cause of concern to assertive outreach teams. Patients with a diagnosis of catatonic schizophrenia or with a severe depressive component in either bipolar affective disorder or schizophrenia may self-neglect during relapse and require increased home visits to monitor and assist with self-care and nutrition. Patients at longer-term risk of self-neglect will be those with pronounced cognitive deficits and negative symptoms. These patients will require continued assistance with daily living skills and monitoring of risk.

Self-neglect is not restricted to patients with psychosis. Those with dementia, learning difficulties, and eccentrics can manifest this behaviour. Diogenes' syndrome (named after the Greek philosopher who lived in a barrel) is characterized by gross self-neglect, social withdrawal, and living in squalor (Williams *et al.* 1998).

Table 14.1 Risk factors for self-neglect

Short-term/acute risk factors	Long-term/chronic risk factors
◆ History of self-neglect during relapse	◆ History of self-neglect
◆ Non-compliance with treatment	◆ Pronounced negative schizophrenia symptoms (social withdrawal, poverty of thought, poor volition)
◆ Psychomotor retardation	◆ Cognitive deficits (schizophrenia or organic disorder)
◆ Severe bipolar affective disorder	◆ Neglect of physical disease (diabetes, hypertension)
◆ Catatonic schizophrenia	◆ Poverty
◆ Financial crisis or problems	◆ Learning disability
◆ Lack of social support	◆ Lack of social support

Assessment

Assessment needs to be sensitive and morally non-judgemental. Many healthy teenagers may be considered to have problems with personal care. Self-neglecting patients are often not ashamed of their lifestyles and offer good reasons for not going out, mistrusting statutory services, and hoarding. The question of whether the patient is putting themself at significant risk is our overriding concern.

The risk assessment format, which follows the case study in this chapter, can be used to clarify and document assessed risk and to formulate interventions (see Examples 14.1–14.3). Failure to eat and drink due to stupor, depression, or catatonia are the main alerts. It is possible to survive for many weeks without eating but only a few days without drinking. Assessment should include a history of food and drink intake in recent days, noting evidence of weight loss, pallor, weakness, or fatigue due to starvation.

Gross self-neglect is fairly obvious, but less extreme forms may be underestimated without a visit to the patient in their own home to ascertain:

◆ Is there food in the house?

◆ What has the patient eaten and drunk today?

◆ Is there a fridge?

◆ Is food rotting and dangerous to eat or attracting flies/vermin?

◆ Is the physical environment of the house safe?

Where gross self-neglect is evident then a full physical examination, using either the resources of the team or by accompanying the patient to the GP, is advisable for new patients.

Assessment of self-neglect presenting less immediate risk needs to focus on activities of daily living such as personal care and household management. The purpose of such assessment is to establish a baseline from which to support the process of change and to gain understanding of the factors that hinder functioning. How often do you bathe and wash? How competent are you with laundry, cleaning of teeth, dress and appearance, shopping, cooking? (See Chapter 24, 'Daily living skills'.)

Formal assessment tools may be off-putting for patients. A patient with a history of being reclusive is not going to readily discuss their personal hygiene routine. A mixture of observation over time and sensitive probing can build a picture from which to formulate a care plan. Accurate and measurable documentation is important for evaluating progress. For example, record the length of time the patient has worn the same clothes without washing them, record evidence of shopping or cooking.

Formal scales do exist but encompass more global daily living activities (e.g. the life skills profile) (Rosen *et al.* 1989). They are often suitable only for in-patients. Assessment in the community must take into account what resources the patient has available. If they have little or no money, no hot water, and no washing machine or iron then this is very relevant to their personal care.

Individual interventions

Managing relapse

In some patients neglect of personal hygiene is part of their relapse signature and not necessarily an ongoing problem. Treatment of the psychosis may be the only intervention needed. Where the self-neglect is life-threatening (e.g. neglect of physical illness, failure to eat and drink) physical treatment takes precedence. Care and risk management plans need to reflect this relapse signature and give clear instructions.

For patients whose mental state changes rapidly, and who are prone to stop eating or drinking, frequent contact with patient and family is critical for safe community care. Patients with severe bipolar illness can sink to this state in a few days and, for these patients, you must know:

- What is their usual pattern?
- Will their relative phone you if they do not see them for a day or two?
- Have you negotiated a relapse plan with the patient?
- Will the patient allow you or their family member to have a key to their home to be used in the event of their being inside, in a manic stupor?

Neglecting physical health care

The key worker must sometimes also take responsibility for the patient's physical health needs, both identifying problems and registering and accompanying the patient to a GP, and often also treating physical illness (see Chapter 22, 'Physical health care').

We regularly monitor patients' blood sugar, supervise somatic medications, and advocate on behalf of our patients to ensure they get the physical treatments and care they require from services. District nurses and hospital specialists can too often see psychiatric patients as unreliable or low priorities for general health care. Where failure to take life-saving physical treatments such as insulin or antihypertensives is clearly due to psychosis, it is possible to intervene, using the Mental Health Act to treat the psychosis. The use of such legislation with patients who have the capacity to understand the implications and consequences of their act is much more difficult. For example, a patient without active psychiatric symptoms who is judged to have capacity and who refuses to have life-saving dialysis for renal failure cannot be forced to do so under the Mental Health Act in the UK.

Social linking and networks

Social linking and rebuilding support networks is invaluable for patients who self-neglect. Neglect of personal care is stigmatizing; people avoid contact with malodorous individuals. This initiates a vicious circle as impoverishment of social contacts and occupation reduces incentives for change in the patient's behaviour. Talking to patients about their personal care is not easy. If we have a friend who smells do we actually come out and tell them? One strategy to avoid offence is to depersonalize the issue by suggesting that if they start attending a resource centre, or if they want to seek paid employment, they will need to tidy themselves up. Otherwise, it is advisable to build up a strong relationship before coming straight to the point!

Daily living skills' training

Teaching patients self-care and hygiene routines will only be successful once the patient is ready for change. Motivational techniques may include pointing out how the patient's appearance or hygiene may negatively influence other people's perception of them. Self-care can be presented as an intermediate step towards stated goals. Daily living skills' training is discussed in more detail in Chapter 24.

Home care

Many patients self-neglect directly as a result of thought disorder and chaotic lifestyles due to psychosis. Practical help with shopping and the provision of meals on wheels can reduce nutritional risks. Direct assistance with household tasks such as laundry and cleaning, plus the provision of home care, can make the difference between the patient being able to keep their own flat and being in residential care.

So called 'deep cleans' for grossly neglected flats needing many hours' work can be arranged through the social services home care department. Regular home care to keep the flat in a reasonable condition after a deep clean is a worthwhile investment as it can enable the patient to survive in the community long-term. Such cleaning needs paying for from the team or social care budget.

Home carers are not mental health professionals, but domestic staff. With difficult patients, chaotic patients, and hard-to-engage patients home care arrangements tend to break down. The same applies to meals on wheels. Regular liaison and problem solving with the home care agency can keep the service going. Often, however, patients refuse to allow access to the home carer or get into disputes after having possessions moved around or items unwittingly thrown out. In these instances, the only option may be for team members to give direct practical assistance to the patient as part of their regular visits.

Team approaches and responses

Some key workers find working with patients who are grossly self-neglecting distasteful, and struggle to hide this in their interactions with patients. They may ask for a reallocation of their case load. Furthermore, new members of staff may find it hard to resist the immediate temptation to tidy up a messy flat.

The needs of the patient dictate that home visits, regular contact, transport, and the whole range of social and medical interventions are offered. Patient choice also dictates that they may not want someone being judgemental about their personal and domestic care and insisting they help them tidy up. These situations are best dealt with through clinical and peer supervision. Similarly, we have had instances of receptionists pointedly spraying air freshener around rooms when malodorous patients have come to the team base. Dignity, respect, and understanding apply equally to patients who self-neglect, and staff may need reminding of this.

The team must respond to more life-threatening self-neglect by assertive efforts to find patients known to stop eating or drinking when they relapse. Well-established relapse and risk management plans and rapid responses to identified risk should be part of the team culture (see Examples 14.1–14.3). We do have permission from some of our patients to hold their door keys, which allows us to establish quickly if the patient is safe. Entering a patient's house with their keys in the absence of a response to knocking needs to be negotiated and is usually only undertaken if the team member feels the patient is at immediate risk. Such negotiated responses, which anticipate and plan for future risk, are the hallmark of good practice.

Case study

Donald is 60 years old and developed schizophrenia late in life, when 43. Always a loner, he had spent brief periods sleeping rough, generally working in unskilled, low-stress jobs. He had moved from rural Scotland at 19 to work in Birmingham. He had no friends, had lost touch with his family, and had never had sexual or intimate relationships.

After 10 years of declining social function, he was referred following a series of hospital admissions precipitated by gross self-neglect and episodes of barricading himself in his flat due to persecutory delusions and auditory hallucinations. The voices told him he was worthless, should not accept state benefits, and that he would be arrested if he went out.

In Donald's home, his gross self-neglect and spartan living arrangements were most evident:

- He had worn the same clothes for many months.
- He had lost approximately 15 kilos in weight; the majority of his other clothes no longer fit him.
- He did not bathe, but did shave and cut his own hair.
- He ate dried potato reconstituted with water but uncooked, tinned fish, biscuits, and cereal with water.
- He had no fridge and tended to hoard packets of food.
- He shopped once a week in the nearest shop when he went out to cash his welfare cheque.
- He avoided going out at any other time for fear of persecution.
- A bed was the only furniture in the flat; Donald had thrown the rest out believing he was going to prison.
- There was no telephone, television, or radio, as Donald believed that 'they' would discuss his personal business over the airwaves.
- He boiled water for tea on a single-ring appliance.

Conclusions

Self-neglect is under-reported and often overlooked in terms of interventions. It is not glamorous as a focus for mental health professionals' attention. The chronic and insidious nature of some patients' self-neglect can lead to therapeutic pessimism or acceptance of the behaviour. This may actually be hindering the integration of the patient into their community. Patients with unstable mental state who self-neglect during relapse are a particular target group for frequent and assertive contact. Long-term self-neglect can result in premature death, particularly from neglect of chronic physical illnesses such as diabetes.

Assertive outreach teams must recognize and assess these problems and provide intensive and comprehensive support over the longer term. Social linking and rebuilding support networks provide scope for enduring improvements in patients' lives.

Example 14.1

ENHANCED CPA/SECTION 117(2)REVIEW (delete as applicable)	
Patient's name: Donald F. Address: Flat6, Fraser House, Wandsworth Phone: 0208 997 xxxx Date of birth: 25/10/40 GP: Jones Phone: 0208 675 xxxx	CMHT: ACT TEAM Phone: 020 8877 xxxx New patient: No If No, date of review: 01/6/01 Diagnosis: 1. Paranoid Schizophrenia F20.0 2. .... F —— ·——

Assessed needs or problem	Intervention	Resp. of
Engagement	♦ Does not tolerate intensive contact. Frequent short visits, minimum two times per week. ♦ Telephone contact as required. ♦ Offer practical assistance with household tasks as engagement tool.	CP
Self-neglect	♦ Frequent contact to ensure not barricaded in flat and obtaining sufficient food and drink. ♦ Monitor weight. ♦ Negotiate bathing, changing clothes and bed sheets. ♦ Practical assistance to obtain fridge, clothes, visit laundrette, obtain furniture. ♦ Encourage healthy diet by assistance with shopping and meals-on-wheels three times a week. ♦ Increase variety of social contact and activity. Visits by different team members. Encourage contact with brother. Accompany to park of café.	CP

Involved in care: Dr✓ Psychologist CPN OT SW Ward nurse CM✓ Support worker✓ Other

Present at meeting: Dr✓ Psychologist CPN OT SW Ward nurse CM✓ Support worker✓ Other

Discussed with the patient?   YES   Copy to patient?   YES   Copy to GP?   YES

Care co-ordinator (print):   Caroline Phillips   Phone: 020 8877 xxxx

Care co-ordinator (signature): .... Date of next review: 1/12/01.

Job title: Clinical case manager   Patient's signature: ....

Supervision register?	NO	Care management?	YES	Risk history completed? YES
Supervised discharge?	NO	Section 117(2)?	YES	Relapse + risk plan required? YES

Example 14.2

CONFIDENTIAL: RELAPSE AND RISK MANAGEMENT PLAN

Name: Donald F.

Categories of risk identified:

Aggression and violence	NO	Severe self-neglect	YES
Exploitation (self or others)	NO	Risk to children & young adults	NO
Suicide and self-harm	NO	Other (please specify}	

Current factors which suggest there is significant apparent risk:
(For example: alcohol or substance misuse; specific threats; suicidal ideation; violent fantasies; anger; suspiciousness; persecutory beliefs; paranoid feelings or ideas about particular people)

Two recent admissions due to barricading self in flat and failing to obtain adequate supplies of food and drink. 15 Kgs weight loss over past six months.

Clear statement of anticipated risk(s):
(Who is at risk; how immediate is that risk; how severe; how ongoing)

Intermittent episodes of self-neglect resulting in starvation. Moderate risk of severe consequences if not discovered quickly.

Action plan:
(Including names of people responsible for each action and steps to be taken if plan breaks down.)

Early intervention in the event of withdrawal from services, barricading self in flat, noticeable weight loss, or failure to eat or drink adequately. Early detection through twice weekly visits and regular telephone contact.

If barricaded in flat, team member discovering this to initiate Mental Health Act assessment after discussion with medical staff and social worker and to contact council immediately to gain access.

Date completed: 01/06/01	Review date: 01/12/01

This risk assessment may contain confidential and/or sensitive information provided by third parties. Such information should not be disclosed to the patient without prior consultation with the informant

Example 14.3

RISK ASSESSMENT DOCUMENTATION

Client's name: Donald F.

RISK HISTORY

Give details of any risk behaviour shown by the patient (actual or threatened). Each entry must be signed and dated
(E.g. previous violence; weapons used; impulsivity; self-harm; non-compliance; disengagement from services; convictions; potentially seriously harmful acts)

1999 April and July: two episodes of barricading himself in flat during exacerbation of psychotic illness. Failed to take adequate food and drink. Gross weight loss evident.

Chapter 15

Schizophrenia and delusional disorders

Introduction

Schizophrenia is the archetypal mental illness; what most people think of when they imagine 'madness'. It affects all aspects of mental functioning—thinking, feeling, experiencing, and even movement. More than any other mental disorder it is the one where the loss of contact with reality is most obvious. It was first described by Kraepelin in 1896 (Kraepelin 1919) who called it 'dementia praecox' to emphasize its long-term, deteriorating course in distinguishing it from manic depressive disorder.

The term 'schizophrenia' was first coined by Eugen Bleuler in Zurich in 1911 (Bleuler 1950) who stressed the clinical picture rather than the course of the disorder. He used the term to draw attention to the disruption (or splitting) of a wide range of mental processes. Bleuler described the core features of schizophrenia in his 'four 'A's'—autism (the withdrawal from close personal contact), associations (their loosening in thought processes), affect (blunting and disturbances of mood), and ambivalence (the inhibition of motivation). He considered that hallucinations and delusions were not core symptoms but secondary results of the patient trying to make sense of their strange experiences.

The focus of diagnosis shifted to these 'secondary symptoms' in the system introduced by Schneider (1959) whose so-called 'first-rank symptoms' described the features of the acute illness that could be often identified at a single interview. These were mainly hallucinations, delusions, disorders of thinking, and passivity feelings. Schneider's approach has persisted, with subsequent diagnostic systems continuing to emphasize the so-called 'positive' symptoms of hallucinations, delusions, and thought disorder (American Psychiatric Association 1994; World Health Organisation 1992). The introduction of antipsychotic medicines (which tend to act on the positive symptoms rather than on the negative ones) and the description of the core features by Bleuler have consolidated this diagnostic approach.

These early pioneers in schizophrenia research worked in large mental hospitals and tended to see only the patients who failed to make a recovery. Not surprisingly, they developed a very gloomy view of schizophrenia—Kraepelin particularly. It is only with follow-up studies of patients outside hospital (Ciompi 1988) that a more balanced prognosis has emerged, reminding us that between a third and a half of patients make a fairly good recovery (Harding *et al.* 1987). Maintaining an optimistic view of the disorder remains a problem for mental health workers in the community as we also inevitably focus on those who do less well.

Classifications

A disorder as complex as schizophrenia (some insist on saying 'the schizophrenias') has been subject to various attempts at subclassification. The purpose of classification in medicine is only to try and improve prediction of prognosis and to target treatments more accurately. It is not an attempt at ultimate truth. There is no logic linking the different classificatory systems as they have replaced each other and various terms persist even when the classification has been superseded. Of the first classification (into paranoid, catatonic, hebephrenic, and simple), paranoid (where the picture is dominated by persecutory delusions) is still in regular use. Catatonic (dominated by disorders of movement, either excitement or stupor) is increasingly rare in the developed world, as is hebephrenic (early onset in adolescence dominated by thought disorder and a strange disconnected mood state). Simple schizophrenia was originally used to describe patients with severe negative symptoms (apathy, self-neglect, etc.) without any history of acute episodes.

Acute and chronic are used to distinguish between florid periods of relapse with prominent positive symptoms (hallucinations, delusions, and disordered thinking) and periods between such episodes where the patient demonstrates mainly negative symptoms (apathy, self-neglect, withdrawal). While still useful terms, they are far from straightforward. An attempt was made to classify schizophrenia on the basis of these positive and negative symptoms (Crow 1980) but it became clear that simplistic ideas that negative symptoms always came after positive ones (as in the old idea of a 'schizophrenic defect state') did not hold up. Positive symptoms can persist for decades, negative symptoms can precede positive ones, and so on.

The current diagnostic system adopted by the World Health Organisation, ICD-10 (World Health Organisation 1992), includes the clinical types alluded to here plus a fifth digit to clarify the course (e.g. episodic, continuous). Paranoid schizophrenia is the commonest type.

Bordering disorders

Many patients present with a picture closely resembling schizophrenia but are not classified as such:

♦ *Persistent delusional disorders* are those where the patient is disabled by usually a single delusional preoccupation (e.g. that they have a misshapen body or that they are the object of a specific plot) which may fluctuate over time but remains for years, without any other features of schizophrenia developing.

♦ *Schizotypal disorder* is rarely used, but refers to an odd, eccentric, and often aloof individual with strange thinking patterns that remind us of schizophrenia, but who never develops any definite features.

♦ *Acute and transient psychotic disorders* are, as their name suggests, brief, with an often rapidly fluctuating clinical presentation.

- *Schizoaffective disorders* are when there is major mood disturbance and schizophrenia symptoms concurrently in the same episode. They can be either manic or depressive. It is still unclear how these disorders overlap with bipolar affective disorder.

- *Schizophreniform disorder* is a commonly used term which, although no longer officially part of the classification, is often used by clinicians who want to defer judgement.

Table 15.1 ICD-10 classification of schizophrenia (World Health Organisation 1992)

Type	Course
F20.0 Paranoid	.0 Continuous
F20.1 Hebephrenic	.1 Episodic with progressive deficit
F20.2 Catatonic	.2 Episodic with stable deficit
F20.3 Undifferentiated	.3 Episodic remittent
F20.4 Post-schizophrenic depression	.4 Incomplete remission
F20.5 Residual	.5 Complete remission
F20.6 Simple	
F20.8* Other	.8 Other
F20.9* Unspecified	.9 Observation <1 year

* '8' is always used for 'other', and '9' for 'unspecified'. Hence, missing numbers.

Family factors in schizophrenia

The role of nature versus nurture has been a highly controversial one in schizophrenia. Initially, the disorder was considered entirely genetic, although Bleuler took a more dynamic approach to it. Genetic explanations dominated until after the Second World War when a period of confusion about diagnosis (predominantly in North America) and the ascendancy of psychoanalytical thinking focused attention on experiential factors—particularly child rearing. Not surprisingly, the families of severely ill patients were noted often to be dysfunctional, and a number of theories were developed. Many attributed the development of schizophrenia to family behaviour. These theories have been fairly conclusively disproved now.

Evidence from twin and adoption studies have clearly demonstrated the importance of inheritance in developing schizophrenia. The Danish adoption study (Rosenthal *et al.* 1971) is probably the most powerful evidence. In this, children adopted at birth were followed up as adults and the incidence of schizophrenia in those who were adopted from mothers with schizophrenia was still about 10%. This is as high as would have been expected had they stayed with their mothers. Even more interesting, the researchers found that some of the adoptive parents with schizophrenic children demonstrated the 'over-protectiveness' thought to be one of the causal factors. It could be that such over-protectiveness is an understandable reaction of a parent to a struggling child. Similarly, twins separated at birth show the same risk for concordance for the disorder as those not separated. It is important, however, to recognize that the genetic risk does not count for everything. There is little doubt that upbringing and experience can help protect against the development of schizophrenia. Even in identical twins, the risk of both developing the disease is just over 50%.

Although these family theories have been effectively discredited within the professions, it is essential to be familiar with them. They live on as part of our culture and few parents of an individual with schizophrenia do not blame themselves. Many harbour continuing doubts, despite reassurance. Often these doubts are sustained by these theories. For staff working with them it is best to acknowledge the theories and explain why they are not correct. Simply saying 'the old family theories of schizophrenia are out of date' will not reassure effectively. Much better to discuss them explicitly and counter them.

Double bind

Probably the most well-known theory is that of the double bind (Bateson *et al.* 1956). This proposes that faulty communication between parent and child confuses the child so that they develop disorganized thinking and confusion about relationships as an adult. The double bind is classically quoted as giving one message with words and another with non-verbal communication: 'That's all right I forgive you, it was nothing important' expressed with a face like thunder.

There is nothing unusual about such conflicts in human relationships. In fact, Bateson was concerned with the conflict of different *categories* of statements, having recently been fascinated by some mathematical writings of Bertrand Russel. He meant that some contradictory statements at different levels were logically impossible and therefore confusing. Although it is a fine piece of thinking, there has never been any confirmatory evidence that double binds are more frequent in families with a schizophrenic member.

The schizophrenogenic mother/ schism and skew

This first is a particularly damaging concept because mothers seem more prone to blaming themselves and feeling guilty than other family members. The term was coined by Frieda Fromm–Reichmann (1948) to mean an overcontrolling but emotionally cold mother. The important thing to point out to families is that Fromm–Reichmann was a psychoanalyst who *never* met the parents of her patients. It is reported that she developed her theory about the schizophrenogenic mother from the analysis of 11 patients with a diagnosis of schizophrenia in the US in the 1950s. (At the time, diagnosis was notoriously 'hit and miss'.). She had no direct contact with these mothers from which to judge for herself.

Lidz, on the other hand, did work with parents and proposed that there was a particular imbalance in the parental relationship in families with schizophrenia (Lidz and Lidz 1949). He suggested that the marriage was characterized by a skewed power relationship or a degree of separation (schism). Remarkably, this is one of the communication theories that has received some empirical verification with Lidz able to identify affected families from listening 'blind' to tapes. Of course, this gives no support for causation. The finding has not been repeated.

R.D. Laing

Although Laing does not have a specific theory attached to him, he has had a powerful effect on the debate about family influences. A brilliant writer, his works caught the mood of the 1960s and 70s, in particular, *The divided self* (Laing 1960). His views changed over time but he is most remembered for his proposal that schizophrenia was the failure of those around the patient to understand the rich and often symbolic communications in which they expressed their view of the world. Laing suggested that society was too rigid and responded with incomprehension and repression when individuals expressed different views.

The image of anxious, rigid parents (and parent figures such as doctors and nurses) trying to deny the true experience of the patient because it challenged their impoverished orthodoxy became a powerful stick to beat the professions with. Again, there was never any empirical evidence and, in his latter years, Laing often permitted routine treatments alongside the 'voyage of exploration' he advocated. In some of his later work he presented schizophrenia as a personal odyssey—but this had little impact. It is the sense of struggle against an uncomprehending world, and the plea to just let the patient be, for which his work is best remembered.

Expressed Emotion

The work on expressed emotion differs from those theories outlined above in that there is no claim for causation. The work of Leff and his colleagues is based on the earlier observations that intense family situations increase the likelihood of relapse in established schizophrenia (Brown *et al.* 1972). This has given rise to a 'family' treatment approach which has been subject to multiple rigorous studies indicating that it does reduce the relapse rate (Mari and Streiner 1994*b*).

Although the expressed emotion approach is usually considered non-controversial in the UK, it is seen as apportioning blame to the family by some groups in the US and Australia. Its applications are discussed in more detail in Chapter 25 and below, but it is important to explore the families' understanding of the approach. Although an important first step is to educate the family about schizophrenia (and hopefully dispel many old myths), we have found that parents can remain feeling very guilty. Despite our protestations that this is not about 'causing the disease', they may still feel that it highlights how they have failed to ameliorate it.

Treatments in the community

We have dealt with schizophrenia at such length because it is such an important and controversial disorder and because individuals suffering from it are likely to form a major part of outreach work. Because it is such a pervasive disorder and can affect all aspects of an individual's life, it is especially important to take a holistic approach. Although different treatments are classified and organized both in this and other chapters, this should not suggest that they are independent of each other. Currently, the most effective treatments in schizophrenia are undoubtedly pharmacological, but this should not imply a simple insistance on drugs. Without attention to the personal and social needs of our patients, the drugs would not be enough—assuming they took them!

It is oversimplistic to decide that because the drugs are more effective than most psychosocial interventions, then most of our time should be devoted to the drugs. Successful engagement using effective psychosocial interventions may take enormous amounts of time and energy but may mean that obtaining consistent co-operation with medication comes that much easier.

Antipsychotic medication

The role of antipsychotic medication is addressed in some detail in Chapter 7 and compliance is covered in Chapter 11. Schizophrenia is the disorder par excellence where persistence with maintenance medication pays greatest dividends. There is no doubt that remaining on medication, whether oral or depot, significantly reduces the risk of relapse. For most patients it also ensures that they can function better in between relapses. They feel less vulnerable and less easily stressed, so there is less friction with family and friends. Concentration is often better, although tiredness and a sense of mental sluggishness is common.

Supporting individuals in continuing with medication over periods of years requires an honest approach. It is no good ducking the issues of how long the patient needs to continue. While it can sometimes be necessary to be vague in the beginning, while developing a rapport, the fact that you will want an open-ended approach to continuation will have to be faced at some time. It is important to avoid being too gloomy but not to be dishonest: *'You will have to stay on them for a long time. I don't know exactly but it's months not weeks.'* *'Things have stabilized now but I wouldn't want to even consider a reduction for at least another year or so.'* *'Yes, lots of people do stay on these drugs for life. Not all need to but it's very difficult to predict. We'll just have to take it one step at a time.'*

As pointed out in Chapter 11, it is best to take a 'normalizing' approach to problems with long-term medication. It is not easy to maintain medication and we should see our role as helping achieve it, rather than uncovering 'the reason' for non-compliance. It is important to explain, as thoroughly as possible, the role of the medicines. Comparisons with physical disorders can help destigmatize the whole process—but it is essential to choose the right comparison. We have often heard staff compare the process with the need for diabetics to take insulin daily. This is not a good comparison. If the diabetic patient misses a dose, they rapidly feel unwell and there can be dramatic consequences. In schizophrenia, if the patient misses a dose then they often feel *better* immediately (the side-effects disappear) and it will be some time, often months, before the relapse. Much better to compare to something like hypertension, where the side-effects have to be endured to prevent long-term problems (Chapter 11). As with all health promotion, this approach is generally more successful with older rather than younger patients.

With such an emphasis on collaboration and an empathy with the normal problems of persisting with medicines, monitoring need not seem like snooping. Much depends on the key worker's own mind set. If you really believe that you are checking how many tablets are left in order to support your patient in taking them, then it will not come across like spying. If you are doing it only to check up, then it will.

Collaboration has been shown to be the key to all forms of treatment compliance, not just medication. Patients who have genuinely been involved in the decision are much more likely to take responsibility for ensuring the treatment happens. Even if the range of options is only which of two very similar drugs to take, presenting it as a choice is better than no choice at all. This issue of choice has become much more real with the advent of the atypical antipsychotics such as respiridone, seroquel, and olanzapine. Whilst the therapeutic effects may be very similar to each other and to the older antipsychotics, there is a genuine difference in side-effect profile.

The most obvious choice in relation to medication is usually that between oral and depot preparations. Depots have not been abandoned since the arrival of the atypicals, with their more acceptable side-effects. For many patients it is simply not possible to maintain regular oral medication and depots are the only way of ensuring cover. A few patients prefer depots because it means they do not have to think about tablets and illness. However, many find them quite demeaning and, even when well established on them, there can often be a real purpose in working towards oral self-medication as a goal, with its greater sense of empowerment and dignity. For patients with severe schizophrenia, anything that improves self-esteem is worth striving for.

Clozapine

Clozapine is the only antipsychotic with a clear advantage over the others in terms of clinical recovery and is particularly indicated in resistant schizophrenia (Kane *et al.* 1988). Both patients and their families report improvements beyond simple symptom control, including a calming effect and improved clarity of thinking (Angermeyer *et al.* 2001).

Well-functioning outreach teams can establish and maintain patients on clozapine in the community. Our team relies heavily on supervised medication, often with daily visits in the beginning. We initiate clozapine for patients, without admission, when there are no serious complications (O'Brien and Firn 2002). Even with very successful results (and we have had several remarkable improvements), patients need ongoing support and encouragement to take the medicine.

Relapse signatures and early intervention

Clinical experience suggests that early intervention may both abort incipient relapses and certainly shorten the duration of the relapse and reduce the severity. As a result, much attention has been paid to identifying the early phase of relapse. For most patients there is a period of mounting anxiety and preoccupation as normal coping mechanisms become overpowered. This may reflect the phase of 'affect dysregulation' that Hogarty wrote about (Hogarty *et al.* 1995). For some patients this can be very specific—old delusional ideas that come to the surface, bizarre hypochondriacal ideas. Helping patients and families recognize these warning signs may be of help although, as yet, there is no convincing evidence that this is the case with schizophrenia, unlike bipolar disorder (Perry *et al.* 1999). However, it is a promising approach that is receiving a lot of attention.

With the emergence of these warning signs the patient can increase the maintenance medication or take other previously agreed steps such as reducing contact with family members or day centres or stepping up prearranged CBT practices. Such planning has the added benefit of reducing the overwhelming sense of helplessness which can be so damaging in this illness.

Psychosocial interventions

Stabilizing the living situation of individuals with schizophrenia by a range of psychosocial interventions is a core function of assertive outreach. If the main feature of the disorder is a vulnerability to psychotic breakdown when overwhelmed by stress and anxiety, then interventions to reduce routine anxieties will help protect the patient (Zubin and Spring 1977). Most of these interventions are directed at reducing interpersonal stressors, helping avoid conflict and friction with family members, neighbours, and acquaintances. While they are of value with the whole range of severe mental illnesses, they are particularly important in schizophrenia where a heightened interpersonal sensitivity is central to the disorder.

Few of the proven psychosocial interventions work in a crisis. They need to be offered and pursued generally when the patient is in remission. For this reason it is essential that there are team mechanisms to ensure that they are routinely offered. It is rare, even these days, for the family of a individual with schizophrenia to ask directly for family work. They may ask for explanations and support but rarely for help in finding new problem-solving techniques to reduce high expressed emotion. We have found it essential to review the provision of complex psychosocial interventions such as family work, CBT, or relapse prevention routinely at our regular multidisciplinary care reviews. Until we did so, our provision of such difficult procedures was very low indeed.

Schizophrenia family work and CBT for patients with psychosis are the subject of Chapter 25.

Example 15.1 (See case study p. 160)

ENHANCED CPA/SECTION 117(2) REVIEW (delete as applicable)	
Patient's name: Jonathon P. Address: 15 Sudbury Walk, Battersea Estate, Battersea. Phone: none Date of birth: 12/10/65 GP: Givens Phone:	CMHT: ACT TEAM Phone: 020 8877 xxxx New patient: NO If NO, date of review: .... 17/4/01 .... Diagnosis: 1 Schizophrenia .... F20.0 2.. F — —ˑ—

Assessed needs or problem	Intervention	Resp . of
Psychotic experiences, mainly paranoid	◆ Maintain on Risperidone 4 mg nocte. ◆ Monitor compliance openly and collaboratively. ◆ Monitor mental state at each visit. Observe for relapse signature signs of suspicion, unusual beliefs, and hostility. Repeat BPRS at 3-monthly intervals. ◆ Relapse plan negotiated that if Jonathon believes his brother or other member of his family has been substituted again, then Jonathon will accept increased dose of Risperidone up to 6 mg nocte. ◆ Ongoing weekly CBT sessions aimed at modifying beliefs of Capgras' syndrome.	AC
Risk of aggression when acutely paranoid	◆ Low threshold for joint visits. See risk assessment and contingency plan.	AC

Involved in care:	Dr Psychologist CPN OT SW Ward nurse CCM ✓ Support worker Other	
Present at meeting	Dr ✓ Psychologist CPN OT ✓ SW ✓ Ward nurse CCM ✓ Support worker ✓ Other	
Discussed with the patient?	YES Copy to patient? YES Copy to GP? YES	
Care co-ordinator (print):	Alison Charles Phone: 020 887 xxxx	
Care co-ordinator (signature):	.... Date of next review: 17/10/0/1	
Job title:	Clinical nurse specialist Patient's signature:	

Supervision register?	NO	Care management?	NO	Risk history completed?	YES
Supervised discharge?	NO	Section 117(2)?	YES	Relapse + risk plan required?	YES

Example 15.2

CONFIDENTIAL: RELAPSE AND RISK MANAGEMENT PLAN			
Name: Jonathon P.			

Categories of risk identified:

Aggression and violence	YES	Severe self-neglect	NO
Exploitation (self or others)	NO	Risk to children & young adults	NO
Suicide and self-harm	NO	Other (please specify}	

Current factors which suggest there is significant apparent risk:
(For example: alcohol or substance misuse; specific threats; suicidal ideation; violent fantasies; anger; suspiciousness; persecutory beliefs; paranoid feelings or ideas about particular people)

No significant risk presently. Currently relatively well and accepting treatment of CBT plus medication. Paranoid beliefs mild and patient does not act on them.

Clear statement of anticipated risk(s):
(Who is at risk; how immediate is that risk; how severe; how ongoing)

No current risk.

Action plan:
(Including names of people responsible for each action and steps to be taken if plan breaks down)

Risk history of hostile and aggressive behaviour when acutely paranoid. Believes members of his family and health care team have been substituted by imposters. Has admitted to violent fantasies in past usually directed at consultant psychiatrists. Has made one threat to kill consultant psychiatrist and has thrown chair at father (see risk history). If acutely paranoid and becoming suspicious of health care staff and family do not visit alone. Joint visits. Relapse plan to increase medication to 8 mg immediately following return of beliefs that people have been substituted with imposters. Supervision of medication may be required. Responds well to medication within period of 2–3 weeks. If becomes increasingly hostile and resistant to intervention institute Mental Health Act assessment with view to compulsory admission.

Date completed: 17/04/01   Review date: 17/10/01

This risk assessment may contain confidential and/or sensitive information provided by third parties. Such information should not be disclosed to the patient without prior consultation with the informant

Example 15.3

RISK ASSESSMENT DOCUMENTATION
Client's name: Jonathon P.

RISK HISTORY

Give details of any risk behaviour shown by the patient (actual or threatened). Each entry must be signed and dated
(E.g. previous violence; weapons used; impulsivity; self-harm; non-compliance; disengagement from services; convictions; potentially seriously harmful acts)

Jan 1996: Threw chair at father after argument over Jonathon's belief that father was a clone who had substituted his real father.

May 1997: Deliberate self-harm, overdose of painkillers after break up of relationship. Did not intend to kill himself.

June 1999: Smashed up property in his house. Relapsing with increased paranoid ideation.

June 1999: Threatened to kill consultant psychiatrist if he was sectioned. Aggressive and hostile to staff.

Case study

Jonathon was referred to the team following repeated hospital admissions with a diagnosis of schizophrenia. The referring CMHT had experienced great difficulty treating him. He was a highly intelligent man from an upper-class background whose relatives sometimes colluded with his paranoid beliefs about psychiatry and society. Jonathon did not believe he was ill and his family did not believe he was receiving the type of treatment that he deserved—namely CBT or psychotherapy.

He was extremely adept at intellectualizing and rationalizing his behaviour (sometimes angry and threatening) and beliefs, an incident of deliberate self-harm, and the Capgras syndrome from which he suffered (a fixed notion that each person he came across had been switched for an impostor).

On assessment by the team, we agreed that CBT may be offered to him as he was intelligent, cognitively intact, and able to discuss his experiences openly and understand psychological concepts. We were prepared to review his medication but maintained that his best chance, given his history, was not to stop antipsychotics as he wished. Intellectually, Jonathan was intimidating. When floridly psychotic, he was also quite threatening. He was allocated to one of the clinical case managers with most experience and training to deliver a formal programme of CBT.

Following a further admission due to non-compliance, we discharged him early, but still on section, and negotiated daily supervised medication with an oral, novel antipsychotic. He responded moderately well to prolonged treatment and his suspicions reduced to the point that he related well to his key worker and other members of the team. He enjoyed the CBT sessions as he was able to flex his intellectual muscles in debate about the nature and veracity of his beliefs.

Some of his beliefs became 'memories' of events that he insisted had really happened but were no longer occurring. In turn, his beliefs about the value of medication began to change and the team reduced the level of supervision. A relapse plan was negotiated which specified thresholds for intervention including increased medication and joint visits (Example 15.1).

He is currently on surprisingly good terms with us and holds down a part-time job. We have not been successful, however, in increasing contact with his family to help them better understand his illness and need for treatment.

Conclusions

We have dealt with schizophrenia at length, ignoring the general format of this book, because it is such a complex and demanding disorder—one that lies at the heart of mental health practice. Because the experiences and symptoms of the patient are so fascinating, they can become the focus of discussion to the detriment of seeing the whole person. Using structured assessments of mental state such as the present state examination (Wing *et al.* 1974) demonstrated that so-called 'non-specific neurotic symptoms' (anxiety, panic, depression) are just as prominent as delusions and hallucinations when schizophrenia patients break down. We simply overlook them.

In intensive community work we find the stress–vulnerability hypothesis (Zubin and Spring 1977) and Hogarty's concept of affect dysregulation (Hogarty *et al.* 1995) a good basis for our work. Rather than focus too much on individual hallucinations and delusions, we try to spot the stresses as they start to build up and intervene to reduce them if possible. In this way, we hope to help our patient stay in control of his or her life and not be overwhelmed by it.

Chapter 16

Bipolar affective disorder

Introduction

Bipolar affective disorder is the term currently used for what was originally called 'manic–depressive psychosis'. Manic–depressive psychosis was one of the major mental illnesses that Kraepelin distinguished in his original studies (Kraepelin 1919) and it affects just under 0.7% of the adult population (Weissman *et al.* 1996). He distinguished it from schizophrenia (then called 'dementia praecox') not so much on the grounds of the symptoms as on the course of the illness. Dementia praecox was characterized by a gradual decline in functioning punctuated by episodes of severe disturbance, but manic–depressive patients often showed full recovery between episodes, although the disturbed periods could be equally severe. French psychiatrists called it 'folie circulaire' (Falret 1854).

The linking of what appears to be such opposite mood states—the elation of mania and the despair of depression—arose from the clinical observation that they were linked in the same patient over time. Virtually all patients who had episodes of mania also had periods of severe depression, sometimes in close proximity. Sometimes even during the episodes of elation patients displayed periods of extreme sadness. These fluctuations in mood were (and still are) quite remarkable with a rapid descent from joy and over-confidence into bitter self-reproach and sometimes suicidal acts.

The term 'mania' and, with it, 'maniac', have pejorative overtones. Hence the pressure to rename the disorder as bipolar affective disorder (BAD). Not all patients with severe mood (affective) disorders experience mania or hypomania. The two terms, mania and hypomania, are used interchangeably now, although hypomania implies a much milder form of the disturbance which need only last a few days and during which the patient retains both psychological and social control. While virtually all patients who experience mania also experience severe depressive episodes, there are many patients who only experience depressive episodes.

A series of family studies of depressed patients in Northern Sweden (Perris 1969) showed that families 'bred true' as either 'unipolar' depressives (they only had depressed but not elated episodes) or as 'bipolar' depressives (they had both depressed and elated episodes). There were no families that had only elated episodes. Any patient who suffers an episode of mania is, therefore, diagnosed as suffering from a bipolar disorder, even if they have yet to experience a depression. Unipolar affective disorder is dealt with along with the wider concept of depression in Chapter 18.

Causes of bipolar affective disorder

There is undoubtedly a constitutional element in bipolar disorder. It runs in families, with the children of affected individuals having about a 10% risk of developing the disorder. This more than doubles if both parents are affected. As with schizophrenia, the risk increases to over 50% in identical twins. The importance of genetics in the development of BAD is now undisputed, although it has been controversial in the past.

Elated and disorganized states have been associated with stimulant drugs (e.g. amphetamines and cocaine) and depression has also been caused by drugs (e.g. reserpine, methyl-dopa) which deplete the brain of neurotransmitters such as dopamine and serotonin. This, combined with the observation that antidepressant treatment can precipitate manic episodes, has given rise to various transmitter theories, often rather simplistically associating mania with raised and depression with lowered levels of the same transmitter. It is rare for such theories to remain unchanged for long and there are regular amendments—which transmitter is involved, adjustments for receptor sensitivities, etc. It is likely, however, that such dramatic changes in levels of energy, affect, and cognition are associated with changes in brain chemistry.

As with all mental illnesses that run in families, the issue of nature versus nurture has been vigorously debated (see Chapter 15, where this is explored in schizophrenia). Psychoanalysts have tried to understand mania as a defence against depression. Melanie Klein (Segal 1983) describes this most extensively. Analysts' patients reported that they often dealt with potentially overwhelming depressive feelings by denying them and behaving as if they were happy. Most of us will have seen this in recently bereaved individuals who seem able to hold their emotion at bay and remain active for a time. This is called a 'manic defence' against depression. This explanation was strengthened by the flashes of misery that are so common in the manic state, by the fact that most mania is preceded and followed by depression, and by the remarkable fact that mania responds dramatically to ECT (the most powerful treatment for depression). The analysts' treatment was to identify and interpret the depression that was being defended against. Few would now advance this as a causal explanation or as a treatment approach, although many of us find it a helpful way of understanding the situation when working with a manic patient.

Clinical picture

The clinical presentation of hypomania is well described in standard textbooks. The patient is usually overactive, with boundless energy and reduced sleep. Thoughts are racing, often with rich and surprising associations (many creative artists (e.g. Handel, Schubert, Spike Milligan) have their inspiration during manic episodes and work on them further when more stable).

While the classical picture is of an elated, over-joyful individual, the more common experience is of someone who is irritable and impatient and who can become frankly hostile or paranoid if their wishes are frustrated. Delusions and hallucinations are not uncommon in mania although, unlike in schizophrenia, they tend to be overshadowed by the mood and to be mood-congruent. Severe mood swings may be associated with life stresses (Paykel 1978). The impact is not immediate, with vulnerability for relapse extending to 2–3 months (Kendler *et al*. 1995). This may become diminished and less obvious over time. For many patients there are specific times of the year when breakdowns are more likely.

If mania was simply restricted to periods of over-activity and poor sleep (often with increased output) there would be little reason for mental health services to get involved. Unfortunately, the most difficult aspect of mania to define—the deterioration in personal judgement—is probably the most damaging. Although the patient may continue to do routine tasks (e.g. make business deals, see friends, form relationships, buy household goods), they often fail to demonstrate the judgement needed in these activities. The result is great damage to themselves and their families, which they bitterly regret when they recover. Foolish financial deals can lead to ruin, reckless sexual behaviour can devastate families and health, and disinhibition (particularly if the patient is also drinking excessively, which is not unusual in a manic episode) can lead to exploitation, abuse, and even prosecution.

Case study

Janine worked for a national newspaper as a researcher in the fashion section. She was keen to become a journalist, and was usually described as 'bubbly' and enthusiastic. She was in her early 20s and still single, always very well presented and sought after by lots of men.

Over a period of some weeks her employers became worried that she was not so reliable about turning up on time and there had been a couple of evenings when she had been 'outrageously' drunk. It was assumed that there were some boyfriend problems and this was, after all, a professional establishment that prided itself on being rather bohemian.

She was seen by her GP who thought she was going high. (Her mother phoned from Wales because she had experienced similar episodes with her late husband.) Unfortunately, Janine laughed off the concern, did not attend her psychiatric appointment, and failed to show for work. The police picked her up in Manchester two weeks later, sleeping rough in a bus station at night. She was cheerful but dishevelled and it became clear that she had run up over £2000 in debts in those two weeks and had been exploited sexually by at least three men.

On admission to hospital in London she rapidly settled with treatment but became profoundly depressed and humiliated, thinking back on what had happened. She refused to return to work (although they were happy to have her) because of embarrassment about how she had behaved in the weeks leading up to her departure.

Treatment in the community

Perhaps one of the most important principles of treating bipolar patients in the community is to remember that admission may be in everyone's interest if the situation is deteriorating fast. There are few psychiatric disorders in which insight is lost so quickly and the 'window' of opportunity for collaborative work can be very narrow.

Bipolar patients, unlike the majority of patients with severe psychotic illnesses, often have jobs and dependants and reputations, all of which can be quickly lost by a few weeks' ostensibly irresponsible behaviour. This is particularly so as the early symptoms of a relapse are not perceived as 'illness' by the general population. The failing judgement may be very obvious to the key worker and family but may be put down to enthusiasm, confidence, or even foolishness or heavy drinking by the outsider.

We will return to the issue of how to set thresholds in outreach work with such patients.

Forming a therapeutic alliance

One of the paradoxes of working with these patients is that there often seems to be little justification for input between relapses since, unlike individuals with schizophrenia, for example, there is usually no established disability or persisting problems that need attention. Although the individual's personality is well preserved, we end up with little opportunity to really get to know them. We have found one of the most powerful advantages of assertive outreach work with bipolar patients is that it gives us a real opportunity to get to know them well and to form an effective therapeutic alliance.

A key component in this process is to have an acknowledged target for frequency of contact. In our team we aim to see all our patients, on average, two times a week. Even if they are well, we expect to see them at least once a week. Making this explicit means that the case manager does not have to keep justifying regular contact with someone who is well, nor does he or she end up feeling guilty about possibly neglecting other patients.

Endorsement of the social care component of the team approach ensures that these contacts can still be meaningful. There is the opportunity to use them for supporting leisure activities and engaging in joint activities (cleaning out the flat, sorting out muddled finances) that the patient would find daunting, even if they were capable of doing them. Repeated hospital admissions can disrupt a patient's ability to plan ahead and to organize their lives, housing, finances, and careers. Given that social and relationship stressors can precipitate relapses, bipolar patients will be more vulnerable in the absence of a stable life. The role of the key worker is often to mediate or advise in stressful negotiations and to help the patient to stabilize housing, finances, work, etc. It is often through these shared activities that greater understanding and trust develop.

Relapse signatures and early intervention

Relapse in bipolar disorder is fast—sometimes only days between normal functioning and a loss of insight and extreme elation. Increased contact with patients and increased familiarity with them means that case managers can often spot and recognize the earliest symptoms of deterioration.

Case study

One of our patients always starts to wear hats when she is becoming unwell—this happens long before there are any other signs of her hypomania. Asked why she is wearing a hat, she will give an utterly sensible explanation, and certainly there is nothing in itself odd about the hats she wears. Long experience, however, has taught us and her family that within days of wearing a hat she will start to sleep poorly and become aroused and erratic.

More often the indicator of an incipient relapse is a preoccupation that becomes prominent before the illness is manifest and continues throughout the relapse. Not all patients, of course, have such specific and reliable 'relapse signatures' but where they do, and where they can be agreed, there is a real chance of being able to intervene very early and prevent relapses altogether.

Poor sleep is probably the commonest indicator of relapse in bipolar disorder, followed by over-talkativeness and increased energy. Even then, it is not too late to intervene with an agreed 'relapse plan'. There is convincing evidence that spending time exploring the early indicators of relapse with patients when they are well can yield both an understanding of the predictors and a plan of intervention that either aborts relapses or substantially modifies them (Perry *et al.* 1999). With many of our patients we talk them through the process of previous breakdowns and identify with them the early signs. When we have agreement on these we write them down (see Examples 16.2 and 16.3) and discuss with the patient what should be done when they happen. For most patients the agreement is about taking added antipsychotic medication for a set period: e.g. 'After two nights of disturbed sleep add 2 mg of risperidone nightly for the next five nights.' It is helpful that the intervention is linked simply to the experience and not to its potential meaning (i.e. 'after two nights...' not 'after disturbed sleep and the start of a relapse...').

All the discussion about the significance of the early signs needs to take place when it is being agreed on. The start of a mood swing is not the time to be discussing the meaning of behaviour if it can be avoided. Similarly, it is essential to agree how long the intervention should last. We err on the side of caution. Taking the risperidone for two nights may be enough sometimes, but it is better to play safe. Inevitably, there may be times when the medicine is taken unnecessarily—there may be alternative reasons for poor sleep (worry over a family matter, even indigestion)—but the consequences of missing the 'window of opportunity' are considerably greater than the discomfort of a few days' medicine.

The balance of risks and benefits of the intervention must be negotiated carefully with the patient. It has to make sense and seem proportionate otherwise it will not be complied with. Although medication is the commonest early intervention agreed (and is invariably one component of our contingency plans), it is not the only one. For some patients, an agreement to stay with a family member for a set period may be part of it, as may giving up their car keys or reducing risks in other ways such as by handing over credit cards to a member of the family for safe-keeping.

On the whole, medication and increased monitoring and contact are the staples of such early interventions. Where there is an involved carer, then assessments and monitoring should include them if the patient allows it. That way, family members learn how we assess the level of over-activity, and they gain confidence in their own ability to judge improvement and deterioration.

Managing hypomania

Early intervention does not always succeed in preventing a hypomanic episode. It may still be possible to manage the patient without admission to hospital and our patients tell us that, on the whole, this is very much what they prefer. Even families prefer it—as long as one remembers that admission should be arranged if things seem to be getting out of hand.

There is no substitute, however, for frequent contact. If a patient lives alone, then daily contact is probably essential to manage a hypomanic episode initially. These contacts do not have to be long. Indeed, it is often best that they are not too long as patients can become irritable if they feel 'trapped' in the interview. Sharing these visits across the team can be particularly helpful, as long as the patient knows those who visit them. Novelty is attractive to patients when high and can be used to gain co-operation when repeat visits may be viewed as 'dull' or 'boring'.

Our ability to manage bipolar disorder has been one of the real benefits of going from a five-day to a seven-day service. Missing medicines for even one day can rapidly escalate to a situation where collaboration is lost.

Negotiating and agreeing the direct care provided for the patient is the core of early intervention and management but need not be restricted to it. In our team we have found it valuable to agree with the patient (during their well period) who else we can inform and work with should they start to relapse. Knowing their routines and what they did in previous episodes can highlight other points of containment. For instance, if you know that your patient always goes to social services and creates a fuss when unwell, or spends his or her time exploring his spiritual experiences with the local priest, it can be invaluable to get their agreement that you can approach these people and give them advice on what to do. Sometimes you may simply want these people to inform you that the patient is there, to save you time searching for them.

On occasions, we obtain the patient's written permission for these extensive interventions. This serves two functions. First, it makes us feel safer about doing it and, second, it is a way of helping the patient focus on the reality of their disorder. This is something that many bipolar patients are adept at avoiding, either by not thinking about the disturbed periods at all or by playing down their severity.

Getting a good night's sleep is essential to managing hypomania. It is both an indicator of recovery and also a prerequisite for avoiding admission. Even when taking antipsychotics, patients often need hypnotics to get off to sleep. Where patients have involved family members, worry about what the patient is doing in the middle of the night while they are asleep can be a major burden. Everything always seems worse in the night! The difficulty of summoning help if things do take a dramatic turn is also, in reality, much greater then. The family's emotional resources are likely to be fairly depleted looking after the patient and without sleep it becomes quite impossible. In general, we feel that if disturbed behaviour continues through the night for more than one or two nights, and we cannot get a handle on it, then a brief admission may be the best solution.

As mentioned in Chapter 7, we have experienced no problems (such as dependency) when using benzodiazepines with psychotic patients. Similarly, concerns about 'disinhibition' seem misplaced. After all, the patient is usually quite disinhibited when such sedation is being considered. We use them liberally with bipolar patients both in the community and in the ward.

Mood stabilizers

The use of mood stabilizers in bipolar disorder (Chapter 7) is an essential part of the job of an assertive outreach team. The evidence is clear that such drugs reduce the likelihood of a relapse, although the impact for an individual patient may be very difficult to demonstrate with any certainty. There is only limited evidence for the superiority of any one mood stabilizer above the others and the choice is usually dictated by patient preference driven by sensitivity to side-effects (Sachs *et al*. 2000). Simultaneous use of more than one mood stabilizer may be more effective (Denicoff *et al*. 1997).

The case manager's task is twofold. He must work with his patient to ensure compliance with the medicines over long periods. This involves early preparatory work explaining the purpose, functioning, and side-effects of the drugs involved. For some patients it will include motivational interviewing (Chapter 11), adapted for compliance enhancement. All patients will need support, prompting, and encouragement. As many patients have complete remission between episodes the value of maintenance prophylactic medication needs to be more convincing. The current range of mood stabilizers also require careful monitoring. Lithium and carbamazepine necessitate regular blood tests to measure therapeutic levels and, for lithium, to monitor thyroid and renal damage. Local agreements and practice will vary about how blood tests are organized. Good general practices are able to monitor lithium in compliant patients, but even the best have difficulty recognizing and following up non-compliance. For patients needing regular outreach it is usual for the case manager to organize these routine blood tests whether through the GP, the team, or by taking the patient to out-patients. It is often better for the patient to take responsibility for this aspect of their treatment if they are capable of it. The case manager is responsible, however, for making sure it happens.

The range of drugs licensed for treatment and maintenance in bipolar disorders is rapidly increasing. Atypical antipsychotics such as olanzapine and clozapine are now recognized as valuable additions. Newer drugs such as lamotrigine and depakote (Bowden *et al*. 1994) are promising.

In some of our more unstable, disorganized, and non-compliant bipolar patients we have used low-dose depot antipsychotics with very good effect. With both antipsychotics and mood stabilizers the patient should be regularly assessed for side-effects. Bipolar patients seem more sensitive to drug side-effects than schizophrenia patients. Training all team members in routine side-effect screening is not that difficult (Chaplin *et al.* 1999) and improves overall drug management (Chapter 7). Ensure that it happens regularly.

Depression

Managing manic episodes in the community is a stressful activity. Not only must one anticipate and respond quickly to the patient, but there is the ever-present worry of them crashing down into depression. The mixture of depressive thinking and mood with manic energy and impulsiveness can be a lethal combination. Sometimes the risk is just too great and admission is essential. Fleeting (but intense) depressive phenomena are frequent and characteristic of hypomania. Similarly, depression after the hypomanic episode is to be expected as the patient falls back to sober reality, often to the memory of foolish and embarrassing exploits. Elated mood and over-activity are also, quite simply, exhausting for both patient and family and there is often a flat, joyless period to follow. Any decision to use antidepressants should be thought through carefully in such circumstances, both because of the natural course of the illness, and also because there is evidence that in some individuals antidepressants can increase the risk of an elevation of mood (Altshuler *et al.* 1995).

Psychological and psychosocial interventions

Bipolar patients often want more explanations of their illness and the treatment than many other patients. This is an illness where understanding and self-management can be central to a significant improvement in the quality of the person's life. Most of us have had the frustrating and demoralizing experience of witnessing an otherwise able young individual stubbornly refuse to make some fairly minor adaptations to their lifestyle for which they pay an enormous price in repeated, devastating relapses. Sometimes it seems that they must learn their own way. On the other hand, remarkable changes can occur when 'the penny drops', after a vivid episode which has included some successful engagement.

Case study

Jamie was the younger son in a family with extensive bipolar illness. His father still managed to work, despite several breakdowns in his early life. He needed to take time off now and then, but remained on his lithium and out of hospital. His elder brother was living a 'hippy' life in a commune, was frequently depressed, refused medication, and had only rare admissions for mania. Jamie's illness was much more severe and, by the age of 25, he had been compulsorily admitted six times and had twice nearly died (once from a drug overdose and once after falling from scaffolding when high). He was a talented musician, played in an amateur rock band, and would neither take the drugs we prescribed nor refrain from those offered by his friends.

Case study (*Continued*)

During one of his admissions he became friendly with another, equally talented, bipolar patient with whom he shared the same key worker. For some reason, all three 'clicked', and by the end of that admission Jamie had acknowledged that he did suffer from a bipolar illness and agreed to continue on lithium and restrict (though not stop) his illicit drug use. He was surprisingly able to balance his anarchic artistic life with his treatment and has now stayed well for several years.

In all previous discussions Jamie had equated treatment with the abandonment of his talent and personality. He had seen it as an 'either/or'. Our protestations that the changes needed to protect him were fairly minor were to no avail—until that last admission. Education and information may simply need to be repeated over and over again.

The importance of relapse signal training and of compliance enhancement skills in the care of these patients has been mentioned above. Psychological treatments to enhance coping skills are also of great benefit. Relapses are often clearly stress related, so any treatment or training aimed at improving coping skills will help reduce vulnerability. Which coping skills are to be the target of such training are highly specific to the individual. For many patients, learning how to manage anger and frustration whilst still being assertive can be particularly beneficial. Social skills' training, though no longer that fashionable, can make a major improvement in an individual's life. How to conduct a conversation and establish and maintain non-intimate, low-key friendships can make all the difference between a rewarding day and brooding loneliness. Outreach teams have the advantage that social skills' training can occur *in vivo*—where, and with whom, the patient wants to use them.

CBT to explore and reduce depressive thinking and vulnerability can be particularly valuable with bipolar individuals. Whatever the exact relationship between elation and depression in this disorder there is no doubt that managing mood and how you feel is central to it. CBT has an established efficacy in reducing depressive thinking (Beck *et al.* 1985). Many bipolar patients have told us that they find the depressions worse than the elations (although their families often do not agree). Help in reducing the self-criticism and pessimism central to their depressive psychopathology is greatly appreciated. It helps protect from full-blown depressions (and perhaps from manic responses) and also cements the working alliance.

Stress reduction lies at the heart of many of the psychosocial interventions common to assertive outreach work used to help bipolar patients. Such interventions include work to protect the social framework around the patient, to enhance community tenure by ensuring that housing is secure, and to prevent the building up of enormous debts. Working with the informal network of social supports in the neighbourhood is especially important because most bipolar patients need company and do not thrive in isolation. The response of individuals within this network can be the difference between a successful early intervention and a compulsory hospitalization.

Example 16.1

ENHANCED CPA/SECTION 117(2)REVIEW (delete as applicable)	
Patient's name: Jamie S. Address: 52 Willerton House, Roehampton Phone: none Date of birth: 12/3/71 GP: Asquith Phone:	CMHT: ACT TEAM Phone: 0208 877 xxxx New patient: NO If No, date of review: 25/5/01 Diagnosis: 1. Bipolar affective disorder .... F31.0 2. .... F — —·—

Assessed needs or problem	Intervention	Resp. of
Frequent relapse; manic relapse can appear over period of few days	◆ Frequent home visits, two visits per week to assess mental state and intervene early. ◆ Relapse signature and plan agreed—if no sleep for two nights and starts to believe he has special powers to take additional Risperidone 2 mg twice daily. Depressive episodes largely managed in the community unless risk (see below). ◆ Provide regular pschoeducation and advice about harmful use of drugs and effect on mental state and risk of relapse. ◆ Liaise with family and friends regularly during high-risk periods. Ensure they know how to access help easily from team and services day or night. Involve family in relapse plan.	BP
Poor compliance with medication	◆ Actively engage Jamie in care. Jamie interested in music. ◆ Reinforce messages of need for maintenance medication. ◆ Medication currently Lithium 1200 mg nocte. ◆ Routinely assess for side-effects, information on side-effects of Lithium. ◆ Ensure Lithium levels monitored by GP 3 monthly.	BP

Involved in care: Dr ✓ Psychologist CPN OT ✓ SW Ward nurse CCM ✓ Support worker Other

Present at meeting: Dr ✓ Psychologist CPN OT ✓ SW Ward nurse CCM ✓ Support worker ✓ Other

Discussed with the patient?	YES	Copy to patient?	YES	Copy to GP?	YES

Care co-ordinator (print): Bill Primo   Phone. 0208 877 xxxx

Care co-ordinator (signature): .... Date of next review: 25/11/01.......

Job title: Clinical case manager   Patient's signature: ....

Supervision register?	NO	Care management?	NO	Risk history completed?	YES
Supervised discharge?	NO	Section 117(2)?	YES	Relapse + risk plan required?	YES

Example 16.2

CONFIDENTIAL: RELAPSE AND RISK MANAGEMENT PLAN

Name: Jamie S.

Categories of risk identified:

Aggression and violence	NO	Severe self-neglect	NO
Exploitation (self or others)	YES	Risk to children & young adults	NO
Suicide and self-harm	YES	Other (please specify}	

Current factors which suggest there is significant apparent risk:
(For example: alcohol or substance misuse; specific threats; suicidal ideation; violent fantasies; anger; suspiciousness; persecutory beliefs; paranoid feelings or ideas about particular people)

Currently moderately depressed. No current suicidal ideation.

Clear statement of anticipated risk(s):
Who is at risk; how immediate is that risk; how severe; how ongoing)

Attempted suicide by overdose when severely depressed.
Risk of accidental self-harm when high due to reckless behaviour.

(Action plan:
(Including names of people responsible for each action and steps to be taken if plan breaks down)

Relapse signature and plan agreed with Jamie that if does not sleep for two nights and starts to believe he has special powers will take additional Risperidone 2 mg twice daily. Provide increased visits and early intervention.

For mild episodes of elation increase contact, consider direct supervision of medication, and liaise with family if they can provide additional support and supervision at Jamie's house.

Depressive episodes largely managed at home unless risk. Assess mental state regularly using both BPRS and Beck depression inventory. If significant suicidal risk such as evidence of planning, hoarding of medication, etc., offer informal admission or assess for formal admission after discussion with team. For mild episodes of depression increase contact and liaise with family if they can provide additional support and supervision at Jamie's house.

Date completed: 25/05/01   **Review date: 25/11/01**

This risk assessment may contain confidential and/or sensitive information provided by third parties. Such information should not be disclosed to the patient without prior consultation with the informant

Example 16.3

RISK ASSESSMENT DOCUMENTATION
Client's name: Jamie S.
RISK HISTORY Give details of any risk behaviour shown by the patient (actual or threatened). Each entry must be signed and dated (E.g. previous violence; weapons used; impulsivity; self-harm; non-compliance; disengagement from services; convictions; potentially seriously harmful acts) 1990: Attempted suicide by overdose when severely depressed. Took 20 tablets of temazepam with bottle of spirits. 1991: Got into a fight when elated and abusive to people in pub. Suffered broken nose. 1993: Accidental self-harm by falling off scaffolding two storeys up when elated and abusing stimulant drugs.

Working with the positives when the patient is well is the secret of assertive outreach with bipolar patients. It gives us insights into their personality and strengths on which we can build a therapeutic relationship. It also can improve the quality of their life directly and thereby increase their commitment to staying well. Only if there is something to get well for, and to stay well for, can we expect our patients to put up with the treatments we offer them. Time and effort devoted to strengthening this is time well spent.

Conclusions

Work with individuals with bipolar affective disorder can be one of the most rewarding and successful aspects of assertive outreach. Initially, it may not seem like that and we were rather despairing of our ability to help this group at the beginning of our service. We have found that the benefits take a couple of years to manifest and have to be built on team experience of relapse. In the period after a relapse, the relationship can be developed using a range of approaches—social, psychological, and also pharmacological. From dominating the 'problem' slots in the team review we now find, some years on, that this group of patients is often surprisingly silent.

Often these patients will have much more to work with—families, interests, even jobs—so that the benefits of even moderate stabilization in mental state are visible and rewarding. The temptation to reduce contact frequency once symptoms recede should be vigorously resisted. Persistence is all. We insist on a minimum weekly contact even when things are going swimmingly. Two years without a significant mood swing (not two years without an admission) is needed before we go below weekly contact and, only then, would we negotiate a transfer of care back to the CMHT.

Chapter 17

Personality problems and disorders

Introduction

Personality is that which makes each of us different and unique. When we speak of someone's personality we focus on those aspects of him or her which make them most memorable. We have an enormous range of terms to describe an individual's personality—strong, fiery, passionate, phlegmatic, intellectual, cold, ruthless, conscientious, etc. If we are to work successfully with long- term relationships, we need to pay due attention to personality. Our patients' personalities profoundly affect how they deal with their illnesses and undoubtedly have a major impact on their overall outcome.

Not only do our patients have personalities, but we do also. Our personality dictates that, despite a thorough professional training, there will be aspects of our work that we are better at than others, some patients with whom we work better than others. Even before we address the thorny issue of whether personality disorders are more than a set of labels, assertive outreach work demands that personality is taken seriously.

The number of theories about personality formation attest to the fact that we really do not know that much about why different people grow up to behave so differently. Earlier, doctrinaire battles of nature versus nurture have generally given way to a recognition that both contributions are important (although individuals still divide according to which they think contributes most!). Family resemblances in personality are equally balanced by the wide variation within families. Most parents are struck by how different their children may seem right from birth—one placid and easy going, another alert, inquisitive, and refusing to go to sleep.

It is probably safe to say that an adult's personality is the result of the interplay between their constitution and their experiences while growing up. This is not the same as saying their 'upbringing'—there is more to growing up than what parents do. Illness, peer-group norms and pressures, and physical development have all been shown to influence personality. Constructing a 'personal narrative' may help to make sense of an individual personality. Presented with an elderly person who was a concentration camp victim in their childhood, and who is now anxious and unable to trust or form relationships, it may be helpful to explore how this earlier horrific experience distorted their life. We have to remember, however, that the vast majority of victims of such atrocities appear to develop normally. We should guard against believing that any explanatory model is conclusive or predictive. We need our models, however, and each of us must have some way of 'understanding' personality if we are to go about our business of working with relationships. When the facts and the theory do not fit though, we must believe the facts.

Diagnosis of a personality disorder

Even if we accept personality as a meaningful construct, do we accept personality disorder? This has long been a highly controversial area in mental health work—never more so than now. In an era of evidence-based practice, the reliability of personality disorder diagnoses has been strongly questioned. The durability of the clinical descriptions of personality disorders is, however, quite striking. Schneider, who considered abnormal personalities to be 'constitutional variants that are highly influenced by personal experience', described ten specific types (Schneider 1923). Eight of these are still clearly distinguishable in DSM-III (American Psychiatric Association 1980).

There is a clear hierarchy of reliability in psychiatric diagnoses. There is good agreement on organic and functional psychoses, fair agreement on neurotic disorders, but only very modest agreement on individual personality disorders. There is, however, concensus on the presence or absence of a personality disorder overall (Merson *et al.* 1994). In many ways this is not surprising as the features of most personality disorders are essentially exaggerations (caricatures even) of the components of most of our personalities. The extreme forms of personality disorders, however, are usually recognized easily.

In the 1959 Mental Health Act (Department of Health 1959) personality disorder had a different status from other mental disorders. Detention was only permitted if there was evidence of danger or 'treatability'. This requirement for 'treatability' reflected the doubts that existed then that it was a 'real' mental disorder. Its inclusion in the Act was to ensure that research into the issue would continue and a resolution hopefully found. It was retained in the 1983 Mental Health Act, still with this difference in status.

Most UK psychiatrists are highly sceptical about the treatability of personality disorders—certainly without the patient's consent and commitment. As a result they are reluctant to use compulsion with this group and will often decline to offer treatment despite strong representations from GPs and families (and sometimes patients). The result is that the diagnosis of personality disorder (PD) may be seen as stigmatizing and neglected.

Current definitions

ICD-10

Current definitions of personality disorder emphasize description and avoid theories of development. The ICD-10 (World Health Organisation 1992) stresses the long-standing nature of the disorders and that they are usually discernible by adolescence but not diagnosed before adulthood. The broad ICD-10 diagnostic guidelines for a personality disorder are:

F60—specific personality disorders

+ Markedly disharmonious attitudes and behaviour involving usually several areas of functioning e.g. affectivity, arousal, impulse control, perception and thought, relating to others.

+ The abnormal behaviour pattern is enduring, long-standing, and not limited to episodes of illness; it is pervasive and clearly maladaptive to a broad range of personal and social situations.

+ The above manifestations always appear during childhood or adolescence and continue into adulthood.

+ The disorder leads to considerable personal distress but this may only become apparent late in its course.

+ The disorder is usually, but not invariably, associated with significant problems in occupational and social performance.

(World Health Organisation 1992)

There are eight major personality disorders recognized in ICD-10. Of these, only two are particularly relevant to work in assertive outreach—dissocial PD (F60.2) and borderline PD (F60.31)

F60 Specific Personality Disorders	
F60.0 Paranoid PD	**F60.1** Schizoid PD
F60.2 Dissocial PD	**F60.3** Emotionally unstable PD
	(**F60.31** Borderline type)
F60.4 Histrionic PD	**F60.5** Anankastic PD
F60.6 Anxious (avoidant) PD	**F60.7** Dependent PD
F60.8 Other Specific PD	**F60.9** PD unspecified

(ICD10, World Health Organisation 1992)

DSM classification

American DSM-III (American Psychiatric Association 1980) and DSM-IV (American Psychiatric Association 1994) personality disorders are broadly very similar to the WHO's ICD-10. There are some differences in terminology (ICD-10: dissocial, anankastic, anxious; DSM: antisocial, obsessive-compulsive, avoidant) and borderline is given its own category in DSM. Both DSM-III and DSM-IV have grouped the personality disorders into three clusters which reflect their broad characteristics:

Cluster A: 'odd' or 'eccentric'
- Paranoid
- Schizoid
- Schizotypal

Cluster B: 'dramatic' or 'erratic'
- Histrionic
- Narcissistic
- Antisocial
- Borderline

Cluster C: 'anxious'
- Avoidant
- Dependent
- Obsessive-compulsive
- Passive-aggressive

(American Psychiatric Association 1994)

Treatability of personality disorders

This is a difficult area. Opinions do vary about the treatability of personality disorder (most particularly dissocial and borderline types). There do exist imaginative but still essentially experimental treatments—democratic therapeutic communities (Jones 1952) for dissocial individuals (Lees *et al.* 1999) and some forms of dynamic psychotherapy (Kernberg 1984; Ryle 1997) and, more recently, adaptations of CBT in the form of dialectical behaviour therapy (Linehan *et al.* 1991) for borderline patients. The status of these treatments and the precise characteristics of who will respond to them are still uncertain. Clinicians may be reluctant to offer such treatments either because they remain unconvinced that they work or, even if convinced, they do not have the skills or resources. The result is that the diagnosis is often seen as an 'excuse' to refuse to take on difficult patients.

We share the scepticism about the treatability of personality disorders as such. That does not mean that we refuse to take on the care of these patients. There is a difference. Just as individuals with psychoses can also suffer from neurotic disorders and personality disorders, so personality disordered individuals have concurrent problems which both warrant treatments and respond to them. Not only that, but people with personality disorder also benefit from a thorough and honest assessment of their problems. An analysis of their behaviours, the likely triggers and risk areas, and difficult relationships can often form the basis for useful advice. Even being told that the issues are to do with personality, and not depression or some other mental illness, can be helpful. It allows the individual to do some sensible planning. Occupational or interpersonal stresses may be the result of failure to recognize the importance of personality (e.g. an impulsive and stimulus-seeking man who had been encouraged to get a clerical job to 'settle him down' began to control his temper much better when he got a job in a fairground). Sometimes, fairly simple advice from a skilled and objective professional can make an enormous difference.

Personality disorder and assertive outreach

We have dealt with personality disorder at such length for two reasons. Firstly, assertive outreach teams are likely to come under considerable pressure to take on patients with dissocial or borderline personality disorders because they are often very high profile, frequently admitted, and cause real concerns about safety. Their general reluctance to be consistently involved with care also qualifies them on the grounds of 'hard to engage'.

We have resisted the pressure to accept individuals purely on the grounds of personality disorder because there is as yet no significant body of knowledge to suggest that outreach has anything specific to offer. Indeed, one of the few North American studies of assertive outreach which failed to find any advantage to it was where the individuals had significant offending behaviour (Solomon and Draine 1995b). As assertive outreach is such an expensive treatment we feel that it should be restricted to those who we know will benefit from it. We also have real concerns about involving staff with people they are likely to disappoint (having no clear clinical advantage to offer them) and for whom they will be held responsible in what is a fiercely blame-oriented culture.

We have also focused on personality problems and disorders because the sorts of issues they present are also very common in individuals with severe mental illnesses. The onset of psychotic disorders in early adult life (and there is increasing evidence that the prodromal phase stretches well back into adolescence) dramatically interferes with normal development. Interpersonal skills, vocational skills, and self-confidence are all disrupted by the onset of the disorders. Not surprisingly, many of our patients display several features associated with personality disorders.

Dissocial personality disorder

Many young men with psychotic illnesses display clumsiness in their interpersonal relationships, relying on bluster and threat to make up for poor self-esteem and deficient social skills. Being socially marginalized they may feel there is little to lose by delinquency, and for many this is the norm of their subgroup. Such delinquency and restricted social conscience should not surprise us given the experiences of many of our patients. This is not the same as a dissocial personality disorder, however. It requires us to steer a path that includes support allied with appropriate confrontation and, where possible, encouragement and training to acquire the missing skills. Dissocial personality disorder is more pervasive and is characterized in ICD-10 by:

F60.2—dissocial personality disorder

- Callous unconcern for the feelings of others.
- Gross and persistent attitude of irresponsbility and disregard for social norms, rules, and obligations.
- Incapacity to maintain enduring relationships, though having no difficulty in establishing them.
- Very low tolerance of frustration and a low threshold for discharge of aggression, including violence.
- Incapacity to experience guilt and to profit from experience, particularly punishment.
- Marked proneness to blame others or to offer plausible rationalizations for the behaviour that has brought the patient into conflict with society.

(World Health Organisation 1992)

There will undoubtedly be a few patients on the case load of any team who suffer both from severe mental illness and from dissocial personality disorder. These patients pose massive problems, both therapeutic and ethical. Most of these issues are touched on elsewhere (e.g. Chapters 8, 10, and 19). Needless to say, issues of safety must be uppermost. Regular team reviews are essential to protect individual workers from placing too much faith on the strength of their engagement with such patients. Realistic goals need to be set and assumptions about the relative contributions of illness and personality to troublesome behaviours should be tested continually.

When to protect the patient from the legal consequences of their actions and when to ensure that they face them is always difficult. Individuals with dissocial personality disorder do not learn well from punishment. On the other hand, failure to allow the law to take its course may mean that the extent of the risk that an individual patient poses is not confronted. There is also the safety of others (both within the team and the public) to consider. On balance we very rarely attempt to prevent prosecutions where there has been physical aggression unless it is clearly associated with an acute psychotic relapse. The problem is more often that the police will not prosecute because they do not consider it in the public interest.

Confidentiality and risk

Issues of confidentiality can be very difficult when the patient has a dissocial personality disorder. If there are risks to a third party because of illness, then the Mental Health Act can be invoked and aggressive treatment initiated. Where callous disregard for others is not part of the illness, it becomes more problematic. For instance, what to do when a patient makes clear, non-delusional, threats against a neighbour and you have little doubt that they mean it? Similarly, we had a patient who worked as a minicab driver despite having no license (and hence no insurance) and without admitting he was on heavy medication. Knowing what is going on, can one ignore it? In neither of the above cases did we. We broke confidentiality and informed the neighbour and the minicab firm. We told both patients what we were going to do, explained our reasons, and had to live with the resultant fury. In the case of the minicab driver our relationship remained strained for over a year and has never really returned to how it was before.

Issues of confidentiality are addressed in Chapter 12. Undoubtedly, this will remain a problematic area in mental health for the foreseeable future. Current professional guidelines are simply not in touch with modern practice.

Borderline personality disorder

Common diagnostic practice is that dissocial personality disorder is overwhelmingly applied to men and borderline personality disorder overwhelmingly applied to women. It is tempting to draw the conclusion that borderline personality disorder is simply used for females instead of dissocial personality disorder. Interestingly, in a process echoing that with psychopathy (dissocial personality disorder), it was only introduced into DSM-III (American Psychiatric Association 1980) after much discussion and scepticism and in order to permit further research (Burns 1986). The same caveats were expressed about entering it into the ICD-10 (World Health Organisation 1992). Although its introduction has led to extensive research, this has mainly been into treatment, not into whether it is a valid diagnosis. Its expression is much more focused on self-harm and in stormy relationships than is dissocial personality disorder.

F60.3—emotionally unstable personality disorder

'A...marked tendency to act impulsively without consideration of the consequences, together with affective instability. The ability to plan ahead may be minimal, and outbursts of intense anger may often lead to violence or 'behavioural explosions'...Two variants...are specified, and both share this general theme of impulsiveness and lack of self-control.'

F60.31—borderline type

'Several characteristics of emotional instability are present; in addition, the patient's own self-image, aims, and internal preferences (including sexual) are often unclear or disturbed. There are usually chronic feelings of emptiness. A liability to become involved in intense and unstable relationships may cause repeated emotional crises with...a series of suicidal threats or acts of self-harm.'

(World Health Organisation 1992)

A therapeutic approach

Clearly helping such individuals is a daunting task, especially if they also suffer from a bipolar disorder or schizophrenia (though the latter seems rare with borderline but not dissocial personality disorder). Maintaining a non-judgemental approach is essential but this can be difficult. Such patients have had more than their fair share of criticism and punishment and have little real ability to make good use of either. Sometimes punishment may be inevitable but, where it is not, an honest but positive and supportive approach is really the only way. Confrontation may make us feel temporarily better but will not help the patient (nor, in the long run, our ability to help them). Trying to distinguish what is personality and what is 'illness' (although this is a highly artificial distinction) can help identify different strategies.

Team approach and reviews

In assertive outreach, patients with personality disorder have particularly benefited from a shared approach to care. The team can 'depersonalize' the relationship and the treatment to good effect. The patients are visited by different members of the team and visits are task-orientated rather than 'psychotherapeutic'. Such an approach requires meticulous care planning, boundaries, and communication to avoid the obvious 'splitting' that could arise.

This rigorous team approach protects both the focus on treatments and the morale of individual team members faced with an emotionally unstable and demanding patient who phones them several times a day and demands crisis visits.

We find it useful to review such patients in detail regularly in team meetings. Reminding ourselves of the multiple disadvantages which most of them endured can help neutralize the moral disapproval that otherwise may develop. It is also essential to acknowledge that, even with the best training, none of us is such a saint that we are immune to judgemental and even, occasionally, spiteful responses when pushed by patients. And pushed we will be—whether by accurately barbed comments about our personality or appearance, racist remarks, or physical intimidation. It is then that the team can support and protect us, and also rehabilitate the patient's reputation.

No team can help a patient if they have decided against him or her. If there is a real personality clash between key worker and patient this should be acknowledged and talked through. Sometimes it will be necessary to change key worker. This should only happen rarely however. It is generally better to work through such differences and learn from them.

Much of our work with personality disordered patients is aimed at reducing overall stress (in exactly the same way we try to stabilize the environment to avoid psychotic relapses). For dissocial and borderline individuals more of the focus needs to be on identifying potential flash points and finding ways of avoiding them. The use of alcohol or drugs is particularly risky in this impulse-ridden group of patients. Where avoidance is not possible, then agreeing some distracting manoeuvres can save the day.

Case study

A very handsome patient, with schizophrenia and an impulsive personality, is prone to violence. He is frequently approached by women and cannot cope with them. We have helped him to find activities that take place in a predominantly male environment (e.g. a gym, a music group that practises but does not perform). When he cannot avoid confrontation we have taught him to excuse himself, and when he begins to get stressed by it, have agreed that he will work off his tension with a particularly punishing set in the gym.

Time spent on such problem solving is well worth it for even short crises can wreak havoc and take ages to repair. It is also experienced by many individuals as an acceptably collaborative approach—one that does not evoke a well-established opposition to authority.

Conclusions

Personality problems and disorders are the daily bread of mental health professionals. We need to have a model of understanding personality that makes sense to us even if we do not necessarily believe that it explains it. One of us (TB) finds psychodynamic models helpful, while the other (MF) relies more on developmental and cognitive models. Whatever model it is, it needs to be robust enough to protect against moralizing. It also needs to survive when the facts do not fit, and to allow for an eclectic, pragmatic treatment strategy.

Arguments about the role of mental health services in the care of individuals with personality disorders (for which read 'dissocial personality disorder'!) are set to rage for the next decade. There is a clear international agenda to explore how we can ensure some form of risk reduction and social policing.

Assertive outreach services are likely to best serve by focusing on what we know that they can do well, what there is evidence for, and avoiding too many forays into speculation and theory. We work with a group of patients who routinely face challenges and problems that the average man in the street would only expect to confront once or twice in a lifetime. Inevitably, this will mean that we learn how to help individuals with troubled and troublesome personalities. While we should not withhold our skills, we should be wary of overstating what we can do or of misdirecting the resources we represent.

Chapter 18

Depression, anxiety, and situational disorders

It is easy to forget that people with severe mental illnesses also suffer anxiety, depression, and grief just as we all do. Although the most prominent features of their illnesses are their psychotic symptoms, careful examination of the mental state of individuals with schizophrenia often betrays very high levels of so-called 'neurotic symptoms' (Wing *et al* 1974). The management of situational and common mental disorders is not the primary focus of this book, as it is unlikely to be a major responsibility of outreach workers. However, a familiarity with them, and a working competence with them, is necessary if we are not to fail our patients. Shy, anxious individuals with psychotic disorders are not easily referred on for specialist help from other services.

Depression

A raised sensitivity to depression is essential in working with individuals with schizophrenia. Depression is common in such a devastating disorder—the loss of future ambitions, the exhausting stress of persecutory delusions and hallucinations, the isolation, and the damage to self-esteem. To complicate matters, depression can be very difficult to diagnose in schizophrenia. It has to be distinguished from the apathy and emptiness of negative symptoms and also from the inertia and sluggishness that result from over-medication. Post-psychotic depression is, however, common and there is increasing evidence that appropriate treatment with antidepressants can significantly improve recovery (Mandel *et al.* 1982).

Antidepressants

The choice of antidepressant can be difficult because of possible interaction between SSRIs and novel antipsychotics. Where antidepressants and antipsychotics are used concurrently in individuals with long-term disorders we have found the use of structured rating scales (Chapter 7) particularly valuable. The Beck depression inventory (Beck *et al.* 1961) is popular, but we find it long and quite demanding for our patients. The Hamilton depression scale (Bech *et al.* 1981) and the hospital anxiety depression scale (Zigmond and Snaith 1983) are shorter and generally easier to use.

Making sure you use a structured assessment is more important than which scale you use. Distinguishing fluctuations in overall mental state, mood, and more general, personal life changes is a challenge for even the most skilled worker. Forcing some objectivity into the rating of mood helps you decide whether there is a response to treatment. Given the risks of long-term polypharmacy in our patients, we must be hard-nosed about the justification for antidepressants.

Cognitive behavioural therapy (CBT)

CBT has been shown to be successful in alleviating depression in non-psychotic individuals (Beck *et al.* 1985) and is increasingly being used in the direct treatment of psychotic symptoms (Kuipers *et al.* 1997). There is as yet no strong published evidence of its value for depression in individuals with psychotic illnesses (Birchwood and Iqbal 1998) but we have found our patients receptive to CBT for depressive thinking and low self-esteem. Indeed, simply attempting such a collaborative approach (for CBT is nothing if not collaborative) can do wonders for a depressed and demoralized patient who for years has 'been done to' rather than 'negotiated with'.

A particular bonus with CBT in such patients is that the technique is broadly the same for the treatment of depression and for the treatment of residual psychotic symptoms. Once the approach has been established, then it can be used across several areas as clinically indicated over time.

Case study

Diana suffered from bipolar affective disorder but had long periods of remission and normal functioning. This functioning, however, was compromised by chronic low self-esteem. As part of the CBT approach to this, Diana was asked to draw up a list of all her negative self-beliefs e.g. 'nobody loves me', 'I am a bad person', 'I am unattractive'. In subsequent sessions the task was to find objective evidence that contradicted or supported these beliefs e.g. a letter or phone call from a friend or relative would contradict the belief that 'nobody loves me'. Each piece of evidence was written in a column for supporting the belief or contradicting it.

The therapist's task is to guide Diana and help her discover that the majority of objective evidence contradicts her beliefs. What supports her beliefs are predominantly her thoughts.

Support and specific treatments

It is easy, with the current emphasis on evidence-based practice, to overlook the importance for depressed individuals of simple support and counselling. It makes a real difference when you are struggling with low mood (even if it may resolve without specific treatments) to have it recognized and talked about. Acknowledging that you, as a key worker, can appreciate what the patient is going through, that this is a particular difficult patch, can make a real difference. Not only does it reduce the isolation and fear that are such a feature of feeling depressed, it can legitimize a more measured approach to dealing with things. If your patient realizes that they are depressed they may not drive themselves so hard and so give themselves space to recover. Often this healthy use of the 'sick role' may be all that is needed.

Sometimes, patients with severe mental illness may need specific counselling, such as bereavement counselling or treatment for post-traumatic stress disorder. The indications for their use and their practice are essentially the same as for individuals without severe mental illness. However, greater sensitivity and judgement may be required to detect their need and generally a slower, more supportive approach is indicated.

Bipolar disorder

In patients with bipolar disorder there can be a risk with using antidepressants, as these may precipitate hypomania (Chapter 16). There is no easy solution to this. Patients may need the antidepressant, so the only approach is to be cautious and highly vigilant in monitoring. After hypomania, a period of depression is almost inevitable. Indeed, there are those who consider it an integral phase of the disorder. It is not normally necessary to prescribe antidepressants immediately.

Several weeks or even months of hypomanic over-activity are understandably exhausting. We warn our patients to expect this and to be optimistic that it will resolve fairly quickly. Side-effects of drugs used to control the hypomania can also result in the patient feeling flat, anergic, and apathetic. It can be very difficult to get the balance absolutely right as sensitivity to both the therapeutic impact and the side-effects of the tranquillizers changes rapidly as the hypomania resolves.

There are also psychological aspects of recovering from hypomania that need to be worked through. Often, when high, the patient will have done things that later they deeply regret and about which they are embarrassed. These feelings will fade eventually but, in our experience, are best acknowledged. There is no formula for how to do this; judge each case individually. Broach the issue too early and it will be too painful to discuss and be hotly denied. Leave it too long and it may be stale and already resolved and you may be accused of exaggeration. It is probably best to mention it fairly early and see how the patient responds.

Avoiding things sets up an unhealthy dynamic, introducing tension into the relationship. We have found that gentle, but penetrating, exploration of incidents that occurred during a period of florid illness can lead to a remarkable strengthening of the therapeutic relationship, especially if they have been lived through by both parties.

Anxiety disorders

Diagnosed agoraphobia and panic disorders seem relatively unusual in the severely mentally ill. Having said that, chronically high levels of arousal and tension are far from rare. Isolation, resulting in becoming housebound, is common but it can be very difficult to be sure if such withdrawal is due entirely to apathy and negative symptoms or fear of confronting the world outside. The published literature on treating phobic disorders is generally unhelpful as individuals with psychotic disorders (or any possible delusional basis for their reluctance to go out) are almost invariably excluded from studies. Our experience, however, is that the same principles of management apply, although they need to be used with discretion and sensitivity.

Most treatment in anxiety disorders is informed by behaviour therapy principles. Fears are understood as normal phenomena, albeit exaggerated in this specific incidence. Time and energy are not expended in an exhaustive attempt to understand exactly how they arose but in helping the patient overcome them. Often support and encouragement are enough—helping the individual face the worry by going with them to a new day centre or accompanying them on the first trip back to a shop where they made a fuss when they were last ill.

Graded exposure

Where this is not enough, then *'graded exposure'* (often called *desensitization* or *reciprocal inhibition*) (Al–Kubaisky *et al.* 1992) can be very successful. This consists of breaking the task down into small, manageable steps, which do not raise the patients' anxiety levels more than they can cope with, and repeating that achievement until it generates no significant anxiety, before attempting the next step. There are self-help books explaining the principles and practice of simple behavioural techniques (Ingham 2000; Juniper 2000; Kennerley 1997). Basically, they offer formalized commonsense.

The important lesson is to think through the steps with the patient, having explained and discussed exactly why you believe the approach to be a good idea and what it involves. The trick is to be very explicit, give clear recognition and praise when each goal has been achieved, and not to rush it. Asking patients to rate their anxiety level on a given scale during each attempt is often recommended but we have found this over-complicated and generally not that helpful. Better, on the whole, simply to make sure that the arousal is tolerable. You should expect the odd bad day and make sure that the patient also expects it so that it is not immediately interpreted as a failure of the treatment.

Most programmes of graded exposure involve a mixture of accompanied exercises and 'homework' where the patient practises on their own what you have achieved together. Your presence works to reduce anxiety, and so doing the same thing alone is still a challenge. Often with severely ill patients in outreach teams we downplay the homework and accompany the patient throughout each of the steps until the goal has been achieved. Only then do we encourage consolidation alone.

Medication

There is no conflict between taking a psychological approach to helping patients manage their anxiety and the use of medication; there is no *'either-or'* about medicine or psychological interventions. Indeed, some early behavioural studies of graded exposure showed they were more successful if augmented by medications (either benzodiazepines or tricyclic antidepressants).

For individuals with psychotic disorders, the mild sedative effects of their antipsychotic medications can be utilized in managing anxiety. It is very common for patients to ask us to increase their dose of antipsychotic temporarily when they are going through a stressful period. We do this often when there are family or external stressors, or even if there is nothing obvious but the patient reports increasing anxiety. The effect is probably both pharmacological and psychological—many patients see their medicine as a shield against stress and simply knowing they are getting more helps.

Benzodiazepines have been severely criticized in the management of anxiety states because of the risks of dependence in long-term use. However, we have increasingly used them with our patient group and so far have not experienced problems with dependence or abuse. (The abuse problems we struggle with come from anticholinergics.) We have used high doses of benzodiazepines in managing acute psychotic episodes in the community (Chapters 7 and 15) and often use them both as sleeping tablets and for short-term management of anxiety without patients insisting on their continuation when the crisis is over. Perhaps our patients are less hedonistic, or perhaps the sedative side-effects of their antipsychotics are enough to contend with. Whatever the reason, we have experienced very few problems either with dependence or disinhibition in the use of benzodiazepines.

Situational disorders

Post-traumatic stress disorder (PTSD)

Individuals with major mental illnesses are prey to stresses and crises as much as other people. They can suffer bereavement or PTSD, and we need to be alert to these risks. Indeed, given the traumatic experiences of many of our patients, it is surprising that there are not more cases of severe PTSD in individuals with long-standing mental illnesses.

Priebe has shown that most of the symptoms of PTSD are present in patients with acute schizophrenia—but as part of the general arousal, not a discrete syndrome (Priebe *et al.* 1998). Memories of traumatic experiences around admission to hospital and also on the ward are sometimes very powerful in determining patients' behaviour, although they may not amount to a fully-fledged PTSD. For some patients it can lead to them avoiding services, while in others, the vivid memory of the consequences of relapse can lead to improved compliance with treatment.

Acknowledgement of the trauma is healing for the individual but also strengthens the therapeutic relationship. We, as staff, may have been part of the trauma, and we need to recognize it and take it seriously. As noted in Chapter 8 on the use of compulsion, we have found our patients well able to relate to us while acknowledging that at times we may do things they do not want. To date, we have not found it necessary to refer on for specific PTSD treatment and have approached the incidents which have occurred with a mixture of ventilation and graded exposure.

Case study

Caroline became acutely paranoid following a protracted period of intermittent compliance with medication and moderate use of cannabis. Within the space of a few days she became convinced that someone was having an affair with her boyfriend. On one occasion she followed him to work after hearing people in the next door flat discussing the details of the affair. When her key worker came to assess her with a doctor, she assaulted the key worker, believing that she was the one having the affair. Caroline was admitted to hospital via the police. In hospital she attempted to hang herself from a window bracket with her tights, seemingly in response to command hallucinations.

Within a few weeks Caroline improved, gained partial insight into what had happened, and had good recall. She was shocked and frightened by it. Her boyfriend had nearly left her as a result of her paranoia, she had nearly taken her own life, and she had assaulted her key worker. Helping her through this difficult time focused on rebuilding relationships and working on preventing such a dramatic relapse in the future.

Looking back, Caroline sees this admission as a watershed that forced her to acknowledge the diagnosis, the treatment, and her vulnerability to cannabis. Her compliance and substance abuse have improved to the extent that she has stayed out of hospital since.

Bereavement

An understanding of the process of bereavement—with its stages of shock and protest (including denial and disbelief), preoccupation, disorganization, and, finally, resolution (Bowlby 1961)—is essential for assertive outreach. Even if your patient does not experience the loss of a family member, the illness itself imposes a bereavement. Having to accept that their aspirations (successful job, close family, etc.) have been profoundly, and often abruptly, changed with the onset of the illness is very similar to grief. Many patients (and families) never get beyond the phases of anger and denial. The result is an inability to adapt to the reality of the disease and the adjustments in their plans and routines that it requires.

Coming to terms with the reality and significance of the disease can be a long and painful process. Probably all of us have dealt at some time with angry young men with bipolar disorder who steadfastly refuse to discuss it, or co-operate with treatment until they have 'learnt the hard way' via several relapses. Usually, it is emotional resistance to the enormity of the change rather than any rational difficulties in understanding the facts or mastering the treatment regime. Recognizing the sense of loss that underlies the anger and denial is the first step to doing anything about it. Premature attempts at compliance enhancement strategies are unlikely to succeed until there has been some working through of these emotions. Patients will usually set the pace and determine when, and how, this can be done. We have to make clear to them that we are aware of what they have lost and are willing to engage with it.

Serious illnesses in the families of our patients can cause great distress. Anticipatory anxiety about impending loss can be as serious for patients as their families. Families (particularly parents, but sometimes siblings) describe a persisting worry about what is going to happen when they die. This is sometimes referred to as the 'WIAG' ('when I am gone') syndrome. Clinical experience is often contrary to the fear and patients often survive the loss surprisingly well. Notwithstanding this, an impending loss can have a major impact on a patient.

We also need to be alert to the effects of a parent's grief, after the loss of a spouse, on the patient. We have a small number of middle-aged schizophrenia patients who live with very aged parents who have devoted themselves to caring for the patient. Often it is predominantly the mother who is involved. This care can be substantially reduced or interrupted when the mother has to cope with her own grief at the illness or loss of her husband. It is also important to ensure that she has the support and space to allow herself her own grief. Her concerns about now being the only one left to support her son or daughter will inevitably be heightened by her loss.

There are a number of strategies to help. One is for us to spend more time with the patient, reassuring the mother that she can concentrate on her own needs. Another is to spend time with the mother, encouraging her to talk through her grief and helping her with it. Alternatively, one might ensure that she gets prompt attention from a local bereavement service. Of course, we are equally likely to do a bit of all three!

Case study

John had lived at home with his parents for over 20 years, since his first breakdown. He led an ordered, if somewhat unexciting life. Without constant support from the team he invariably stopped his medication and relapsed—neither he nor we could understand why as he was generally satisfied with things when well.

His father suffered from severe asthma and hypertension and was housebound. He was taciturn, rather critical of his son, and otherwise had nothing to do with him. His mother was an energetic and outwardly happy individual who did everything for John. She said that she had long since come to terms with his illness, thought he was a 'lovely lad', and took pride in how she and her two daughters supported him.

His father died suddenly (though not unexpectedly) and John seemed unperturbed by it. In the months following the funeral he began to deteriorate and we had difficulty understanding this—he denied any worry or grief. Only slowly did it dawn on us that, although his mother was still as committed, she was struggling to deal with her own grief and loneliness. Whilst John was still getting his meals cooked and his washing done, he was not getting the same level of interest and support he was used to.

Helping his mother to accept her own needs was not at all easy. Only by engaging his sisters were we able to make any progress at all. Even then, things remained rocky for over a year and John had his first admission for several years.

'Neurotic disorders'

We have emphasized in this chapter that individuals with psychotic disorders are prey to most things that can befall those who do not suffer from them. Not surprisingly, they may be less concerned about symptoms that would worry us—they have much more serious problems to contend with. They can, however, display a range of 'neurotic' symptoms, either the so-called 'non-specific' neurotic symptoms embodied in depression and anxiety or more specific problems such as obsessive–compulsive symptoms, somatization, or eating disorders. Again, the treatment literature is rarely that helpful as most specialist units exclude patients with severe mental illness from their studies.

Obsessions and compulsions

A significant proportion of psychotic patients display repetitive thoughts or actions. For most, these cause no distress and are often considered 'mannerisms' or, occasionally, 'stereotypies'. For a smaller group, the repetitions and intrusions are distressing and have the quality of obsessions or compulsions, although they may not be resisted as strongly as in purer forms of the disorder. There is a small group of schizophrenia patients whose hallucinatory experiences demonstrate obsessional features (i.e. *they are obliged* to hear the voices repeatedly).

We take a pragmatic approach to trying to help with such complications. For a couple of patients we have found some improvement with SSRIs, but it has not been spectacular. The behavioural approaches we have used have been aimed more at reducing the impact of the thoughts and actions on the patient's life and minimizing their impact on those around them. If the patient is not distressed and there is no social impact from the symptoms we generally think it is best to leave well alone.

Eating disorders and diet

Patients can develop all sorts of strange eating habits—but then, so can any of us. We have a number of patients with very specific diets, some of which are quite healthy and some of which are not. Some of these have delusional origins—we have one patient who has delusions about China and will only eat what he considers to be 'Chinese' food, although most of us would not recognize it as such.

Concern about weight and diet is increasingly common in our patients, particularly women, because of weight gain from atypical antipsychotics. One has developed a form of bulimia nervosa as a consequence of trying and failing to diet. Dietary and exercise advice is clearly necessary in these instances, although we have had little success with it so far in our female patients. We have had some modest success with younger male patients who can use exercise both as a control for their weight and as a source of self-esteem.

Case study

Marie suffers from severe bipolar affective disorder, manic type, and requires intensive interventions to manage her at home during periods of elation. She sees her main problem, however, as her attempts to control her weight and the consequent binge eating. It took two years of working with Marie, around her 'core' psychiatric symptoms, before she first discussed her eating disorder. She describes binge eating, vomiting, guilt, and use of stimulants (coffee, smoking, and procyclidine) to excess—all to reduce her appetite.

Anorexia nervosa can occur with psychosis (Hsu *et al.* 1981) and is difficult to treat. We have not yet had experience of working with someone with this problem in our assertive outreach team but have come across it previously in a CMHT. Help from specialist units is recommended, although many will not be well set up for such patients.

Weight maintenance and harm minimization are probably the only short-term goals that can be added to drug treatment of the psychosis.

Drug treatments can be very difficult with individuals who restrict their diet severely. One of our patients (driven by persistent delusions of personal worthlessness) has a hopelessly inadequate diet, mainly restricted to breakfast cereals. His blood pressure is hardly measurable so antipsychotics (which certainly improve his mental state) have to be in tiny doses and cautiously monitored.

Conclusions

Working in assertive outreach with the severely mentally ill requires us to achieve a fine balance. We must develop and maintain the specialist skills appropriate to our target group but must also not lose sight of the fact that our patients are more like the general population than they are different. Our main task is to help them manage their psychosis so that they can take advantage of as normal a life as possible. For this reason we must focus on the complexities of these long-term disorders. We must use techniques such as structured assessments to ensure that we do not become so embroiled in their day-to-day existence that we fail to see the wood for the trees. On the other hand, we need to have a sensitivity to the problems and to the often time-limited disorders (such as depression and anxiety) that affect the severely mentally ill also.

We would argue that being alert to these 'less technical' aspects of management serves another purpose besides making sure our patients get the treatment they need. It constantly reminds us that we are dealing with *people* not *disorders*. It reminds us also that the people we are dealing with are more like us than they are different from us. The history of psychiatry teaches us that even the best-intentioned staff can lose sight of this when constantly working with dependent and disabled individuals.

Chapter 19

Substance abuse

Introduction

Psychotic illnesses are increasingly complicated by alcohol and drug abuse as patients no longer spend long periods in hospital. Treated in the community the benefits of social inclusion can be offset by greater exposure to drugs and alcohol. Dual diagnosis patients will be used throughout this chapter to refer to patients with a psychotic illness plus significant alcohol or substance abuse.

Assertive outreach provides the opportunity to accept dual diagnosis patients and work towards resolving the cumulative problems that both conditions bring. Dual diagnosis carries additional problems for both patients and services. Integrating both substance abuse strategies and more traditional mental health interventions in the same team is an essential response for such chaotic individuals.

Service responses

One very real problem for these patients has been the reluctance of either CMHTs or addiction services to work wholeheartedly with them. The response of services has often been one of 'passing the buck'. Interviewing key professionals and reviewing local strategies in the UK, Rorstad and Checinski (1996) concluded:

> Where major disabling mental health problems co-existed with an addiction problem, intervention strategies appeared to be based on the assumption that until the mental health problem had been addressed there was little or nothing that could be done by a substance misuse service to help the patient. The problem with dealing with psychoses or other major and disabling mental health problems was seen as beyond the training and resource competence of a substance misuse service even where that service was staffed by qualified mental health nurses and medical personnel.

Patients with dual diagnosis straddle the divide between general and addiction services. Treatment in parallel systems appears to be ineffective and inefficient with a failure of clinicians to modify their models of working (Drake *et al.* 1995).

The conflicting assumptions of the models of care that traditionally operate in addiction and assertive outreach services are outlined in Table 19.1. These differences are poorly understood, they hinder the establishment of partnerships, and patients have great difficulty finding their place within the system even when motivated. The most fundamental conflict arises if addiction services use clinic-based treatment programmes, partly to ensure that patients are motivated. Attendance at appointments is expected and discharge from the service will follow repeated non-attendance.

Table 19.1 Differences in approach between addiction services and assertive outreach

Substance misuse services	Assertive outreach services
◆ Confrontative approach	◆ Emphasis on engagement and collaboration
◆ Clinic-based	◆ Outreach is standard
◆ Motivation important element of entry criteria	◆ Optimistic about developing motivation
◆ Psychotropic medication is discouraged	◆ Antipsychotics actively prescribed
◆ Treatment episodes are focused and time-limited	◆ Comprehensive and not time-limited
◆ Defaulters not normally followed up	◆ Assertively follow up patients who do not engage
◆ Compulsory treatment not used	◆ Compulsory treatment a common feature
◆ Group therapy is widely used	◆ Groups poorly tolerated by severely ill psychotic patients

In the wider social care context, dual diagnosis patients are often excluded from housing and residential facilities, especially where illicit drug use is involved. Possession or use of cannabis in a mental health hostel is unlikely to lead to the involvement of the police but is likely to jeopardise that placement because the hostel needs to protect its legal status. Conversely, drug rehabilitation programmmes rarely tolerate residents with severe mental health problems. Homelessness or prison are frequent consequences (Lehman and Dixon 1995). This reluctance of other services to provide the same flexible response to need as assertive outreach, can cause frustrations for team members and patients alike.

Incidence

Dual diagnosis patients make up 20–50% of the case loads of assertive outreach teams in the UK. Most of the experience and research in this field comes from the US, where 40–60% of patients with severe mental illness are estimated as also having a problem with alcohol and drug abuse (Mueser *et al.* 1995). A South London study identified substance abuse in 36.3% of 171 psychotic patients in contact with services (Menezes *et al.* 1996). Alcohol abuse was most common at 20.5%; 4.7% had a problem with drugs only, and 11.1% with both. Cannabis was the most common of the drugs abused. Men were twice as likely as women to suffer substance abuse. Among men there was a trend for drug use, but not alcohol use, to decrease with age. Both decreased with age for women. The authors acknowledge that these findings cannot be widely generalized but they give a benchmark to compare local experience. We have seen a rise in the use of 'crack' cocaine by our patients in recent years, with stable levels of cannabis and alcohol use.

Table 19.2 Distinguishing characteristics of dual diagnosis patients

Characteristic	Study findings
◆ Greater use of in-patient services	Mean number of admissions the same in preceding year but: 30% more likely >60 days as in-patient 3 times more likely >120 days as in-patient (Menezes *et al.* 1996)
◆ Worse clinical outcomes	Greater symptom severity (Lehman *et al.* 1993)
◆ Worse social outcomes	Poorer housing and occupation stability, greater offending (Lehman *et al.* 1993)
◆ Greater incidence of violence and aggression	Significantly more likely to report history of offending or recent hostile behaviour (Scott *et al.* 1998)
◆ Greater incidence of suicide	Alcohol use correlated with depression and suidical behaviour in two independent studies of schizophrenia (Bartels *et al.* 1992)
◆ Demographically younger and male	Male patients are twice as likely as female to have dual diagnosis. Drug abuse diminishes with age in men, but not alcohol abuse (Menezes *et al.* 1996)
◆ Poorer compliance with prescribed medication	Medication non-compliance significantly higher (Owen *et al.* 1996)
◆ More contact with the criminal justice system	Offending generally of low severity— theft, alcohol offences, driving offences (Scott *et al.* 1998)
◆ More use of A&E services	Greater utilization by current abusers (Bartels *et al.* 1993)
◆ Increased costs for services	'Core' psychiatric costs increased by £1046 per annum (McCrone *et al.* 2000)

Characteristics of dual diagnosis patients

Table 19.2 sets out the key characteristics associated with a dual diagnosis. Many, if not all, echo usual referral criteria to assertive outreach services and reinforce our willingness to accept these challenging patients.

Assessment

Structured assessments for the presence and degree of substance misuse, of harmful use, and of dependence will help target interventions appropriately and guide possible treatment. Inadequate assessment can lead to both a neglect of substance abuse interventions (e.g. education, detoxification, and counselling) and also over-treatment of the psychotic illness through misdiagnosis (Drake and Mercer–McFadden 1995).

A brief drug and drink history carried out in a non-judgemental and confidential manner will maximize disclosure. Acutely ill patients, or those with cognitive deficits, may significantly under-report use. We find that well-engaged patients will acknowledge alcohol and cannabis use but rarely admit to the use of 'crack' cocaine, opiates, and amphetamines. Although we know our patients well, we are still surprised by revelations of covert drug and alcohol misuse. Urine drug screens for patients admitted to hospital can often provide unexpected information. Similarly, liver enzymes can indicate recent heavy alcohol use. Simply smelling alcohol on a patient's breath is a cheap guide to alcohol use as is the observation of pupillary changes, behaviour changes, or drugs paraphernalia and empty beer cans in the home. Family and friends are often keen to provide information on drug and alcohol use and to express their concerns.

A realistic approach to sensible drinking and harmful use of illicit drugs is necessary. Many of our patients regularly use alcohol and cannabis and describe broadly positive effects of reduced arousal and improved social interaction and mood. Others patients show clearly detrimental effects from alcohol abuse such as aggression and disruption of relationships, gastric problems, impulsive behaviour, depression, and forgetfulness. Cannabis is clearly associated with a worsening of psychotic symptoms, especially paranoia, for many vulnerable patients.

For alcohol, one unit is equivalent to half a pint of ordinary strength beer or lager or one small glass of wine or one single measure of spirits. Current guidance for safe drinking for men is 21 units per week and 14 units for women. It is now considered more helpful to view this guidance in daily terms. Men consistently drinking four units a day and women consistently drinking three units a day incur a progressive health risk.

Comorbid substance abuse disorder is diagnosed not only on quantity of intake but on the basis of the adverse social, psychological, vocational, or medical consequences (Drake and Mercer–McFadden 1995). With dual diagnosis patients, the drug history may need to be brief and tailored to what the patient can reasonably tolerate. Given that the patient is already with an assertive outreach team, details of psychiatric history, treatment, and social circumstances will already be well understood. A simple guide is the mnemonic 'CAGE' (cut down, annoyed, guilty, eye opener) (Mayfield *et al.* 1974). This very quick oral or written questionnaire is much used in general practice to detect alcoholism:

CAGE questionnaire

- Have you ever felt you should cut down on your drinking?
- Have people annoyed you by criticizing your drinking?
- Have you ever felt bad or guilty about your drinking?
- Have you ever had a drink first thing in the morning to steady your nerves or to get rid of a hangover (eye opener)?

Scoring: 0 for each 'no', 1 for each 'yes'—2 or greater is clinically significant

(Mayfield *et al.* 1974)

The following list outlines the areas relevant to any substance abuse, but need not be covered with all patients. Many patients would find such a detailed enquiry exhausting. All should, however, be borne in mind when assessing a patient who abuses one or more substances.

Elements of a full drug history

Past and current alcohol/drug use

- Age when started misuse (including nicotine)
- Types and quantities of alcohol/drugs taken
- Frequency of misuse
- Awareness of effects on mental state—positive and negative
- Routes of administration, use of clean equipment and sharing habits if injecting, HIV/hepatitis B or C status and knowledge of modes of transmission, use of condoms, supply of needles and syringes
- Experience of overdose
- Periods of abstinence and triggers for relapse
- Symptoms when unable to obtain alcohol or drugs
- Cost of use

Medical history

- Complications of misuse—abscesses, gastric and liver problems, hepatitis B or C/HIV
- Accidents or head injuries
- Cognitive effects of alcohol—Wernicke's encephalopathy, Korsakoff's syndrome, peripheral neuropathy
- Diet
- Previous addiction treatment or rehabilitation

Social history

- High-risk peer group
- Drug or alcohol misuse in partner or family
- Effect of use on relationships, family, work, housing

Forensic history

- Currently offending
- Past contact with criminal justice system

Assertive outreach for dual diagnosis

Assertive outreach is a good foundation for developing specialized interventions aimed at addiction. Patients with alcohol and drug abuse are invariably poor at attending outpatient clinics (Burns *et al.* 1993b). This is not surprising given periods of intoxication when good intentions are easily forgotten. Further barriers arise if the patient has a chaotic lifestyle and disorganized thinking from a psychotic illness. At its very least, assertive outreach can help the patient deal with the practical problems that prevent them getting treatment. In addition, stable living conditions, symptom management, daytime activity or distraction, and development of a non-abusing peer group are part of a comprehensive approach to harm minimization and treatment.

The New Hampshire model (McHugo *et al.* 1999) incorporates these elements of assertive engagement, attention to basic needs such as housing and finance, and harm reduction delivered through case management. Non-confrontational approaches to the management of substance abuse are preferred and supported by experience and research. Treatment goals are often limited to harm reduction and compromising on drug or alcohol use rather than abstinence. Principles of collaboration fit the needs of dual diagnosis patients well. This integrated model consists of a self-sufficient assertive outreach team set up to work exclusively with dual diagnosis patients. Expertise in addiction is incorporated into a team that has a clear remit to focus equally on substance abuse and psychosis. The approach rests on the assumption that dual diagnosis patients should be treated within the mental health system and not the addictions system.

The New Hampshire model uses a four-stage approach to individual and group treatment of substance abuse:

1. Engagement stage
2. Persuasion stage
3. Active treatment.
4. Relapse prevention (Osher and Kofoed 1989)—similar to the motivational interviewing approach (Miller and Rollinick 1991)

Motivational interviewing

Motivational interviewing is particularly useful for dual diagnosis patients in that it guides interventions with those who lack 'insight' and motivation to change their behaviour. (The model refers to this as the 'pre-contemplative phase'—the patient is not yet considering reducing or stopping harmful use.) The process is similar to compliance therapy which is discussed in Chapter 11 (Kemp *et al.* 1998). The goal of the therapist is to guide the patient from pre-contemplation towards a readiness to change and beyond to reduction and possibly eventual abstinence.

The emphasis is on helping the patient review their beliefs and behaviours and to expose cognitive dissonance between their goals and their current substance abuse in order to generate motivation. The 'pre-contemplative' patient is given information and education to help him or her contemplate change and move to the 'preparation stage'. One method is to ask the patient to draw up a list of positive and negative aspects of their drug or alcohol abuse. When the ratio of perceived costs and benefits tips towards costs (e.g.

crisis or hospitalization resulting from drug abuse), the patient may be motivated to change and is then guided to the 'action stage' of how to proceed with changing their behaviour. Finally, the 'maintenance stage' is about securing abstinence and positive behaviours.

Stages in motivational interviewing

1. **Pre-contemplative stage**—the patient is not ready or interested in behaviour changes.
2. **Contemplative stage**—the patient is uncertain or ambivalent about change.
3. **Preparation stage**—the patient is ready for change.
4. **Action stage**—change is occurring; interventions assist change.
5. **Maintenance stage**—interventions aimed at maintaining healthy behaviour.

Such sophisticated approaches are hindered by the cognitive deficits that impair many patients with severe mental illness. Impairments of memory, attention, and information processing put the onus on key workers to make the intervention process clear and unambiguous, with frequent repetition of educational information and checking for understanding. We all suffer from denial of the future consequences of our current behaviour—paying tomorrow for what we can have today. Making these links between the present and future may be difficult for our patients. Living marginalized and impoverished lives they may have less to lose. Potential losses can act as motivating forces for others (Carey 1995).

Further substance abuse interventions

Alcoholics Anonymous

The classic intervention for addiction is the 12-step approach of Alcoholics Anonymous (AA) and Narcotics Anonymous. AA groups are underused by persons with dual diagnosis and mental health professionals are cautious about referring patients to AA because of fears that the AA group will discourage them from taking prescribed medication (Meissen *et al*. 1999). In addition, AA is founded upon a self-help, moral and spiritual model, which can seem out of step with mainstream psychiatric practice. Advantages of the model, however, include a powerful support network available to members. New members can obtain a 'sponsor' from the group and experienced members act as guides. We have one patient who attends AA regularly, who self-referred.

Pharmacological

The use of medication in the management of dual diagnosis can be for the clinical management of detoxification, to prevent relapse, or to treat any causes of substance misuse such as depression or control of side effects.

Detoxification using substitute medication is necessary for patients with physical dependence. Substitute medication (usually tapering doses of benzodiazepines and anticonvulsants) reduces the risks of delirium tremens and grand mal convulsions associated with alcohol withdrawal. Traditionally, detoxification is achieved in hospital with a one- to two-week regime. Outreach provides the option of a home-based detoxification with frequent or daily visits, supervision of substitute drug administration, and longer detoxification time scales. This may not be a safe option for all patients. Poorly motivated patients may need to get away from the home environment. Availability of carers at home may be a critical factor. Psychological support of the patient during and after detoxification is vital to prevent relapse into addiction and for the concurrent mental illness. In-patient detoxification may be safer for those with severe physical problems.

The pharmacological treatment of cocaine and amphetamine abuse and craving has not been established. A number of compounds have been attempted, including antidepressants for the treatment of depressive episodes associated with stimulant abuse, but this remains an area for further research. Benzodiazepines for alcohol detoxification and methadone (a synthetic opiate agonist) for opiate dependence, are safe and effective. The current guidelines are beyond the scope of this book and will vary between clinicians.

Antabuse (disulfiram) has been widely used in the treatment of uncomplicated alcohol abuse. It causes uncomfortable headache and flushing if the patient drinks alcohol. It has little place in the care of dual diagnosis patients as it can exacerbate psychosis and can be dangerous. Patients can drink safely only several days after stopping treatment with antabuse. It is therefore most effective in highly motivated patients or where daily supervision of the medication is available from the assertive outreach team or a family member (Schwartz and Lehman 1995).

Relapse prevention

Relapse is a hallmark of addictive disorders, and is the rule rather than the exception after a successful course of treatment.

(Carey 1995)

'Keep away from people, places, and things related to addiction' is a slogan used in AA as a relapse prevention technique. Identify the relapse scenarios and triggers, and rehearse coping strategies. In our work we can turn talking into behaviour by enacting situations and asking the patient to say how they would refuse an offer of drugs or alcohol or an invite to the pub. For dual diagnosis patients this involves contingency planning for how to cope should their mental health deteriorate, and inhibitions or judgements become affected. Unstable bipolar patients will have particular problems when going high. Family education and support will be an integral part of both treatment and relapse prevention.

Harm minimization

This approach concentrates on reducing the damage that substance abuse brings to the patient and their networks. The concept originated from helping opiate abusers with strategies such as needle exchanges, where the abuse is tolerated but assistance given to reduce very serious associated risks. For the 'pre-contemplative' patient this may be the only approach possible. Intervention on behalf of a patient to protect their tenancy, diffuse a conflict, or prevent offending behaviour likely to lead to prosecution helps to minimize complications and preserve supportive networks still available to the patient. Even helping a patient change from spirits or high-strength lager to normal-strength beer, or providing meals on wheels and vitamins, are potent harm minimization strategies.

Case study

David drinks 20 cans of Guinness a day, suffers from schizophrenia, has a poor diet, diabetes, liver damage, severe tremor, memory loss, and is vulnerable to exploitation. The team had never known David when he was not drinking this amount.

David's main concern was the amount of money he spent on alcohol, and this functioned as the key motivating factor. Individual counselling and motivational approaches got us nowhere because of his cognitive damage. After lengthy negotiation, David agreed to in-patient detoxification, as he believed he would save money. We felt that a routine detoxification and return to his flat, even with daily contact, would not make a lasting impact, as he lived alone and had no other activities besides drinking. However, he was someone who would follow 'no drinking' rules in day centres, hospital, hostels, etc.

We delayed admission and detoxification in order to explore the option of residential accommodation on a permanent or rehabilitative basis with David. We started taking him to a mental health resource centre daily, where he could get a meal and a bath and spend periods of time, up to five hours, abstinent.

Given his level of psychiatric illness, a rehabilitative 'dry' house was difficult to find. David was ambivalent about leaving his flat, even for a few months, fearing he might lose it.

Eventually, we were able to identify and finance a three-month residential placement in a dry house. David was detoxified in hospital and went directly to the dry house. We were able to assess his mental state, physical health, and tremor more accurately once he had dried out. The assertive outreach team continued to be intensively involved throughout. Whilst David was in the hostel we applied for appointeeship of his benefit money. This acted as a further safeguard against relapse as money to buy alcohol was controlled and limited.

The team continues to see David daily now he is back at home. We supervise his psychiatric and physical medication, check his blood sugars, help him maintain his flat and finances, and support him in staying off alcohol. David still has periods of binge drinking but has not returned to regular use or physical dependence. His physical health has been stabilized and his mental health, ability to retain information, and interaction with others has improved somewhat.

Example 19.1

ENHANCED CPA/SECTION 117(2)REVIEW (delete as applicable)		
Patient's name: David G. Address: 21 Harvest House, Savona Estate, Battersea Phone: 0207 622 xxxx Date of birth: 30/7/51 GP: Alexander Phone: 0207 535 xxxx	CMHT: ACT TEAM Phone: 020 8877 xxxx New patient: NO If NO, date of review: .... 22/5/01 .... Diagnosis: 1 Schizophrenia .... F 20.0 2 Alcohol dependence syndrome F 10.2	

Assessed needs or problem	Intervention	Resp. of
Poor compliance with medication and treatment due to cognitive deficits	◆ Daily supervised medication. ◆ Psychiatric and physical medication dispensed in dosette box. Supervise on each visit. ◆ Monitor blood sugar by BM stick on each visit.	AC
Risk of relapse of severe alcohol abuse	◆ Accompany to resource centre 2–3 times weekly to develop non-drinking environment and activities. ◆ Liaise with appointee to manage David's money, limiting amount available to buy alcohol. ◆ Reinforce psychoeducational and motivational messages about risk to health of alcohol binges or return to regular use. ◆ Give practical assistance with maintaining accommodation, dealing with correspondence, personal care, and household tasks.	AC
Difficulty managing personal and household affairs	◆ Home help once per week.	AC

Involved in care:	Dr✓ Psychologist CPN OT SW Ward nurse CCM✓ Support worker Other
At planning meeting:	Dr✓ Psychologist CPN OT SW✓ Ward nurse CCM✓ Support worker Other
Discussed with the patient? YES	Copy to patient? YES Copy to GP? YES
Care co-ordinator (print):	Alison Charles Phone: 020 8877 xxxx
Care co-ordinator (signature):	.... Date of next review: 22/11/01......
Job title:	Clinical nurse specialist Patient's signature: ....

Supervision register?	NO	Care management?	NO	Risk history completed?	YES
Supervised discharge?	NO	Section 117(2)?	YES	Relapse + risk plan required?	YES

Example 19.2

CONFIDENTIAL: RELAPSE AND RISK MANAGEMENT PLAN

Name: David G.

Categories of risk identified:

Aggression and Aggression and violence	NO	Severe self-neglect	NO
Exploitation (self or others)	YES	Risk to children & young adults	NO
Suicide and self-harm	NO	Other (please specify}	

Current factors which suggest there is significant apparent risk:
(For example: alcohol or substance misuse; specific threats; suicidal ideation; violent fantasies; anger; suspiciousness; persecutory beliefs; paranoid feelings or ideas about particular people)

David has been exploited by local drinkers who have threatened him, used his flat, and taken money from him.

Clear statement of anticipated risk(s):
(Who is at risk; how immediate is that risk; how severe; how ongoing)

David is at risk of assault from other residents of his estate who abuse alcohol and have intimidated and extorted money from him. Low risk to staff of assault by these people during home visit to his flat.

Action plan:
(Including names of people responsible for each action and steps to be taken if plan breaks down)

David encouraged not to allow access to these people. Police to be informed when further incidents of extortion occur. Allocated team member not to visit alone when it is known others are in his flat, phone to check this before visiting each day.

Date completed: 22/5/01	Review date: 22/11/01

This risk assessment may contain confidential and/or sensitive information provided by third parties. Such information should not be disclosed to the patient without prior consultation with the informant

Example 19.3

RISK ASSESSMENT DOCUMENTATION

Client's name: David G.

RISK HISTORY
Give details of any risk behaviour shown by the patient (actual or threatened). Each entry must be signed and dated
(E.g. previous violence; weapons used; impulsivity; self-harm; non-compliance; disengagement from services; convictions; potentially seriously harmful acts)

April 2001: David threatened and exploited by group of three local men who abuse alcohol. These men persuaded David to let them in and proceeded to threaten him and extort money and cigarettes.

Conclusions

Unfortunately, people with severe mental illness have an increased risk of developing substance abuse and dependence disorders compared to the general population (Regier *et al.* 1990). This is particularly evident for young, male patients. Reasons for this are complex and include social isolation and high rates of unemployment. Some develop substance abuse because of the distress from their psychiatric symptoms or due to cognitive impairments. Involvement with substance abuse peer groups may also be less stigmatizing than involvement with psychiatric patients.

Psychotic patients appear to be more sensitive to drug and alcohol use—smaller amounts destabilize them. Furthermore, individuals with psychotic illness may suffer greater consequences of substance misuse such as more frequent hospitalization and difficulties finding a place within separate treatment systems for dealing with the two disorders.

Accepting responsibility for this group of patients within one treatment team offers more promise. Most substance abuse treatments can be incorporated into assertive outreach with appropriate training and commitment. These include harm minimization strategies, relapse prevention strategies, housing protection, motivational interviewing, individual counselling, practical assistance, pharmacological treatment of withdrawal, and family work. This is a difficult task and means coping with often contrasting models. Many mental health workers think of psychosis as beyond an individual's control, but substance abuse a foolish exercise of free choice. Such a simplified dichotomy has to be abandoned in this work.

We should, however, be cautious about assuming that substance abuse interventions are unambiguous, evidence-based strategies with a high success rate. Real life is more complex and many of our patients have established freely chosen patterns of drug or alcohol use for which they do not want our help—however much hardship and conflict arises from their use. We have a responsibility to offer help and to seek out both practical and more sophisticated interventions.

It may be the willingness of assertive outreach teams to accept these patients (who are otherwise all too easy to exclude from services) for comprehensive, routine care that makes the most difference.

Chapter 20

Personal finance

Introduction

Many patients with severe and persistent mental illness will identify money as their main problem in surviving in the community. If the key worker and team can help with this problem, then they have a head start. It is an invaluable engagement tool, as well as ensuring the patient can survive outside hospital.

In assertive outreach one soon recognizes that financial crises are a frequent cause in themselves for patients to self-present at hospital, or that the stress they impose increases the risk of relapse. We neglect finances at our peril. Do not assume that because the patient has not informed you of any problems, that they are receiving their full benefit entitlement or that the rent or electricity is being paid. Look out for unopened brown envelopes by the door and make sensitive enquiries—especially with patients with a history of neglecting to pay bills or to reapply for benefits.

Much of a case manager's time will be spent assisting and advocating for patients' personal finance. High rates of unemployment, due to the disruptive effects of frequent illness and hospitalization, limit independent means of support. Complex, frequently revised, and often bewildering rules for eligibility and applications for welfare benefits require intervention or advocacy for even the most able of our patients.

This chapter will describe the broad sweep of benefits, other sources of help, and practical interventions to protect community tenure and entitlement. Because of national specificities and frequent amendments to state benefits we will not attempt to describe the fine detail, apart from some detailed discussion about one UK benefit, disability living allowance. This has made a huge impact on the financial status of many patients with severe mental illness.

State welfare benefits

The state offers financial protection for people because of either low income (means-tested) or against specific criteria such as disability, maternity, age, and/or previous contributions through taxation (non-means-tested).

Means-tested benefits

Means-tested benefits are designed to ensure an individual's or family's income does not fall below the poverty line. Income support and housing benefit are both means-tested.

When applying you are required to declare savings and any other income. Depending on this assessment, payment can be either a 'top up' or meet the entire cost of living or rent. The following examples from England and Wales indicate the complexity:

- If a person is on a low income with savings below a set limit, and is working less than 16 hours per week or not working, they may be entitled to either **income support** or income-based **jobseeker's allowance**. For our patients who are not working because of sickness or disability, they will be able to claim income support. If, however, they or their partner works 16 hours or more per week, they may be entitled to **working families' tax credit** or **disabled person's tax credit**. For working patients or those who have been off work due to sickness or disability and are returning to work on lower earnings, they may be entitled to disabled person's tax credit providing they have been getting a benefit for sickness or disability.

- For those on a low income with savings below a set limit (whether or not they are working) who pay rent and council tax, applications for **housing** and **council tax benefit** should be made. This may help pay all or part of their rent and tax.

- The **social fund** is a system of loans and **community care grants** aimed at helping people on low incomes stay in, or return to, community living. The social fund helps people in need with certain important expenses. Applications to the social fund are decided in different ways, depending on the type of payment.

- Payments for maternity, funerals, and heating in cold weather are made automatically if a person meets the entitlement conditions. Eligibility for discretionary social fund payments, however, will depend on the priority of the person's need and whether that level of priority can be met from the local office's budget. Discretionary social fund payments are community care grants and **crisis loans**.

- Community care grants are aimed at people on income support who require money to either prevent a return to institutional care or who will be leaving institutional care within the next six weeks and require money to establish themselves in the community. These grants are means-tested in that they will not be paid to people with even modest capital.

- Where grants are refused, a **budgeting loan** may be offered. These will then be repaid in instalments from the person's benefits.

- Etc . . . etc!

Community care grants are a vital resource since they are for people at risk of readmission to hospital or patients being resettled from hospital. These grants can be used to buy beds, cooking utensils, domestic appliances, and so forth. For patients who have difficulty managing their finances (or who might spend the money on alternatives), it is often possible to get the cheque sent directly to the team. The key worker can then accompany the patient when buying the proposed items and help him or her to get them back to the flat.

The difficulty with community care grants is their discretionary nature. Patients may not make repeat applications within a set time period and local benefits offices have a limited budget for these claims. If the budget is low, even the most worthy claims may not be met.

The role of the key worker is to make as good a case as possible, ensuring that the items relate to the conditions (i.e. resettlement or exceptional difficulties which might lead to hospitalization). Most patients will be offered a budgeting loan from the social fund. However, this must be weighed against the weekly deductions from their benefit and their ability to afford this. Some loans take many months to pay off.

Whereas budgeting loans and community care grants take at least ten days to process, crisis loans can be paid quickly and often collected at the local office the same day. It is best to go to the local office with the patient and explain the nature of the crisis and fill in the form. The patient will require acceptable identification. Crisis loans can be applied for if money has been lost, stolen, or gone missing in the post or if they are waiting for a claim to be processed.

Non-means-tested benefits: disability living allowance

Most non-means-tested benefits (such as sickness, maternity, or disability benefits) are designed to compensate individuals for an inability to work. In England and Wales, incapacity benefit is a contributory non-means-tested benefit for people unemployed through long-term illness and who have a history of working and paying national insurance contributions. Perhaps the most important non-contributory and non-means-tested benefit for patients likely to be treated by outreach workers in the UK is disability living allowance (DLA).

DLA has made a tremendous difference to people living with long-term physical and psychiatric disability since its introduction in 1992. Familiarity and expertise with the application form and eligibility criteria are essential. To claim DLA for psychiatric disability you must be:

- Under 65.
- Unable to work due to mental health problems for the last three months.
- Expect that these problems will continue for at least the next six months.

The form is predominantly designed with physical disability in mind and many patients will be put off by questions like 'are you able to move around in the house or outdoors?' or 'how far can you walk?'. It is important to reassure patients that 'difficulty going outdoors alone' may be because you need prompting to do things due to poor motivation, you need support because of anxiety and poor social and daily living skills, or because you might get distracted by voices, feel paranoid, or get lost. It does not only relate to arthritis or heart failure! The form covers aspects of daily activities such as:

- Ability to take medication.
- Ability to stay safe and to know when the condition is getting worse.
- Preparing and cooking a main meal.
- Washing, dressing, and looking after your appearance.
- Getting out of bed.
- Social and leisure activities.

Payments for DLA are made up of assessed need in two categories: first, the need for personal care; second, the need for help with mobility.

DLA focuses on a person's requirement for assistance in performing the activities outlined above. The purpose of DLA is that extra money will compensate for these difficulties by allowing patients to pay for assistance in the form of nursing care, meals on wheels, take-away food, taxies, and so on. In reality, most psychiatric patients do not use their money directly for these purposes—though we did have one patient who placed an advert for someone to watch over her and keep her company through sleepless nights. Help with psychiatric problems for DLA purposes may comprise:

- Prompting and reminding.
- Accompanying a patient to an activity or place.
- Supervision to ensure the patient remains safe or takes prescribed treatment.
- Emotional support.
- Practical help with shopping, eating, paying bills, reading mail, etc.

The forms ask how many days a week and for how long each day help is needed with a particular activity. This can be very difficult to quantify. Generally speaking, the more often you need help (and especially if you need help day and night), the higher the rate awarded.

DLA is discretionary and assessed by civil servants who may know almost nothing about psychiatric disability. The clearer the case you can make, the easier it will be. The form does ask that descriptions are made in the patient's own words. The key worker should add more technical supporting information on a separate sheet of headed paper. It is worth spending some time on this, emphasizing that this patient has been referred specifically because of their high level of needs, frequent hospital admissions, poor compliance with medication, etc.

DLA can be awarded at three different levels for personal care and for mobility:

Lower-rate care and/or mobility
- Inability to cook and prepare a main meal through disability may qualify for lower-rate care. Lower-rate mobility may be awarded if supervision and support are needed when the patient is out of the house. If help is needed with both of these, both payments can be made.

Middle-rate care and/or mobility
- Awarded for more global deficits.

Higher-rate care and/or mobility
- Seldom awarded to patients able to live in the community. Intended for those who need almost constant supervision, day and night.

In practice, most patient of specialized assertive outreach teams get DLA at middle-rate care and lower-rate mobility. This reflects the targeted group of patients with relatively severe illness but who can live in the community with support.

Benefits for carers

Caring for a friend or family member with severe mental illness clearly has financial costs, not least in reduced hours in paid employment. The state recognizes this with benefits aimed at carers. Carers also provide a valuable service, which would otherwise cost the state many times what they may claim in benefits.

In the UK, carers who look after an individual for at least 35 hours a week may be entitled to **invalid care allowance** if the person they care for is entitled to DLA or attendance allowance. The carer must not be earning more than a set amount. They should also be aware that receiving invalid care allowance can affect the amount of any income support, housing benefit, or council tax benefit the person they care for receives.

Local sources of income and help

Despite the plethora of state benefits, they are inflexible and often paid infrequently. DLA is paid monthly, and budgeting across a long period can prove difficult for many patients. Teams need ready access to a small fund of money to help patients out in difficult situations, as well as to provide for cinema trips or meals as part of the engagement process. We have also used team finances to pay for a patient's dog to be boarded in kennels whilst he was in hospital. We have undertaken with a local day centre that certain patients from our team, who cannot pay for meals, will still get them, and the team will be invoiced periodically. This money can be reclaimed easily if the patient is subject to appointeeship.

Our knowledge of other external sources of financial assistance will help patients both to survive and to have a better quality of life. Examples are disabled travel permits, holiday grants from charities, and voluntary organizations able to give and deliver furniture at minimal or no cost. Many leisure centres and cinemas give concessionary rates at off-peak times to people on benefits. Knowledge of such local resources should be shared with the team. Constructing a resource file at the team base containing charities' digests and information on local organizations and funds is a valuable investment of time.

Helping patients to manage their own money

In keeping with a comprehensive model of assertive outreach, the key worker is often directly involved in giving advice and practical help in personal finances to patients. Along with relatives and carers, they are in the best position to know the needs and circumstances. Referral to welfare rights can represent a fragmentation of the service for those patients who will find negotiating the system difficult. The key worker must, however, be aware of their limitations and, where there is a possibility of the wrong advice being given, they should update themselves before simply passing the case to a welfare rights' organization.

Whilst the team may nominate a specialist to keep up to date in welfare benefits and charitable sources, the responsibility for helping patients to fill in application forms and phone benefits agencies lies with the key worker or person allocated to visit. This is so, regardless of professional background or training. As many benefit applications and appeals are tedious, complicated, and protracted, we have found that the key worker, rather than a whole team approach, works best. Initiative, continuity, and accountability could be compromised if this activity was shared.

The twin aims of rehabilitation and training in community daily living skills mean that, where possible, we should encourage patients to fill in their own benefits forms and give support, and advice. Even if the patient just fills in their name, address, date of birth, and personal details, this is preferable to the patient just handing you every brown envelope that comes through their door, unopened, for you to deal with. Spend time going through letters with patients so that they come to understand, and be less scared of, the jargon used. Similarly, teaching people how to communicate with the benefits agency over the telephone and accompanying them to the benefits office to show them how to apply for a crisis loan in person, enhances survival skills and encourages growth and responsibility.

Budgeting

Help with budgeting is a common and helpful intervention. Few patients, however, will be receptive to written budgets involving excessive calculations. Making the complexity of financial management easy by reducing budgeting down to a set amount to spend on a daily basis can be helpful. For example, if a patient's total disposable weekly income is £120, they can afford to spend £17 per day. A written daily or weekly shopping list may be of more value than a written budget, in monetary terms. Daily disposable income can be broken down further to represent one packet of cigarettes, one take-away meal, purchase of bread and milk, and money towards weekly toiletries and clothing or luxuries.

In vivo daily living skills' training (see Chapter 24) is the most effective way to teach daily money management. This involves accompanying the patient to their local shops and advising them on how to solve the problem of buying necessities from a limited budget. Staple food items and the use of appropriate shops make the money go further. The patient should be encouraged to prioritize and delay gratification for some items. For example, although a patient may want a mobile phone, it may not be possible to get it from one weeks' money and still have money for food. Spreading the cost over several weeks and, for instance, suggesting they buy a 'pay as you go' phone will ensure that crises over bills and food are less likely to occur.

Helping the patient to set up standing orders for any rent or bills means they only need to manage disposable income. Problems arise for patients without bank accounts where benefits are paid in the form of a giro or order book. This means outgoings such as rent and bills have to be paid manually and that money is left over in order to do this. Banks will often refuse to allow people on benefits to open accounts. Building societies, however, are much more accommodating and often have current accounts so that standing orders and direct debits can be set up to ensure regular outgoings are paid. It is possible to have money deducted and redirected at source from people's benefits. This is often done by housing departments for rent arrears.

Another good reason to encourage and assist patients to have benefits paid directly into a bank account is because it avoids the possibility of order books or giros being stolen, lost, or going missing in the post. Lost order books are not easy to replace and require explanations and further form filling.

Patients who continue to use an order book can purchase savings stamps for television licences, gas bills, and so on, at the post office when they get their money. Gas and electricity can be paid for on a 'pay as you go' basis through key and card-based meters. This system avoids arrears but may also leave patients without necessary utilities at times.

Debt

One or two debts for overdue utility bills are not uncommon and can generally be dealt with by asking the company to accept payment by instalments. Banks and companies operate confidentiality policies for personal finances. The company will generally ask for written requests for payment by instalments signed by the patient, and often a letter from the patient authorising the company to discuss details with the key worker, before they will even consider the matter.

Multiple and more complicated debts will require an intervention plan. The following checklist is suggested by Letts (1998):

- ◆ Check that the money is really owed and the amounts correct. Was there a valid contract? If the patient was clearly mentally ill and the creditor aware of their incapacity to understand the transaction, then there is no binding contract and the debt cannot be enforced. For example, a manic patient displaying multiple bizarre behaviours and delusions orders a wedding dress and a pram from a department store.

- Contact the creditors and explain the situation. Do this before the debt is passed on to bailiffs if possible.
- Collect details of all the debts. Has the patient started the process of paying any of them?
- Work out the priority for dealing with each debt. Where creditors have started legal proceedings, these will need rapid attention. If a notice of eviction or seeking possession has been served for rent arrears, then the consequences of failing to resolve this situation will be drastic.
- Investigate sources of income. Is the patient getting maximum benefits? Will family members help out? Can bids to charities be made?
- Work out the payment proposals, ensuring they are affordable by offering payment over time. It may be possible to defer payments without incurring interest.
- Finally, whatever arrangement is reached, make sure the patient keeps up the regular payments.

(Adapted from Letts, 1998)

Appealing against a decision

If you think that any decision by the benefits agency is wrong (e.g. your patient has been turned down for a community care grant or has been awarded too low a rate), you can appeal. However, you must do so within a set time period, usually one month. And remember, an appeal against a DLA rate runs the risk of the rate being revised downwards as well as upwards! It is generally possible to ask the agency for detailed reasons for their decision. You can then submit evidence challenging these reasons.

DLA appeals can be either by oral hearing or written submission. The chances of success are greater with an oral hearing (especially if the patient takes their key worker or a relative as their representative)—but they are stressful and formal.

Hospital downrating

One impact of hospital admission is that state benefits will be reduced after four or six weeks (dependent on the benefit), because patients' living needs are deemed to be met, in part, by the hospital. The patient is responsible for informing the benefits agency about admissions and discharges, but they often forget and are still paid at the lower rate after discharge. It is possible to have the unpaid benefit backdated by supplying written confirmation of admission and discharge dates. A patient who is on leave from hospital is entitled to the full rate, and again leave dates must be given to the benefits agency for the full payment to be activated.

Fraud

Benefits agencies take a tough line on fraud, which can easily be committed unintentionally by our patients. Failing to tell them that you are in hospital, failing to declare other income for means-tested benefits, and, especially, working whilst claiming benefits all constitute fraud. In general, we will advise a patient on their obligations when it becomes apparent that they have not fully informed the benefits agency of their activities. We will also advise them of the legitimate methods of returning to work and ways of preserving their benefits such as therapeutic earnings (Chapter 23). They must also be advised that they run the risk of losing their benefit altogether if they deliberately mislead officials.

It can be tempting to turn a blind eye to benefit fraud—after all, our patients are often poor and disadvantaged—and some case managers have even described it as an aspect of advocacy. It is risky for the patient and risky for the therapeutic relationship (which only flourishes in conditions of honesty and trust). Whilst we do not actively report on our patients' exploitation of the benefits system, we do make it clear that we will not collude. At times this has created tension but, usually, in the long term, we have been able to work through this, very much like the process of accepting differences about sectioning.

Case study

Roger started working casually for a bicycle courier company. He did not declare his income or work to the benefits agency and continued claiming both income support and DLA. Roger received middle-rate care and lower-rate mobility DLA.

He informed his key worker of what he was doing and asked his advice. Roger was advised that he should declare the small amount of income and that this would be deducted from his income support. He was also advised that the nature of his work was in conflict with his claim for DLA. Whilst we might assist him with therapeutic earnings in a more sedentary job, it would be very difficult to justify supporting his continued mobility claim for DLA with the courier job! If he wished to pursue this job he would have to earn enough money to effectively replace the benefits. Furthermore, any subsequent claim for DLA, if he lost the job, would be jeopardized.

Eventually, the benefits agency found out about his earnings and his benefits were stopped. Roger then asked his key worker to write supporting letters asking for the benefits to be reinstated, saying that the work had only been voluntary. We had to say to Roger that we could not write letters that were not factual. Once Roger gave up the courier job, we did assist him in getting his benefits reinstated.

Managing other people's money

Appointeeship

Where a patient is mentally incapable of managing their own affairs, another person can become their appointee for the purposes of their state welfare benefits. The appointee can make claims, collect or receive payments, and spend the money on behalf of the patient. This person can be a relative, friend, hospital or local authority administrator, or nursing home manager. In our locality, the local authority administers the appointee arrangement and the patient's key worker liaises closely with the appointee to request money or make adjustments as circumstances change.

The appointee is responsible for paying rent and bills, collecting benefits, informing the benefits agency of changes, and for allocating spending money to the patient. The appointee role is quite time-consuming and involves setting up bank accounts and standing orders. It may be easier if the appointee and key worker are different people, as conflicts inevitably arise over the withholding of spending money.

The advantages of appointeeship are considerable, not least that it ensures financial and housing stability. The removal of these two potential sources of crisis and stress allow the key worker and patient to concentrate on finer points which make life more satisfying. Patients subject to appointeeship often build up savings which can be used periodically for holidays, televisions, and other luxuries. On a more prosaic note, appointeeship can be used to restrict access to income that would be spent on harmful drug or alcohol use.

Powers of attorney

The powers of attorney extend beyond the management of state benefits. This is a legal intervention, appointing another person (the attorney) to act in respect to property and financial affairs. It can be general or limited to certain aspects. The patient must be capable of understanding the consequences of delegating these tasks, even if they may not be capable of performing them themselves. In short, a power of attorney cannot be made by a patient incapable of understanding what they are doing.

Court of Protection

The Court of Protection is for people deemed mentally incapable of managing their financial affairs. As an office of the Supreme Court, it is a real court, capable of resolving legal disputes. The court must be satisfied, by medical evidence, of mental incapacity and that appointeeship or powers of attorney are not sufficient or possible. The court can authorize someone to look after property, financial affairs, and the day-to-day needs of the patient and their dependents. Applying to the Court of Protection is a protracted and expensive process and seldom used in adult mental health. More often it is restricted to elderly persons with assets.

Conclusions

Helping patients with their finances is a vital part of our job. Nothing is as important to most of our patients as their money. Most patients do not have savings to fall back on when claims are delayed or giros go missing. The most important piece of advice, when dealing with the benefits agency, is to always keep copies of correspondence and to always ask for the name of the person that you are speaking with. Files and claims go missing with alarming regularity and promises of action often fail to materialize. Likewise, if you tell the patient that you will contact the benefits agency for them, or post a letter, do not forget.

Whatever a patient's source of income, teaching them more effective budgeting skills will be a worthwhile investment. Clearly, we all learn from our mistakes, and we must not be over-prescriptive in a person's personal financial choices. We do have a duty, however, to ensure that, as far as possible, major arrears and debts do not occur through simple neglect. Having access to some regular, disposable income is an essential component of anyone's quality of life. Our patients usually have precious little. So, the more we can increase it and help them to manage it, the more we improve their lot.

Chapter 21

Housing and homelessness

Without affordable housing for the mentally ill we have little foundation for care in the community. Yet housing, or the lack of it, is a source of frustration to professionals working in the field of mental health and contributes to the debate about shortcomings in this policy. In the past, the responsibility for seeking out this scarce resource lay with social workers and local authority departments. Nowadays, this is seldom the case, and generic working means that regardless of our profession we need to assist our patients when they find themselves in a housing crisis. Housing is high on the patient's agenda, and also because homelessness causes major difficulties, frequently leading to admission. These may have to be extensively prolonged despite patients being clinically ready to leave hospital.

Incidence of homelessness among the mentally ill population

The prevalence of homeless mentally ill people is highly political and figures quoted by the media and lobby groups should be judged sceptically. The Mental Health Foundation (1996) states that among homeless people, 30–40% have a mental health problem (though this includes substance abuse, depression, experience of child abuse, and other situational disorders). The same paper estimates that 8% of homeless hostel residents have a psychotic illness and estimates a 25% prevalence of schizophrenia among homeless people.

It is a myth that the closure of psychiatric institutions has dumped long-stay psychiatric patients on the street. Although many people sleeping on the streets have mental health problems, they are not a consequence of the closure of long-stay psychiatric hospitals (Leff 1993). An Audit Commission report has suggested that the problem relates to a combination of the decline in acute psychiatric beds, agencies failing to work together, and community mental health services failing to provide adequate support (Audit Commission 1994). A study by Bines (1994) found that 28% of homeless single people living in hostels and bed and breakfast accommodation reported mental health problems. These were overwhelmingly male. High figures of self-reported mental health problems were also found in day centres for the homeless (36%) and at soup runs (40%). These figures are surprisingly similar to those reported from Edinburgh in the 1960s and Chicago in the 1930s—long before community care initiatives.

A census of patients occupying adult acute and low-level secure psychiatric beds in London in 1994 (Koffman and Fulop 1999) recorded 20.5% (817) as homeless. Of these, 306 were identified by ward staff as inappropriately located, of whom 52% were suitable for discharge, and the majority required housing in their 'package of care'. The other 48% needed regular health input but not on an acute ward.

Types of housing and residential provision

Assertive outreach teams generally work with patients living in independent accommodation. Indeed, the rationale for assertive outreach is partly to provide that extra input to enable people to survive in their own homes. If a patient is referred to us who is living in staffed residential accommodation, we generally do not take them on. This is simply because the majority of their needs should be met through the hostel staff. In effect, they are already receiving an intensive service from the hostel and the likelihood of assertive outreach being able to provide added benefit and value is small. This rationale is stated in our operational policy and guidelines for referrers.

There are, however, different levels of staffed residential provision. A 24-hour staffed hostel certainly should be capable of meeting patients' daily needs. A hostel with a non-specialist peripatetic worker, who calls in every few days, will probably not manage a severely ill and unstable resident. Such a patient, living in a very low-input hostel, as are often provided by the voluntary sector, would not be excluded from assertive outreach. Similarly, patients who we place permanently in high-input, staffed accommodation are discharged from assertive outreach after a 'step-down' and settling in period. This usually takes about six months. The types of accommodation shown in Fig. 21.1 are arranged in a hierarchy according to input and intensity of the residential care provided on site.

Assertive outreach would concern itself with patients living in levels one and two in this hierarchy. Patients living at level three may be considered if the residential input was by untrained, non-specialist staff and the patient had wide-ranging needs. This emphasis on independent accommodation is one of the defining characteristics that differentiates assertive outreach from rehabilitation services. Rehabilitation services provide long-term 'hospital hostel' accommodation and group homes for more chronically disabled patients. We have an agreement that patients who require intensive support but who live in, or require such staffed residential care, would be referred to our rehabilitation service.

Independent accommodation

In terms of patient choice, self-determination, empowerment, and our model of care, ordinary, mainstream housing is the ideal for most patients. In the UK, decent, appropriate, and affordable housing is a scarce resource even for the working population. Increasingly, local government has become reluctant to be directly involved in housing and the 'right to buy' policy resulted in the sale of a large proportion of state-owned social housing to tenants in the 1980s. At the same time, successive governments have sought to promote housing associations as alternative major providers of social housing. All local authorities are required to operate a housing register through which

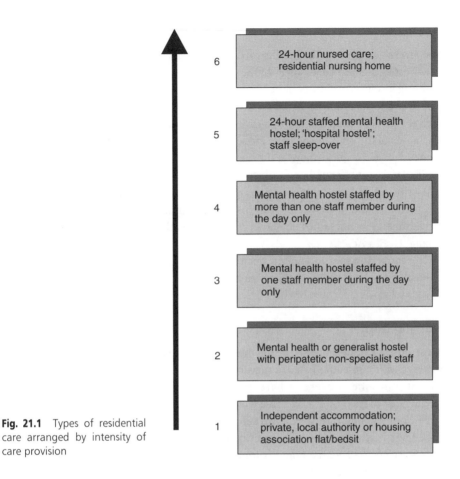

6 — 24-hour nursed care;
residential nursing home

5 — 24-hour staffed mental health
hostel; 'hospital hostel';
staff sleep-over

4 — Mental health hostel staffed by
more than one staff member during
the day only

3 — Mental health hostel staffed by
one staff member during the day
only

2 — Mental health or generalist hostel
with peripatetic non-specialist staff

1 — Independent accommodation;
private, local authority or housing
association flat/bedsit

Fig. 21.1 Types of residential care arranged by intensity of care provision

social housing is allocated. They must give priority to certain categories of people, including people with mental health problems, if they require settled accommodation on welfare or medical grounds.

Nevertheless, the process is not quick. In our locality it takes up to a year from application to an offer being made. Fortunately, applying is relatively simple and key workers nominate patients and complete application forms, detailing the patient's preferences and needs. For example, if a patient needs to be in a certain area to be close to family supports or cannot negotiate stairs, this can be stated. Details can be passed to housing associations and offers made through them. Housing associations generally buy up large properties and convert them into flats for social housing. Often these can be rather grand houses in nice areas and many patients see these flats as preferable to 'council' high-rise or estate properties. Single people generally get offered a bedsit or studio flat.

Patients who are dissatisfied with their accommodation can apply for transfers through mutual exchange schemes with local councils.

Hostels

The level of care offered by hostels varies considerably, as does the range of providers. Few hostels are provided solely by health services, except in rehabilitation services. Housing is a local authority obligation in the UK and many mental health hostels are run by the local authority social service departments or by the voluntary sector. This means that hostels are staffed by residential social workers or by non-specialist staff. The needs of the severely mentally are sometimes not well understood and hostels have tended to 'cherry pick' more stable and co-operative residents. Substance abuse, in particular, is not tolerated or addressed in many hostels.

A criticism of hospital hostels run by health care staff (usually nurses) is that they can become 'mini' institutions, with institutional practices transferred from the ward. An advantage of these hostels, however, is that patients can be detained under the Mental Health Act.

The move towards integrated health and social care agencies will mean greater co-ordination and sensitivity of provision for local mental health needs. There are already hostels set up as a partnership between the local health trust and local authority.

Nursing homes

Most nursing homes are set up to meet the long-term needs of elderly and infirm patients with dementia. Few are registered to take patients under the age of 65. Our patients can suffer a stroke or have nursing care needs (such as dressing, bathing, or feeding due to frailty) beyond those which can be met in a mental health hostel.

24-hour nursing care is expensive and if the local authority is to pay for this care then there is usually a lengthy application and assessment process. This process can only start once a suitable home is found. Local authorities keep lists of care homes registered for mental health and for under 65-year-olds. It is then a case of arranging a visit to such a home with the patient.

Patients in this situation can easily remain on an acute ward for extended periods. A full package of home care, meals on wheels, district nurses, and daily visits can be attempted if the patient retains some mobility or has family support. One alternative for less frail elderly patients is sheltered accommodation. These are independent flats with warden supervision and alarms.

Emergency accommodation

Housing crises are common with patients referred to assertive outreach. Knowledge of immediate resources for the homeless patient, in the form of bed and breakfast accommodation or night shelters, is essential. The use of these resources is a last resort and proper risk assessment is a prerequisite. Short-term bed and breakfast can be arranged in a day. If a patient is unintentially homeless, the local authority homeless persons' unit may agree to place them. They will not place patients who they deem to have made themselves intentionally homeless through eviction for rent arrears. Neither will they place patients with more severe support needs under specialist care. They regard these patients as the responsibility of the mental health social work department and look to them for both funding and placement.

Patients can self-refer to a homeless persons' night shelter. These are usually run by charities and offer dormitory-style accommodation for those sleeping rough. They tend to be rather intimidating places and our experience is that patients often get exploited or assaulted. Most large cities run a homeless persons' telephone line which offers information, on a daily basis, on available night shelter places.

Team approaches

Craig (Craig and Timms 1992) consider that many homeless people with persisting mental health problems have been lost to psychiatric care. Many find themselves home-less as a result of their symptoms and behaviour, eviction for rent arrears, substance abuse, self-neglect, or by persistent, active choice. The impact of services in helping the patient who is engaged to maintain optimal health, finances, and social functioning is then the focus of care. Much can be achieved by retaining people in contact with spe-cialist services and by engagement in assertive outreach.

Lehman *et al.* (1999) demonstrated that the ACT case management model with home-less persons with serious mental illness in Baltimore, Maryland, was both clinically effective and cost effective in promoting stable housing and reducing in-patient and emergency room utilization. ACT patients spent 31% more days in stable housing. In a review by Mueser *et al.* (1998) of ACT and intensive case management, 9 out of 12 studies showed significant improvements in housing stability.

Dual diagnosis patients are highly likely to become homeless, often because their substance abuse results in disruptive behaviour, loss of social support, and financial problems (Drake *et al.* 1997). Drake describes an integrated case management team for dual diagnosis homeless patients with severe mental illness in Washington DC. Over a 18-month period, the integrated treatment group had fewer institutional days and more days in stable housing and made more progress toward recovery from substance abuse than a comparison standard treatment group. Drake suggests that integration of mental health, substance abuse, and housing services within a single clinical team, staffed by mental health professionals, is the important factor for this patient group.

Closer to home, the Nottingham Dispersed Intensively Supported Housing (DISH) Scheme is described in *Keys to engagement* (Sainsbury Centre for Mental Health 1998). Essentially a strengths' approach case management team, DISH worked with severely mentally ill patients, providing accommodation in council or housing association flats for about 50% of its case load. DISH was able to engage patients well by directly offering the housing. It is an excellent example of co-operation between housing departments, housing associations, and health services, effectively giving nomination rights to their flats to DISH.

Another variation is the 'crash pad'. The team rents a flat and agrees with the agency that patients in urgent housing need can be temporarily placed there while more permanent accommodation is arranged. In this alternative to bed and breakfast accommodation, the team have keys and daily access to the flat in order to provide intensive support. We have tried to establish a crash pad for our team through a local housing association but, surprisingly, it is the inflexibility of the association and not health department bureaucracy that has held up this development.

It would seem that fidelity to the model, assertive engagement, and the availability of substance abuse interventions are particularly relevant to helping patients to keep their home. Lehman (Lehman *et al.* 1997, 1999) suggests that well-functioning assertive outreach teams, with continuity of care, shift the emphasis away from crisis resolution towards therapeutic interventions with the homeless and dually diagnosed. He suggests this high-risk group should be a priority for assertive outreach teams.

Individual interventions

The advantage of flexible assertive outreach is that the intensity of care delivered in the patient's own home can be stepped up at times of need, rather than the patient having to move to different locations and levels of care as described above. Assertive outreach is not only an alternative to hospital admission, it also reduces the need for other institutional residential services. The UK700 study (UK700 Group: Burns *et al.* 1999*b*) demonstrated that utilization of costed services such as home care and meals on wheels is reduced in intensive care, compared to usual care.

Key workers give practical help to assist patients in shopping, cooking, and cleaning. We do have patients who receive regular home care due to severe motivational, physical, or behavioural difficulties but we try not to lose entirely the emphasis on rehabilitation and acceptance of some responsibility. We have seen that continued engagement and symptom management help preserve tenancies in ordinary housing, as does substance abuse intervention.

The value of home-based interventions and assessment and frequent home visits means that housing difficulties come to light quickly. Many difficulties are financial and are dealt with in Chapter 20. Other difficulties are repairs and faults. Broken windows and faulty or insecure door locks require prompt attention. We will generally attempt to repair locks if there is likely to be unreasonable delay. Light bulbs and curtains can also easily be replaced and repaired by the key worker prompting and working with the patient. Patients often ask for help with redecorating and, in terms of engagement, setting aside time to do some repainting with a patient is time well spent. We do have an ACT tool kit with basic tools such as drills and screwdrivers. We also have an ACT Hoover that we can loan to patients.

It is worth getting to know the housing officer in the housing association or council who deals with your particular housing area. Explanation of the patient's circumstances usually produces a more sympathetic or rapid response.

Furniture schemes are a good resource for cheap second-hand furniture. The Wandsworth Housing Support Project provides cheap starter packs for single people, to aid resettlement. For a patient moving out of hospital or bed and breakfast accommodation into their own flat a starter pack includes a second-hand bed, cooker, fridge, chair, etc. Furniture is donated, then collected and delivered by volunteers to the patient. Many such schemes exist across the country to put unwanted furniture to good use. Chapter 20 describes the process for applying for a community care grant to facilitate resettlement.

Case study

Tony had lived in a succession of hostels and temporary accommodation since the break up of his marriage. His wife had no longer been able to put up with his increasingly unstable mental state and manic episodes, during which he would drink and sing Elvis songs all night. He was 50, and had had a traditional marriage where he was unaccustomed to cooking, paying bills, or looking after himself. Having lived in a family home for most of his life he could not settle in a hostel and became demotivated and depressed. As his mental health became more stable he started asking for independent accommodation. At the time of referral to the assertive outreach team he was within a few months of being offered his own flat. His previous key worker had made the application to the mental health housing register.

An assessment of, amongst other things, daily living skills and finances, was made in readiness for the resettlement. Tony was motivated to move but knew little about the practicalities of running a home. He had done some preparatory work with the hostel staff—learning to iron, shop, and cook basic meals. Since the hostel did not allow drinking on the premises and most of his money went in contributions to the rent, he seldom drank but was looking forward to having more money and being able to drink at home. Tony was advised to try and save some money in the intervening weeks for moving expenses and in anticipation that his benefits would be disrupted with changes in address and circumstances.

Once the offer was made, Tony and his key worker went to view the flat. Some minor repairs were needed and these were arranged before the move date. A community care grant was applied for and a starter pack from the housing project obtained so that he had a bed and a cooker from day one. On the day he moved in, he was assisted in contacting the benefits agency to notify them of his new address. An application for housing benefit was also made.

Over subsequent visits Tony was introduced to local shops and facilities, whilst basic plans were agreed for weekly expenditure and shopping lists. His key worker helped him to put up curtains and pictures. Both Tony and his key worker spent time trying to work out the complicated key-meter system for the electricity and where to charge up the key. He was registered with a local GP that the team knew had a good understanding of mental health problems.

Tony enjoyed having his own place and his self-esteem improved. He tended to eat out more than cook, and kept the flat in a reasonable condition. He did get drunk occasionally but it did not lead to a more unstable mental state or any behavioural disturbance for the neighbours.

Conclusions

Most people consider moving house a stressful event. Homelessness is more stressful. Stable and secure housing really is a basic need. Morgan (1993) outlines how the stress-vulnerability and social-drift models apply to housing, with unstable housing increasing the stress on vulnerable patients. For psychotic patients, unstable housing is rarely the cause of their illness but can exacerbate arousal and precipitate relapse. Patients with severe mental health problems drift into deprivation and bad housing. Bad housing usually means socially isolating and dangerous estates, inter-tenant disputes, and damp or poor conditions—all with negative consequences for long-term outcomes.

Because assertive outreach employs a direct and comprehensive approach to care, allowing frequent and daily contact, patients can be maintained in their own homes much longer than would otherwise be the case. The root causes and the consequences of bad housing can be tackled in a co-ordinated manner. Problems arise when patients are of 'no fixed abode' and must be placed in whatever hostel or temporary accommodation is available in the locality. This is the traditional brokerage problem of fitting a square peg into a round hole. That is, if there is anywhere available at all! We resist the temptation to place people outside the team's geographical boundary, however temporarily, as flexibility of response and particularly the availability of support may be limited.

Clinical teams that are able to nominate patients directly for housing, such as DISH, are the ideal. We often try and negotiate with housing associations that if one of our patients moves out of a flat, we can move another of our patients in.

Housing is one area of practice which is entirely dependent on local knowledge. There are no structured assessment tools or theoretical models to guide novices. The team as a whole contains much expertise through contacts with bed and breakfast owners, hostel staff, and other patients. Patients will tell you which hostels provide the better service. We stopped using one hostel in the borough, despite a chronic shortage of places, due to poor standards reported by successive patients. The impact of an appropriate housing placement on a patient's satisfaction, well being, and community tenure can be immense. We only wish there was more housing to choose from.

Physical health care

People with severe mental illnesses suffer worse physical health than the general population. They are significantly more likely to die early: the 'standardized mortality' of schizophrenia is 1.6, which means that for any given age, their risk of dying is raised by 60% (Harris and Barraclough 1998). Their overall life expectancy is correspondingly lower than the norm. Some of this increased mortality and lowered life expectancy is due to suicide—but not all. The main causes of this increased mortality are respiratory and cardiovascular deaths. Kendrick (1996) found that a quarter of 101 severely mentally ill patients, studied in 16 general practices, were significantly obese, over half were regular smokers, 11 were hypertensive, 21 had persistent cough or sputum, and 24 suffered shortness of breath! Changes in lifestyle or earlier and better treatment could prevent much of this. Working closely with this patient group means that we need to understand more about why their health is so poor and what we can do about it.

It is not a problem that severely mentally ill patients do not register with a GP or do not visit them: Kendrick's findings related to patients registered with predominantly good practices. The severely mentally ill attend their GP more than the average—about eight contacts a year compared with an average of three for an age-matched control group (Kendrick *et al.* 1994). Most of these appointments are for repeat prescriptions however, rather than specific treatments. We also know that the level of preventive health care (e.g. blood pressure checks, cervical smear, advice on smoking or weight) is very low for individuals with psychosis (Burns and Cohen 1998). These failings of medical care are particularly striking as these individuals are in such regular contact with doctors in both primary and secondary care. There are a number of contributory factors to such poor care.

Help-seeking behaviour

Clinical experience is that individuals with psychoses do not complain about physical illnesses. They appear to tolerate in silence signs and symptoms that would alarm most of us. Why this should be so is unclear, but it is very striking. It is probably one of the reasons the 'annual medical' was a routine in long-stay wards in mental hospitals. Occasionally, patients may tolerate manifestations of diseases for delusional reasons. One of our female patients has refused to have a benign ovarian cyst operated upon because of the belief that she is pregnant. This is rare, however, and the inactivity seems more often to be simply to do with overall self-neglect and shyness in seeking help.

It is easy for us in mental health to forget that, in most medical practice, if the patient does not ask for help, they are assumed to be well. Studies in primary care demonstrate very clearly that consultations are patient-driven. It is the patient who sets the agenda, not the doctor. 'Open-ended' questioning has been strongly promoted as a desirable consulting style. Even in secondary care, where the approach is often more structured, the doctor will not actively pursue the patient if they do not attend for treatment. The responsibility for seeking help is left entirely to the patient, except in the case of mental health and some infectious diseases (e.g. tuberculosis) (Chaulk and Pope 1997; Fujiwara *et al.* 1997) and sexually transmitted diseases (Deren *et al.* 1994).

Failure to register with a GP

The vast majority of severely mentally ill people in the UK are registered with a GP who is responsible for ensuring their general medical care. Nonetheless, the rate of non-registration is higher than for the general population and for a number of reasons. Frequent geographical mobility is common in the mentally ill—they drift around, particularly within cities. This makes remaining registered very difficult. They may also fall out with their GP and be removed from the list. Although there are mechanisms for allocating a new GP, this relies on the patient pursuing the issue. The most important reason for non-registration is that they simply cannot be bothered, either because they do not see the point or because of the inertia and apathy that can be part of their disorder. They also lack many of the social prompts which bind adults to their GPs (e.g. getting insurance medicals, taking the children for vaccinations). Given the high rate of physical ill health that has been shown even in those mentally ill patients with a good GP (Kendrick 1996), being without one is clearly a disaster.

Homeless patients

One group of patients who are rarely registered with a GP are the homeless. These have very significant physical health problems and there are often local initiatives to try and reach them. Many night shelters and drop-in facilities for the homeless and those sleeping rough have clinics providing assessment and treatment by visiting GPs. There are particular problems relating to infectious diseases (e.g. tuberculosis and hepatitis) with this very morbid and disadvantaged group. In assertive outreach teams that target the homeless, trying to get the patient to register with a GP can be one of the most important early interventions. Where this proves impossible, then the use of outreach clinics in shelters or attendance at an A&E department may be the only feasible alternative.

Causes of increased physical ill health

In working with individuals with severe mental illnesses, we therefore need to be alert to the risks of poor physical health and, particularly, untreated problems. Some form of structure helps in assessing the risks and spotting problems. There are generally three main problem areas—although it will be immediately obvious that there is considerable overlap and many causes.

Consequences of self-neglect

The most obvious of these are poor teeth, obesity, and respiratory problems. Many of our patients have very poor dental health simply because they do not brush their teeth. However, good dental hygiene is particularly important in our patient group who are at increased risk of caries because of the dry mouth caused by many of our drugs. This is not just a cosmetic issue—bad teeth can lead to abscesses and pain. They can also add to the social marginalization of our patients if they look off-putting and have foul breath. One of our more rewarding experiences recently was of a man who, after a couple of years coaxing, responded well to clozapine. As a consequence, he allowed us to help him get his massive inguinal hernia repaired and have several months' dental work completed. This has quite transformed his appearance and delighted his long-suffering mother.

Obesity is increasingly common in our patients. Much of it is, of course, because of the drugs we use which increase their appetite. It is also driven by poor eating habits, especially a reliance on fast food in younger patients. In such a deprived group, obesity also can lead to marginalization because clothes do not fit, and self-respect falls even further.

Individuals with psychoses start to smoke as much as the general population. The difference is that a sizeable proportion of adults stop smoking, whereas our patients rarely do. Often their smoking is ignored either because helping them stop is considered too difficult or because there is an unspoken assumption that smoking is trivial compared to their mental illness. There was even a mistaken belief in the past that schizophrenia patients were at lower risk of lung cancer! Cigarettes were also a common currency of social exchange sanctioned by staff, in mental hospitals, in the past. Given the grave health consequences of heavy smoking and the impact of smoking on pharmacokinetics—the fact that smokers need higher drug doses (Taylor 1997)—there is no excuse for ignoring this problem.

Even when conditions have been diagnosed and treatment prescribed, patients may simply not comply. We have experienced the tragic consequences of a relatively young schizophrenic woman who was inconsistent in her compliance with antihypertensives and has now had a series of strokes, leaving her permanently dependent on nursing care in her 30s. Disorders such as diabetes, which require diet or careful management, may be beyond our patients. Unless they are helped, they may suffer excessive complications.

Consequences of treatment

Most psychiatric drugs have side-effects. A dry mouth, increased appetite, and variable degrees of sedation are common. All three contribute to obesity. Patients often drink high-calorie soft drinks because of their dry mouth (which also increases their risk of dental caries), they eat more, and they are more inactive. It is not surprising that they put on weight which is bad for their health and self-esteem. Individual drugs have risks attached to them—the thyroid and renal problems associated with lithium being perhaps the best-known. Tardive dyskinesia is an obvious health consequence of antipsychotic drugs, although we often forget to think of it as such.

Comorbid conditions

Comorbid use of alcohol and drugs is a major cause of poor health in individuals with psychoses and is associated with a range of infections from HIV and hepatitis through to local abscesses from unhygienic syringes. Intoxication is associated also with a raised risk of trauma, whether this is falling down stairs when drunk, getting into a fight in a pub, or being threatened and assaulted by drug dealers when debts have not been paid. Long-term consequences of chronic use, such as neuropathies, cognitive impairment, and deteriorating liver function, are easy to miss. Life-threatening conditions such as delirium tremens or a chest infection presenting with confusion and irritability can be misdiagnosed as relapses of the psychotic disorder. The consequent delay in instituting appropriate treatment increases the risks.

Role of the assertive outreach worker

Most mental health professionals take a holistic and inclusive view of their obligation to their patients. Whether we are social workers, nurses, doctors, psychologists, or occupational therapists, we recognize that if the patient is physically unwell then something must be done about it. Members of assertive outreach teams accept a commitment that stretches beyond their basic professional training. In our team, physical health care is a sizeable component of our work. It is regularly addressed in team reviews and features as an identified need on at least 15–20% of our CPA documents.

Attending appointments

Encouraging patients to attend their GP for routine health care is an essential part of the process. Taking patients to appointments, both with the GP and at the hospital, is often essential. Waiting in out-patients can be a very time-consuming activity, but we regularly do it. The level of support needed to ensure attendance is an individual clinical decision based on how daunting the prospect is, the patient's abilities, and on the strength of the therapeutic relationship. Agreeing to phone on the morning of the appointment may be enough for some. For another patient, a lift to the clinic may be necessary and sufficient. For some, you may have to wait with them. Sometimes workers feel they are being exploited: 'He can perfectly well get the bus there. It's only two stops and he knows the out-patient nurse. Everybody else has to hang around in that clinic for ages.'

We take a soft line generally on this issue of 'dependence' or 'exploitation', giving our patients the benefit of the doubt. We remind ourselves, in team reviews, that they have rarely had the comfort of being able to rely on others as most of us have and do, and that what may seem a fairly straightforward appointment to us may be frightening for them. Waiting rooms, with large groups of people, are nearly always intimidating for anxious or paranoid individuals.

Taking people to hospital appointments also promotes a less professional, more normal interaction. Sitting together, reading a magazine, getting a drink, and so on, are all opportunities to be free of the need to 'treat'. They are greatly appreciated by most patients and very beneficial to engagement.

Monitoring and supporting ongoing treatments

Just as we encourage, monitor, and supervise medicines for the primary psychiatric condition, we see no reason not to help in the same way with physical treatments. Most of our patients need support and supervision for their treatment because they are chaotic and forgetful (Chapter 11), not because there is something special about our psychiatric drugs. If we consider a dosette box necessary for the psychiatric medicines, then it is probably equally necessary for the antihypertensives. Similarly, if we need to visit daily to supervise clozapine administration, then we will supervise administration of glibenclamide.

The principles of encouragement and motivational enhancement transfer equally to other long-term medications. We have two patients with chronic renal failure under our care. For one, we have to supervise all the medicines and often take him, grumbling and resentful, into the hospital for his dialysis. For the other, we encourage her to tolerate what is a demanding regime, but only need accompany her to consultant appointments.

Using the team doctors

Sometimes patients simply will not go to their GP or to hospital for an assessment. It is important to remember that psychiatrists are trained doctors. While consultants may have lost touch with many of their general medical skills, trainee psychiatrists should be able to diagnose and, if necessary, treat most common minor physical disorders. We try and avoid this where possible. Receiving comprehensive health care from a GP is one of the benefits of life in the community that we want to achieve for our patients. It also helps in affirming their normality, reducing stigma and isolation. Emphasizing their common needs reminds all involved (patient, doctor, and the other patients in the waiting room) that the mentally ill are more like the rest of us than they are different. However, we would consider a doctrinaire refusal to treat, say, a chest infection or hypertension in a patient with no GP unacceptable.

Where the patient has a GP but will not go to them it is, of course, essential that the plan of action is agreed. We have rarely found GPs to be resistant to this approach. Where we have had to treat physical health problems directly, patients have usually been very positive. It makes their lives easier and they know that it is not something they would routinely expect from us. They often experience it as us having made a special effort for them.

Problems with providing physical health care directly

Mental health workers often get considerable satisfaction from helping patients with their physical health care—and so they should (in our opinion). There are immediate and obvious benefits to the patient's comfort and quality of life. Family members are often very appreciative and, in a quieter way, so are the patients. There are, however, some problems which need to be thought about. These relate mainly to how to manage the relationship with general health care services but also touch on ethical and professional issues.

Confidentiality

The position of the case manager as advocate and support can be a tricky one. Most clinicians are quite flexible about family members being present during consultations and answer their questions directly. It is surprisingly uncommon for a physician to ask an adult patient if they mind their relative being present—they take the patient's acquiescence as permission. We are much more likely to ask about it in mental health work where family relationships can be very complex.

Where the person attending with the patient is not a family member there does not seem to be any accepted practice. We tend to ask our patients if they want us with them for support. For those who have real difficulties understanding the nature of their physical illnesses and their treatments, we definitely want to be present. We want to know what is involved because we will be responsible for delivering it. We negotiate this with the patient beforehand and explain it to the doctor or nurse they are consulting. Usually it is fine, but sometimes it causes uncertainty and discomfort to which some doctors respond with a dogmatic 'no' and exclude us. We have never found it useful to challenge this. If we cannot be present then we may have to wait for the letter to the GP to find out exactly what is the problem.

Withdrawal of support by primary care

One unwanted effect of intensive community support may be that the primary care team withdraws from engagement with the patient. They may see us as more competent—especially if the patient is very difficult or hostile. Knowing we have general medical skills, they may wish to pass over some of their responsibilities to us. In some cases this is fine, but in others it may be unfair to the patient and to us.

Case study

Ed is a 45-year-old man of Italian extraction who suffers from long-standing paranoid schizophrenia. He has responded well to an atypical antipsychotic and no longer experiences active hallucinations or delusions. He is, however, very isolated and self-neglecting and requires visits on alternate days to ensure his treatment and also to keep his flat acceptable and to 'turf out' local drug addicts who exploit him. His current major problem is that he drinks to excess (his father died of alcoholism) and has developed moderate cognitive impairment and diabetes which he totally neglects. Because we visit him three or four times a week, the local district nurses have refused to visit him and administer his insulin. They insist that as he gets out to buy his vodka, he is not 'housebound' and therefore does not warrant home visits. Since we see him regularly, we have become obliged to manage his insulin, and the district nurses refuse our request that they visit on the three days of the week when we do not. The result is that we now have to visit daily to manage the insulin.

While we were flattered by the GP insisting that without our input this patient would be dead, we are unhappy that he is denied visits from a district nurse. The arguments they present are fairly strong but we remain convinced that had this man less support from us he would, in truth, be getting more appropriate support from primary care. The reality, of course, is that we will simply have to accept the responsibility. We cannot visit him and manage his antipsychotics and insulin one day, knowing that he will not take his injection the next.

Ethical dilemmas over compulsion

The UK Mental Health Act allows us to compel someone to have treatment for their mental illness but gives no authority whatsoever to compel treatment for a physical condition. Knowing this does not necessarily make it easy to work with a patient who is neglecting their physical health. It can be one of the most difficult aspects of our work to suffer the frustration of watching someone we know well and care about, deteriorate, and to be unable to intervene in the way we could if the deterioration was psychiatric. Team support and discussion is essential. It provides the opportunity to ventilate some of these frustrations and reaffirm the realities of our position. We have usually found families fully understand our position (they may for years also have experienced a stubborn refusal to take simple advice). Other professionals are sometimes not so understanding. The primary care team involved with Ed were very critical of us insisting that we should move him to a nursing home. Perhaps to spare their own consciences, they consistently refused to recognize that we could not force him when he was so resolutely unwilling to go.

Maintaining skills

What would we do for a family member? That is the rough benchmark we use in the team when we discuss what is an appropriate level of support to offer our patients. There are few 'professional' guidelines established for these decisions. This rather simple benchmark works well when deciding how active to be in taking patients to and from appointments, but it does not help with deciding on which specific medical interventions we are competent to provide.

Even if a family member often takes responsibility for direct care, society expects (and will insist upon, if anything goes wrong) higher levels of accountability from us. If mental health staff do deliver physical health care, they need to be certain that they have received the appropriate training to do so. More important is to make sure that the skills learnt are adequately maintained. Most nurses will have been trained in diabetes care, but those working in mental health care will not be delivering such care very often. Our memories of the implications of the different blood levels will be rusty. What is the level to test for ketones? What is the level to omit the insulin injection?

Each professional member of the team is responsible for ensuring that they keep their skills and knowledge up to date. The team leader has a responsibility to make sure that each of the team is competent in what they are asked to do. If a team does not have a culture of openness and trust, it is possible that one member may not admit that they 'aren't up to' a procedure that most of their colleagues are comfortable with. Making sure that such concerns are acknowledged and addressed—and not seen as failings—is an essential task for a team leader.

Conclusions

Help with physical health care is a core component of assertive outreach with the severely mentally ill. They have greater than average needs and the barriers to them getting adequate care are daunting. Insisting on a very rigid demarcation of our 'mental health role' is neither in their interests nor, as we have found, in ours. Help with overall health care improves engagement and delivers an often immediately obvious improvement in quality of life that is mutually rewarding for key worker and patient. There are complex 'border' issues that come with this work, often raising important ethical and resource concerns. Honestly handled, we have found these challenges strengthen the team's understanding of its function and also can improve our relationships with wider health care providers. All of this can only be in the long-term interests of our patients.

Chapter 23

Employment and activity

Introduction

Vocational programmes are not new. Victorian asylums recognized the moral and constitutional benefits of work. It is only in the last decades that large psychiatric hospitals in the UK have moved away from having industrial therapy units where patients performed repetitive tasks for pocket money and lunch.

It is evident in both the American literature and practice of assertive outreach that real employment is very much higher on their list of priorities than in the UK. Many US teams have a vocational employment worker with the remit to develop opportunities and support patients in jobs. The successful clubhouse system (Beard *et al.* 1982) demonstrates how dynamic the work-oriented and self-help culture is in the US. Employment law and welfare provision differ there.

In the UK, a rather fatalistic attitude has developed to seeking mainstream employment for people with severe and enduring mental health problems. A number of factors contribute to this apathy, including the role of European employment law, which provides better safeguards for employees. The downside of such legislation is that employers may consider it risky to take on workers with long-standing health problems, since it is not easy to sack people on health grounds once hired. Also, state benefits for the unemployed and disabled are relatively generous and inflexible in the UK and many parts of Europe. This means that there is often little or nothing to be gained financially from seeking employment if you qualify for middle or higher rates of disability living allowance. The inflexibility of the benefit system creates a 'Catch-22' situation where if you become employed you lose your benefit. Then if your employment is terminated, or you leave on health grounds, your case for having disability benefits reinstated is undermined by having worked! Transitional schemes, such as therapeutic earnings and disabled persons' tax credit, do not seem to have a high take-up rate within our patient group.

This chapter seeks to inject renewed enthusiasm into the quest for employment for the severely mentally ill, using assertive outreach. Positive strategies and case studies are presented, together with an example of an assessment tool to help target this intervention on the patients most likely to succeed in either the free market or work schemes.

Helping our patients to structure their day through non-work activity will not be covered in depth. Much can be done to support social and recreational activities. We favour a direct approach, such as regular trips to the cinema or involvement with a snooker club, and avoid a too self-consciously professional approach. Being too organized about such activities can deprive both the key worker and the patient of the pleasure from them. Our patients tend to use mental health day centres for their lunch rather than for group activities. This 'low-tech' approach to leisure and activity does not, however, mean that we regard them lightly.

There are very real effects of discrimination and stigma which impact on employers taking on people with mental health problems. An immediate practical dilemma that arises from this prejudice is whether we advise our more preserved patients not to inform prospective employers of their mental illness. Most often the patient's illness is overt and inroads are best made with employers in a realistic and open manner.

It has been estimated that 50–90% of people with ongoing mental health problems wish to return to work (Grove 1999; Rinaldi and Hill 2000). Surveys of relatives report that structured daytime activity is viewed as the most pressing unmet need in this patient group (Steinwachs *et al.* 1992).

Current approaches to work-related activity

> In the past, extensive resources have been directed towards pre-vocational activities, with little demonstrable impact.
>
> (Bond 1992)

Training schemes abound in catering, computer skills, and administration for people with mental health problems and other disabilities. We refer patients sparingly to such schemes because of high drop-out rates. Patients report that such training too often caters for the lowest common denominator and rarely leads on to real work opportunities. Table 23.1 arranges work-related interventions in a hierarchy, ranging from one-to-one assistance with mainstream employment to groups at mental health day centres. These are described below.

Specialist programmes

Specialist one-to-one work programmes exist purely to help individuals find and keep appropriate work. They may exist in the voluntary or statutory sector and availability varies markedly. The best programmes are usually integrated into mental health services. They are very popular and able to pick patients according to their capacity and possibilities. It is certainly worth visiting and finding out about them before referring patients, or get the vocational worker to come and talk to the team.

Schemes may offer a range of placements from voluntary to fully-paid mainstream work. The programme will have developed a circle of employers who have learnt the benefits of hiring through the scheme. The most successful programmes simply take patients 'as they are' and develop or find suitable jobs. This approach is preferable to trying to mould the patient to fit an existing job. Such schemes rely on direct contact with employers, rather than on advertised vacancies.

Table 23.1 Hierarchy of work-focused interventions

Intervention	Description	Examples
Specialist programmes	Intensive one-to-one assistance with finding, starting, and maintaining real work placements	Individual placement and support program (Drake and Becker 1996); Pathfinder user employment programme (Perkins et al. 2000)
Vocationally focused assertive outreach	Intensive one-to-one assistance with finding, starting, and maintaining real work placements as part of a wider care plan delivered by an assertive outreach team	Training in community living (Test 1992)
Clubhouse model	Mental health day facilities focused on work and user/member involvement	Fountain House, New York (Beard et al. 1982)
Sheltered employment	Social firms or workshops run in partnership with health or social care agencies and with explicit remit to employ disadvantaged groups	Industrial therapy units; Remploy
Voluntary work	Voluntary placements often consisting of only a few hours per week within charitable organizations	Volunteer bureaux
Work training	Courses in basic skills aimed at the long-term unemployed or people with disabilities	Restart; New deal for disabled people
Vocational counselling	Individualized job, interview, and career advice	Disablement Employment Officer at job centre
Work groups at day centre	Job clubs providing advice, support, and resources for job search and application; also work activities such as gardening, typing, word processing, secretarial skills' training, etc.	

The individual placement and support (IPS) program (Drake and Becker 1996) is one American example of such an approach. Extensive links with local employers are built up. The programme uses techniques such as job shadowing, where the patient can follow a regular employee for a day or two, observing and learning the job. There is no obligation for the employer to hire at the end. The targeted jobs' tax credit acts as an incentive for employers in the IPS locality. If the patient is hired on a permanent basis and is disabled, the employer can 'write off' the first $2400 of wages. IPS employment specialists join case management teams and directly assist in searching for jobs. On securing employment, they provide such follow-up assistance as counselling, transport, and intervening with employers. Employment specialists have a case load of 25.

Drake *et al.* (1999*a*) conducted a randomized trial of IPS compared to enhanced vocational rehabilitation (EVR). EVR provided referral to external rehabilitation agencies through a vocational counsellor in the mental health service. All the EVR agencies endorsed competitive employment as a goal but used a 'step-wise' approach, involving pre-vocational training and transitional training through a sheltered workshop. Over 18 months, 60% in the IPS programme became competitively employed against only 9% in EVR.

The Pathfinder user employment programme (Perkins *et al.* 2000) is a modified approach that places patients in existing clinical and non-clinical positions within our local mental health trust. Mental health services are major employers and if other employers are to be persuaded to offer work to people with severe mental health problems we have to lead by example. The trust includes personal experience of mental health problems as a desirable quality on all job specifications. This integrates the concept of expertise by experience into working in mental health. The community support worker with one of the assertive outreach teams in the trust has been employed full-time and on a full salary through this programme. This will undoubtedly be an increasing trend in this country and is already well established in the US.

Vocationally focused assertive outreach

In the absence of such dedicated employment specialists, encouraging a team member to take on a responsibility for the vocational focus will enhance the priority given to seeking work placements. This works best where that person is self-selected, since it can be daunting and frustrating using direct sales tactics with local employers! One of our team (with an occupational therapy training) has successfully developed work placements with a local supermarket. The advantage of identifying these placements in-house is that we can assess and nominate our patients exclusively and continue to support them in the job with a key worker and team that they already know:

Case study

Marion is a young woman with schizophrenia who was highly motivated to get back to work. She had gone on training courses and attended day centres for a number of years but wanted mainstream employment. She presented as a likeable and co-operative patient with noticeable movement disorder side-effects from medication. These had the effect of exaggerating the perception of her functional difficulties.

Marion was highlighted as being motivated for work at her review meeting. Her key worker and the team's vocational worker carried out a formal assessment. Issues highlighted on assessment were:

♦ Marion's unrealistic and over-enthusiastic expectations.

♦ Limited work history, which included loss of jobs, associated with relapse.

♦ Her sufficiently high functional capability to try mainstream work.

The team's vocational worker approached a local supermarket and arranged an appointment with their personnel manager who was having trouble motivating and keeping staff in specific jobs (e.g. putting shopping into bags from individual internet shopping orders prior to delivery). Marion liked the sound of this job—it was not that different from doing her own shopping. The vocational worker on the team spoke to the personnel officer about the maximum number of hours and pay that would enable Marion to still qualify for welfare benefits.

On the day of the interview Marion was smartly presented and excited. She had worked on presentation and practised interview questions with her key worker. The vocational worker who was familiar with the personnel manager took her to the interview. Marion got the job and continues to work at the store 16 hours a week. She has recently started working on the checkout tills. The personnel officer is delighted to have at least one person who actually wants to be there!

Given the success of the IPS model, it would make sense to have a vocational worker or specialist within assertive outreach teams, as is more common in the US. Their recommended PACT standards require one or more team members to be designated as vocational specialists (Allness and Knoedler 1998).

The clubhouse model

The early clubs, such as Fountain House in New York (Beard *et al.* 1982), were set up as self-help psychosocial centres in large cities in the US. One of their chief aims (aside from mutual support) was to provide employment opportunities for the members through pre-vocational work groups operating from the clubhouse itself (e.g. gardening and catering) and also through external work placements. Clubhouses incorporate a belief in empowerment and the potential for productivity of the most disabled.

The success of the model has been studied by controlled trials demonstrating a reduction in hospitalization (Beard *et al.* 1978; Dincin and Witheridge 1982). Mary Ann Test (1992) summarizes well the outcome evidence for and against the Clubhouse model:

> Only one of these studies considered broader outcomes; results suggested that while the psychosocial center led to the development of stronger social networks, it did not result in greater employment, more participation in leisure time activities, or less symptomatology relative to controls (Dincin and Witheridge 1982). Also of relevance is a study by Bond and Dincin (1986), which examined employment rehabilitation methods. This study revealed that accelerated participation in *in vivo* supported employment was more efficacious than transitioning through clubhouse pre-vocational activities.

The clubhouse model has been replicated across the world using a modified franchise approach. Staff at new centres are trained by those from existing sites according to an agreed set of standards. In the UK, a handful of clubhouses are established and, bearing in mind the reservations expressed above, they appear to constitute a valuable resource to complement and enhance assertive outreach services for referral of selected patients.

Sheltered workshops

Remploy was set up by the UK Government in response to the 1944 Disabled Persons (Employment) Act mainly to serve people with physical disabilities sustained in the Second World War. Remploy is very much a traditional, manufacturing-based sheltered workshop. The same ethos can still be seen in industrial therapy units run by hospitals

Example 23.1

ENHANCED CPA/SECTION 117(2)REVIEW (delete as applicable)		

Patient's name: Marion W.
Address: Flat3, 49 Smith Square

Phone: 0208 645 xxxx
Date of birth: 22/6/75
GP: Morgan
Phone: 0208 767 xxxx

CMHT: ACT TEAM
Phone: 0208 877 xxxx
New patient: NO
If NO, date of review: 29/5/01
Diagnosis:
1 Schizophrenia   F 20.0
2 .... F— —·—

Assessed needs or problem	Intervention	Resp. of
Unemployed, lacks structure to day	◆ Assess for mainstream employment with team vocational specialist. ◆ Active assistance with job hunting and application subject to assessment. ◆ Approach appropriate employers directly and explain advantages to them of employing Marion. ◆ Support Marion through process but give realistic appraisal of difficulties involved. ◆ Provide advice on impact of work on benefits.	JF Voca-tional Specialist
Dystonic side-effects of medication	◆ Encourage compliance with anti-muscarinic medication. ◆ Provide education on medication and side-effects. Give written information. ◆ Link impression she gives with prospects for mainstream work.	JF

Involved in care: Dr Psychologist CPN ✓OT SW Ward nurse ✓CM Support worker Other

Present at meeting: ✓Dr Psychologist CPN ✓OT ✓SW Ward nurse ✓CM Support worker Other

Discussed with the patient?   YES   Copy to patient?   YES   Copy to GP?   YES

Care co-ordinator (print):   Judy Fraser   Phone: 0208 877 xxxx

Care co-ordinator (signature):   ....   Date of next review: 29/11/01....

Job title: Clinical case manager   Patient's signature: ....

Supervision register?	NO	Care management?	NO	Risk history completed?	NO
Supervised discharge?	NO	Section 117(2)?	YES	Relapse + risk plan required?	NO

for people with chronic mental health problems and severe mental impairment. Over the years, social firms (now called social enterprises) have developed this idea (often with joint funding from health and social services) setting up small mainstream businesses (e.g. cafes, printers) specifically to employ people with disabilities.

One disadvantage of sheltered workshops is that they do not embody a philosophy of social inclusion. Sheltered workshops are not part of mainstream competitive employment even if they are moving towards being more competitive in business. Most of us now favour mainstream activities where possible, both in the nature and setting of interventions, but this does not deny the value of sheltered workshops.

Voluntary work

Voluntary work can be a valuable strategy during an initial period of a work placement. The employer can assess the employee's competencies and motivation before starting paid work. More often, voluntary work consists of donating a few hours a week to a good cause such as a charity or public service. The idea of working for a few hours a week for altruistic reasons with only expenses paid is, however, anathema to many of our patients! One advantage of voluntary work is that it does not affect volunteers' welfare benefits. Also, valuable skills and social contacts can develop in a non-threatening, non-contractual environment.

Volunteers are free to leave, arrive late, and work to their abilities without sanction. Most areas have a local volunteer bureau, often linked to the local council for voluntary services that helps co-ordinate local charitable organizations. The volunteer bureau acts as a job centre for voluntary work. The patient or key worker phones up the volunteer bureau, is invited for a simple interview to ascertain skills and interests, and local opportunities are discussed. Many volunteer bureaux are skilled in developing places for people with mental health problems and providing some form of support for the duration of the placement. Activities vary from helping at childrens' adventure playgrounds and youth or OAP clubs, to filling envelopes for charity fundraising or lobbying.

Work training

Work training is offered by the employment service for the general unemployed as well as by voluntary organizations aimed at providing assistance to groups with special needs. If a patient is in receipt of disability benefits and no longer providing medical certificates or 'signing on', they are unlikely to be called up by the benefits agency for retraining aimed at the long-term unemployed. Vocational training represents what the Americans call a transitional or 'step-wise' approach, since it is indirect. Competitive employment outcomes are poorer than when direct assistance is given in seeking and maintaining employment.

The employment service's 'work preparation' aims to help people with a disability return to work following long periods of sickness or unemployment. People on incapacity benefit can access this individually tailored programme of work preparation without their benefits being affected. It is short-term, with funding available for six weeks training. Access is through referral to the Disablement Employment Advisor at the local job centre.

In the UK, referrals can be made to voluntary organizations providing training courses for people with special needs, including severe mental illness. Typically, such training is in catering, horticulture, or administration and word processing skills, with national vocational qualification accreditation. There is an abundance of courses offering basic computer training. However, although popular, training in computer skills rarely translates into employment.

Vocational counselling

Most of us are familiar with the drawbacks of vocational counselling from our encounters with careers officers whilst at school. If we want to be a teacher, then chances are that the careers officer will look at our school reports and then suggest that plumbing would be more realistic! Local job centres employ disablement employment advisors (DEAs) whose role it is to assess employment prospects, advise on job opportunities, develop placements, and provide advice on how work will affect welfare benefits. The DEA is part of the local network into which assertive outreach teams can link. DEAs have access to certain training schemes and are up to date with changes in the benefits system.

Work groups at mental health day centres

Gardening and activity groups are often recreational in nature. Groups that have a more mainstream work focus provide telephones and stamps to assist in job searches, practice interviews, and foster self-help and advice among participants. The disadvantage is the remoteness from the labour market and the potential lack of an individualized or highly motivating environment.

Work assessment

Many of the advances in functional and work assessment come from work conducted in psychiatric rehabilitation settings and from the field of occupational therapy. Functional assessment tools vary from focusing on grooming, meal preparation, and ability to use public transport up to specific competencies and behaviours relevant to mainstream working. We will concentrate here on assessment for mainstream work since this represents our biggest challenge.

Perhaps the most comprehensive assessment tool (and certainly the one with the thickest manual!) is the Occupational Performance History Interview, version 2.0 or OPHI-II (Kielhofner *et al.* 1998). This American psychometrically based tool is the product of many years of development and research and is applicable, but not exclusive, to people with severe and enduring mental health problems. The OPHI-II consists of three subscales:

- Occupational identity
- Occupational competence
- Occupational behaviour settings

These scales are scored on a four-point rating system from 1 (extremely occupationally dysfunctional) to 4 (exceptionally competent occupational functioning) with free text to clarify and enhance the scoring system.

The following case history illustrates items from the scale.

Case study

Ian is a 40-year-old man who lives with his ageing mother and who developed schizophrenia insidiously from the age of 19. He had worked for two years after leaving school at a printers but lost his job after his first hospitalization.

The **occupational identity** subscale contains 11 items and is concerned with the patient's sense of self and roles. Item 1 enquires whether Ian has personal goals and projects. Ian scores 3 in that he is motivated to work towards goals and his projects fit his strengths and limitations. However, for item 3 (self-expectations of success) he only scores 2 as he has difficulty sustaining confidence about overcoming obstacles, limitations, and failures.

The **competence subscale** covers nine items. Item 1 asks whether Ian currently maintains a satisfying lifestyle with regard to the level and balance of roles and projects. Ian structures his life rigidly around washing, shaving, reading the newspapers, and occasionally playing snooker. He used to have a regular voluntary job doing basic administrative tasks. He performs his role as a son and family member well. From the anchor points on the scale Ian scores 3, as he is involved in a variety of roles and responsibilities, which generally express a direction or meaning. He scores the maximum 4 points for item 5, as he organizes his time and routine around his roles and responsibilities. For Ian, his routine represents a healthy adaptive coping strategy countering the effect of distracting voices and a tendency to circumstantiality and over-inclusive thinking. He has interests and hobbies consistent with scoring a 2 in item 6. Despite poor concentration, he reads and plays snooker, but has some difficulty finding the energy to participate regularly.

The **behavioural setting** subscale relates to the current, everyday environment and has nine items. Item 4 concerns the home-life social group. Does Ian's interaction with his elderly mother generally support positive functioning? In Ian's case, whilst the mother is over-protective, her emotional and care needs do not keep him at home. The climate supports limited functioning but Ian's mother does not believe that he should be exposed to stress or challenge, or have to be financially or domestically independent. In this respect he scores 2, and the rating points the team towards future intervention in the form of schizophrenia family work in support of the work goals.

In summary, Ian's strengths are his motivation, interests, and his ability to keep to a routine of low-skill tasks. His weaknesses are his lack of confidence and his family environment which does not encourage greater independence and challenge.

The purpose of the assessment is to identify those high-scoring patients for whom real or supported work is a possibility either in the short, medium, or long term. From the complexity of the OPHI-II it can be appreciated that readiness for work is multifactorial and highly individualized.

Welfare benefits and work

Benefits often represent the biggest psychological and practical obstacle to switching to competitive employment. Uncertainty and change in the UK benefits system mean that assertive outreach key workers need to keep abreast of developments. In the first case history in this chapter we described Marion's return to work. In Marion's case she is able to work 16 hours per week and earns over £200 a month, which she declares to the Department of Social Security. Because the doctor on the team wrote to the DSS confirming that Marion's work is part of her rehabilitation and requesting therapeutic earnings, she only loses £20 from her benefits.

Currently, you may be able to do some work while you are sick and claiming either incapacity benefit or severe disablement allowance, provided your therapeutic earnings from work are less than £60.50 per week. You are restricted to less than 16 hours per week and therapeutic earnings will last for six months, with a six-month extension for those working with a personal advisor or DEA. Letters of support from doctors or key workers are vital in supporting therapeutic earnings. Voluntary work and work as part of a hospital treatment programme are also allowed, with no limit on the number of hours. Any person receiving incapacity benefits can earn a maximum of £20 with no limit on time or hours.

Disabled person's tax credit replaced the old disability working allowance. It covers people with an illness or a disability which puts them at a disadvantage in getting a job and who work at least 16 hours per week. Receipt of one of a number of qualifying benefits for disability, currently within six months prior to the date of application, is required, and there are restrictions on savings. Incentives to employers also exist. The job introduction scheme pays a £75 grant to employers for the first six weeks that they employ a person with mental health problems.

Working to strengths

Factors relevant to work can be conceived in terms of a patient's strengths or by their impairments. The strengths' model of case management (Rapp 1992) is particularly helpful in working with a patient's aspirations and goals, since it emphasizes abilities over deficits and collaboration over brokerage. Furthermore, people with severe and enduring mental illness are seen as possessing the ability to learn, grow, and change. The local community is viewed not as an obstacle but as a resource containing many opportunities. Even if the aspirations of the patient to work seem remote, or the choice of work somewhat grandiose, there are worthwhile shorter-term steps on the way to these ultimate goals.

> It is likely that the client generally regarded to be unmotivated is more likely to respond to a positive focus than to a negative focus which highlights the problems.
>
> (Morgan 1993)

Case study

One patient with severe bipolar affective disorder has aspirations to be a supermodel. In many respects, Gloria is well suited. She is slim and has no appetite, she is offhand and belligerent with people, and she smokes and drinks heavily—the characteristics perhaps of an established rather than an aspiring supermodel.

Initial work with Gloria involved not dismissing this aspiration but breaking it down into more achievable goals—healthy eating (as opposed to not eating), negotiation and presentation (as opposed to making demands of other people), and establishing a daytime pattern of activity mirroring that of a working day.

Gloria did eventually participate in a charity fashion show organized by the local mental health day centre.

The strengths' approach does not ignore the assessed needs of the patient but starts from the patient agenda and list of 'wants'.

Conclusions

The evidence consistently favours direct and rapid exposure to mainstream competitive employment over 'step-wise' pre-vocational activities (Drake *et al.* 1999*b*). Such supported employment is more effective than pre-vocational training in helping patients find and maintain competitive employment (Crowther *et al.* 2001). Studies that have looked at whether the potential stress of rapid exposure to competitive employment increases the risk of relapse have shown no association (Bond *et al.* 1997; McFarlane *et al.* 2000).

The value of targeting and assessing patients for exposure is less clear but would seem sensible where jobs are scarce. Studies of 'employability' show that patient characteristics such as diagnosis, severity of impairment, and social skills have relatively little impact on employment outcomes (Grove 2000). Having a history of employment, being motivated, and believing that employment is achievable are positive predictors of employment outcomes.

Assertive outreach teams have the resources, especially if enhanced by an employment specialist, to provide individualized placement and support as part of an overall care package. There are significant differences affecting the UK labour market that may appear to make our job harder compared to our US counterparts. Major unemployment of patients with severe mental illness and patients' desire to work are, however, almost universal challenges for us. We should remember how important work is for everyone's self-esteem and well-being and also the surveys of patients' and families' views that put work top of their aspirations.

Chapter 24

Daily living skills

Introduction

In assertive outreach the teaching and development of daily living and social skills takes place with each patient in the context of their own home, family, and community. We are no longer dealing with institutionalized patients moving out of long-stay wards who may never have used a pedestrian crossing or supermarket. We are, however, often working with people who might find cooking or shopping difficult due to motivational, cognitive, and information-processing deficits. Helping patients to develop and practise daily living skills means that we must resist the temptation to simply do everything for them, as happened in long-stay institutions. This involves listening to the patient's agenda and encouraging decision making and problem solving.

What we now call the programme for assertive community treatment (PACT) was originally called training in community living (TCL). Stein and Test (1980) saw the core task of their outreach team as teaching patients the skills to survive outside hospital, and believed this task would be time limited. Teaching medication management, shopping, cooking, and other household and interpersonal tasks were taught '*in vivo*'. Unless comprehensive psychosocial help was delivered directly to the patient in their own environment, patients often did not link with services. Furthermore, the skills learned in one context, such as a day centre, did not transfer to the context of their home.

Stein and Test felt strongly that traditional aftercare services underestimated the range of skills and assistance that severely mentally ill people needed to survive. The term TCL has not survived because of the experience of continuing to follow up the patients who had received intensive care after the service was withdrawn. Patients improved community tenure, employment, social relationships, symptomatology, and satisfaction with their lives during the 14-month experimental service, but lost most of these following discharge from TCL (Stein and Test 1980). It is an important finding. Stein and Test recognized the importance of ongoing community support and skills training for these patients:

> It must be concluded that even very intensive community treatment models do not provide a cure for severe mental illnesses, but rather provide a support system within which persons with persistent vulnerabilities can live in the community and grow. It appears these supports must be ongoing rather than time limited.

(Test 1992)

Daily living skills' training follows from an understanding of patients' difficulties based on the stress vulnerability model (Zubin and Spring 1977). For vulnerable individuals, interventions aimed at reducing the stresses of coping with money, relationships, transport, isolation or the inability to shop or cook adequately will ultimately reduce arousal, symptomatology, and relapse rates.

The impact of cognitive deficits

The most important principle in support of *in vivo* training is the recognition that many patients with severe psychotic illness have difficulty transferring skills learned in a therapeutic setting to their natural environment of the home, family, and community. The extent to which neurocognitive deficits in schizophrenia affect people in their daily lives is not well known or studied. Undoubtedly though, these can have a profound outcome on the ability to acquire new skills and problem solve, and on prospects for community living. The following aspects of cognitive functioning have been shown by Green (1996) to impede functional and community outcomes.

Neurocognitive factors associated with poorer outcome

- Poor verbal memory
- Poor concentration, vigilance, or attention
- Difficulty processing information
- Poor transfer of learning
- Poor concept formation
- Poor cognitive flexibility
- Negative symptoms

Some of these deficits relate to specific outcomes, for example verbal memory and vigilance are required for skill acquisition. The ability to remember instructions or stories both in the short and long term are necessary when learning a new skill or task. Negative symptoms may reduce the ability to form social networks but they do not appear to hinder skills acquisition. Information-processing deficits are likely to hinder communication and social behaviour. Poor cognitive flexibility can mean that patients transferred to settings where they have more choice and challenge become more symptomatic. Green's review failed to find a relationship between psychotic symptoms and community outcome.

These findings can be applied to individual patient care programmes and Green (1996) provides good examples of how this would work with two patients in similar situations but with different cognitive abilities:

> The patient with good vigilance would probably benefit from skills training programs as they are currently designed, whereas the other patient may need a form of training that is slower

paced, is offered in shorter segments, or includes more redundancy. Likewise a patient with relatively poor verbal memory who is about to enter a community placement may need additional mental health support services to achieve and maintain optimal social and work outcome. In these examples, the focus is on predicting the individuals need for support.

Assessment

Before we embark on individualized and *in vivo* interventions we usually need to establish some baseline through structured or semi-structured assessment. We prefer a naturalistic assessment over time to establish a patient's strengths and weaknesses in daily and social living skills. Frequent home- and community-based contacts soon make these apparent. There may, however, be value in exposing newer patients to routine functional assessments to gauge global abilities and deficits.

Table 24.1 Assessment of social and daily living skills from the social functioning scale (adapted Birchwood *et al.* 1990)

Functional area	Sample questions
Social withdrawal	On average, what time do you get up?
	How often will you start a conversation at home?
	How often will you leave the house for any reason?
Relationships	How many friends do you have at the moment?
	How easy or difficult do you find talking to people at present?
	Do you feel uneasy with groups of people?
Social activities	Over the past three months, how often have you participated in the following activities— going to the cinema; visiting places of interest; visiting friends; sport; going to a pub; eating out; visiting relatives; etc.?
Recreational activities	Over the past three months, how often have you done any of the following— reading; gardening; a hobby; shopping; listening to music or the radio; watching television;etc.?
Independence (competence)	How able are you at doing or using the following— public transport; handling money; budgeting; cooking; shopping; washing clothes; personal hygiene; etc.?
Independence (performance)	How often have you done the following in the past three months— buying an item from a shop alone; washing up; washing own clothes; looking for a job; doing the food shopping; cooking a meal; using buses or trains; etc.?
Employment	Do you think you are capable of some kind of job?
	How often do you make attempts to find a job?
	If not employed, how do you spend your day?

Treatment goals should be articulated and documented in the care plan and based on the patient's expressed desires for role functioning. The purpose of assessment is to guide the process of change. For example, the patient expresses a desire on prompting to meet more people and expand his range of social activities. The key worker then enquires about social and cultural preferences or norms and establishes with the patient agreed and achievable treatment goals. For example, a patient may express a desire for mainstream social activity rather than attendance at a 'drop in' centre for mental health patients. Cultural norms may be going to the pub or going to a snooker club. A treatment goal may be going for a Sunday pub lunch with a parent or key worker. Single-issue treatment goals such as the use of public transport or using the launderette will not require the use of a structured assessment tool as progress can be readily evaluated.

There is no single definitive assessment tool or interview process appropriate for comprehensive functional assessment of daily living skills (Vaccaro *et al.* 1992). One particularly thorough scale is the social functioning scale (Birchwood *et al.* 1990). This scale was developed for assessment of social and daily living skills as a baseline for schizophrenia family work. Table 24.1 summarizes the areas covered in this scale.

In assertive outreach the responsibility for assessment lies with key workers. Occupational therapists have the background knowledge and training to assist team members. We would suggest that managing medication is also best presented to the patient as a normal activity of daily living that requires training, practice, and support.

Specific interventions

Activity analysis

All activities that we wish to teach or rehearse with patients are best broken down into their constituent parts in order to understand what is involved, identify critical elements that may require reinforcing, and in order not to overwhelm the patient with too much information at once. Information on materials needed, time required, the suitable environment, and stages to completion for the activity are all relevant. For example, in order to use a washing machine at a launderette:

- Which is the nearest or most appropriate launderette?
- When is it open?
- What materials are necessary—powder, conditioner, laundry bag, newspaper to read while waiting, the correct coins for both washer and drier?
- Which clothes can be washed together—whites and coloured, cotton and synthetic? How can you tell from the label?
- Where do the coins go in the machine?
- How do you select the correct cycle?
- How long does it take?

This task demands physical ability, numeracy, organization and preparation, patience, and motivation. The patient needs verbal memory and information-processing skills. Stage one of an intervention programme with the treatment goal of helping the patient to learn how to use the launderette may be simply to identify the location, opening times, and coins needed by going with the patient. Stage two might be helping them sort out their clothes into appropriate categories for washing, and so on.

Daily living skills

Following Maslow's (1954) hierarchy of needs, the most important skills for community living are the ability to cook and feed oneself, keeping safe, maintaining stable housing, and maintaining financial security. We do not overly prioritize the physical tidiness of our patients' accommodation since it is often a matter of patient choice and poses little or no risk. We are often reminded of this deviance from social norms of cleanliness or tidiness when taking visitors or students on home visits. They often comment that we are too tolerant!

Many people are poor at cooking for themselves and a whole industry of convenience food has grown up to service this need. Convenience and take-away food is often unhealthy as a sole source of nutrition however. Helping patients investigate their choices and to use their local convenience shops, supermarkets, take-aways, and food delivery services may be all the patient wants. Encouraging the patient to acknowledge that cooking may be more cost effective and an enjoyable skill, using the principles of motivational interviewing (see Chapter 11), may be the starting point for cooking. Often patients may lack the materials necessary to cook for themselves. Obtaining community care grants to buy cooking implements and crockery may act as further encouragement. Cooking does require patience and concentration in order to be a safe activity. If the patient is not prepared to wait until an item is cooked or forgets to turn off the hob or leaves the pan unattended, then interventions aimed at improving attention and delaying gratification will be required before trying to cook.

For some patients it may be best to accept the inevitable and organize meals on wheels, especially for more elderly and frail patients. Likewise, home care, from once to several times a week, can be organized to help patients with cleaning the house, shopping, collecting benefits, etc. These costed services, however, represent a fragmentation of service delivery. Some patients do not allow others into their home; some behave in such a way that home carers are reluctant to provide the service. Patients who are hard to engage are unlikely to be suitable for such external services.

We generally find that direct service provision from the team or utilization of the patient's family, plus daily living skills' training where appropriate, works best. Doing everything for the patient does not motivate them to acquire new skills. A balance between direct support, prompting, and training is required. We refer to this as developing realistic interdependence. We are all dependent on others to some extent for affection, company, or money. The aim in assertive outreach may not be complete independence in all functional areas.

Social skills

Returning to Maslow's hierarchy, teaching patients the basic assertiveness skills to avoid exploitation by others can be a priority. We have encountered a number of patients who are often exploited by others for money or the use of their accommodation. Persuasive and socially skilled acquaintances (often met in hospital) talk their way into the home and then use it for drug-taking activities, at the expense of our patient. Motivational techniques would encourage the patient to recognize the negative consequences on his or her housing tenure, safety, liberty, and finances. If the patient can rehearse assertion strategies denying access, then these consequences may be avoided. At the same time, practical interventions enable and support the skills training. We can ensure that the patient's doors and windows are secure, they have not lost their key, and they have a spy hole and chain fitted. Role play in the patient's home is one method of rehearsing responses. The key worker can play the drug dealer at the door, and the patient is then required to respond assertively to requests to come in.

Social skills' training can, for some patients, include more basic skills such as establishing normal eye contact and other non-verbal behaviour, reducing the amount of 'psychotic talk', asking leading questions and responding to questions, or asking for additional information. The principles of activity analysis, teaching, and rehearsal are the same.

The setting of homework tasks in social and daily living skills' training is common. The patient can then report back how the homework went and how they felt. For example: 'When you go to the post office tomorrow, as we did on our last visit, practise looking at the counter clerk and establishing normal eye contact. Also take your gas bill and ask if this can be paid out of your benefit money.'

Efficacy

Liberman *et al.* (1998) conducted a randomized control trial of social skills' training compared to occupational therapy. Eighty community patients with persistent schizophrenia were randomly assigned to one of the two conditions (social skills training and occupational therapy), each of which lasted for 12 hours a week for 12 months, followed by two years of case management follow-up. Social skills' training modules included medication management, symptom management, and relapse planning, use of recreation and leisure, and basic conversational skills. Case management follow-up encouraged the use of these learnt skills. The occupational therapy condition consisted of expressive, artistic, and recreational activities individually and in groups, with the therapist encouraging discussion of feelings and personal goals. Case management follow-up comprised encouragement to use the expressive activities in the community. Both conditions received help with maintaining housing, crisis intervention, and medication. Patients who received social skills' training showed significantly greater independent living skills during the two-year follow up. The skills learnt in the intensive phase were transferred into the everyday life of the patient. This study also showed that such training can be delivered by support workers without professional mental health qualifications. Liberman (Liberman *et al.*1998) states that the efficacy of socials skills' training in schizophrenia is well established.

The Cochrane database meta-analysis of life skills' programmes in chronic mental illness is less optimistic (Nicol *et al.* 2000). They found only two randomized controlled trials within their criteria and both had small sample sizes. They stated that no firm conclusions can be drawn from their review. They restricted life skills to those skills associated with independent functioning such as budgeting, communication, domestic, personal care, and community living skills.

Case study

Jerome had lived in a low-support hostel for many years and wanted his own flat. Because of the predominance of negative symptoms of schizophrenia he displayed, and the lack of any skills' training in the hostel, it was not felt that this was a realistic proposition. Jerome spent most of his time in bed, would often appear confused, had difficulty managing his finances, and showed little motivation to change. He was referred to assertive outreach as a council flat offer had recently been made through the mental health housing register.

Functional assessment showed that Jerome often stayed in bed until early afternoon, he only went out to the hospital to play pool or to visit patients on the wards, had a few superficial relationships with other patients, had no hobbies, did not use public transport, wash his clothes, cook, or manage his money well. Jerome did not want to work but wanted to manage and keep his own flat and to develop his daytime activities. He had poor concentration, motivation, and verbal memory.

The initial work centred around the priorities of ensuring he made his flat safe, locked the door, knew how to use the heating, and that his finances were kept in order. Jerome was introduced to local shops and places to buy food. He liked West African food and with the help of his key worker they were able to locate a shop that sold some African vegetables and products. This enabled work to begin on showing him how to prepare and cook basic rice and vegetable dishes and to clean up after himself. In order to cook he needed gas, and a lot of time was spent going through bills and showing him how, and where, to pay them, as well as how to budget and save money for future bills.

Unfortunately, while this skills' training was going on a group of associates starting visiting Jerome, taking money off him and using his flat to abuse drugs. This necessitated a shift in priorities to teaching Jerome assertiveness strategies to refuse access to these people.

Example 24.1

ENHANCED CPA/SECTION 117(2)REVIEW (delete as applicable)	
Patient's name: Jerome D. Address: Flat 2, Eden House, Kampala Estate Phone: none Date of birth: 17/08/71 GP: Reynolds Phone: 0208 228 xxxx	CMHT: ACT TEAM Phone: 0208 877 xxxx New patient: NO If No, date of review: 6/6/01 Diagnosis: Schizophrenia .... F20.0 2.. F — —.——

Assessed needs or problem	Intervention	Resp. of
Maintain housing and household security	◆ Skills training to ensure that Jerome maintains his home safely. ◆ Frequent visits, every day in initial resettlement period. ◆ Ensure finances are in order to pay rent through housing benefit and utility bills. ◆ Programme of assertiveness training to provide the skills to refuse access.	BJ
Gaps in daily living skills.	◆ Introduce Jerome to local facilities, shops, leisure facilities, day centre, cafes, post office. ◆ Structured programme of daily living skills training: Activity analysis into component parts. *In vivo* training of managing money, budgeting, shopping, cooking, medication management, relapse planning. Take into account Jerome's poor concentration, and verbal memory. Training to be brief and repeated. Ask Jerome to practise tasks as homework and report back at next visit. ◆ Practical assistance where necessary to resolve difficulties.	BJ

Involved in care:	Dr Psychologist CPN OT SW Ward nurse CCM✓ Support Worker✓ Other
Present at meeting	Dr✓ Psychologist CPN OT SW✓ Ward nurse CCM✓ Support Worker✓ Other
Discussed with the patient? YES	Copy to patient? YES Copy to GP? YES
Care co-ordinator (print): Bill Johnson	Phone: 0208 877 xxxx
Care co-ordinator (signature):	Date of next review: 6/12/01
Job title: Clinical case manager	Patient's signature:...........................

Supervision register?	NO	Care management?	NO	Risk history completed?	YES
Supervised discharge?	NO	Section 117(2)?	YES	Relapse + risk plan required?	YES

Conclusions

We have discussed the foundation and application of daily living skills and social skills' training as one topic because they are both part of the adjustment, adaptation, and rehabilitative process of maintaining patients in their own homes. Assertive outreach eschews traditional group approaches to the training process in favour of direct provision of *in vivo*, individualized intervention. We believe that this form of psychosocial intervention is valuable in teaching patients how to cope with the additional demands of community living. It uses primarily the stress vulnerability model to conceptualize how this may produce beneficial outcomes in terms of reduced relapse, arousal, and symptomatology. Research evidence for significant improvements in community functioning, however, is not yet robust.

We must also recognize the cognitive demands that such complex interventions and skills require of our patients, leading us to provide intervention packages that are not time limited, are realistic, and include reinforcement and rehearsal. Ultimately, such interventions must also be aimed at improving the quality of life of community patients by opening up doors to mainstream activities and opportunities.

Chapter 25

Psychosocial interventions and work with families and carers

Introduction

Psychosocial interventions are much talked about in modern mental health services. They match the mood of the times. They emphasize the broader, non-drug approach to helping individuals with mental health problems while, at the same time, distancing themselves from the older, ideologically overburdened and 'less scientific' psychotherapies. The term is as much a statement of intent as a description of a method of working or an easily identified set of procedures.

What all psychosocial interventions seem to have in common is a commitment to working together (staff, patients, and carers) to understand problems better and develop strategies to reduce their impact. These strategies can be psychological (such as challenging automatic thoughts in cognitive behaviour therapy), behavioural (avoiding expressing criticism in response to symptoms), or even pharmacological (taking increased medication in response to an agreed relapse signature). The procedures and interventions vary between the approaches and for individual patients within approaches. All, however, build on dialogue and collaboration.

Although a simple, satisfactory definition of psychosocial interventions may not be readily available, most of us recognize the areas and the individual techniques attracting interest and research. There are three broad areas of activity which are implied by 'psychosocial interventions':

1. Psychoeducation
2. Behavioural family management
3. Cognitive behaviour therapy

Three equally broad areas of activity which are often overlooked or subsumed into the three above, require attention also:

1. Family engagement
2. Counselling and psychodynamic understanding
3. Supportive psychotherapy

The gulf between theory and practice

The vast discrepancy between what is preached and what is practised is striking. In no other area is the failure of research findings to translate into routine practice so obvious. The volume of high-quality research in some areas (e.g. behavioural family management in schizophrenia) (Mari and Streiner 1994) is remarkable. Yet even in the centres of excellence (and even where much of this research has been conducted), the interventions are rarely part of routine local service. Surveys of nurses with comprehensive training in these approaches, on specialised post graduate schemes such as Thorn courses (Gournay and Birley 1998), rarely find them routinely applying them (Fadden 1997). This is frequently blamed on resource limitations. One problem is that many Thorn graduates are rapidly promoted out of the direct clinical arena. Positive outcomes from training are maximized by ongoing supervision of staff following such courses (Brooker *et al.* 1994). There is a resource issue, but we doubt that it explains the extent of the gulf between theory and practice and think the reasons are more complex.

Efficacy and effectiveness

Firstly, there is the difference between treatment efficacy and clinical effectiveness. Treatment efficacy is how successful a treatment is under optimal experimental conditions (e.g. all the staff are excellent, all the patients get all the treatment, the patients only have one problem, and there are no drop-outs). Clinical effectiveness, however, is how the treatment fares in the real world (where patients may not comply fully with treatments, staff may vary in skill, and other confounding factors complicate the process). Even with simple drug treatments there is a significant difference between treatment efficacy and clinical effectiveness.

Resistance

Secondly, psychological work takes motivation from both sides. These are labour-intensive interventions which require us to enter formal programmes with patients structured over many sessions. In classical psychodynamic psychotherapy, the patient brought the commitment—the therapist's job was to understand and interpret what was brought (even if it was silence!). In most of the current psychosocial interventions, patients and their families may be convinced that it is the right approach but they will rarely seek out the treatment and insist on it. It is we who are usually pushing the intervention. Patient and family resistance can be considerable—and for quite understandable reasons. Families may, over time, have achieved an uneasy truce with the patient and do not want it disturbed. Both they and the patient may be exhausted and demoralized by years of struggle with the illness.

Modern psychosocial interventions, with their emphasis on behavioural change, homework, and targets are hard work. They also give the therapists more control over the pace of change. It should not be forgotten that even the most diplomatically phrased exercise implies a tacit criticism of previous functioning and can cause resentment.

Think about it. How do you feel if someone suggests you change one of your habits? Traditional psychotherapists took understanding resistance to change very seriously and had complex theories about it and strategies to deal with it. In modern teaching it is often glossed over, implying that the obvious benefits from the treatment will overcome any doubts. Drop out is high and early in CBT approaches in psychosis.

Supporting psychosocial interventions in assertive outreach

Despite the problems outlined above it is possible to work towards more routine provision of evidence-based psychosocial interventions for patients with severe mental illnesses. A first step is to make sure that they are taken seriously within the team. The most effective way of ensuring this is to provide high-quality teaching and supervision. Where possible, staff should be encouraged to attend Thorn courses (Gournay and Birley 1998) or their local equivalent. We have established a day-release course locally which is based closely on the Thorn syllabus and we ensure that all new staff go on it within their first two years. Such courses are equally applicable to case managers from non-nursing backgrounds and we have had both social workers and occupational therapists on our course as well as mental health support workers and nurses. For non-nurses, the benefits (in terms of career enhancement) may not be so clear-cut but most have enjoyed the course and found the skills applicable in their daily work.

Access to such a course may not be readily available for all staff (as it was not in the first few years of our service). Ensuring that one or two staff attend and then using professional development slots within the team to share skills and supervise ongoing work can still raise the profile and quality of work. Taking time to review the psychosocial management of individual patients during routine reviews continues to reaffirm their importance. For most mental health nurses, these skills carry high professional status and there is a real hunger to discuss them and improve them. Making sure they are discussed in detail in reviews is rarely a problem.

Keeping up with the literature

This is an area of rapid research and service development. Papers and books on the range of psychosocial interventions are published at a furious pace—particularly in the area of CBT. It is not the place of a volume like this to try and communicate the state of the art in such techniques. Even if we tried, we would be probably out of date by the time the book was published. Having acquired skills in this area it is important to keep up with developments and to refresh practice.

One way of ensuring that our patients do benefit from this range of approaches, however, is to be honest about which ones work for us and which we can deliver. There is a tendency for the most complex and demanding treatments (those that require the highest level of skill) to have the highest status. Scanning current conferences demonstrates the interest in CBT for hallucinations and dialectical behaviour therapy for borderline personality disorder, but little attention to illness education and compliance enhancement. We have decided, as a team, to emphasize the simpler, more feasible interventions that should be routinely available to all our patients and their families. Once they are being consistently applied, then there is scope for the more recherché treatments.

Being honest and realistic about what you can achieve is much more likely to produce results than exaggerated claims about cutting-edge practice. What follows is an overview of what we do. It is not comprehensive and other teams will go further. We consider some of the interventions, however, to be essential components of acceptable practice, without which we would be failing our patients.

Family and carer interventions

Before any successful psychosocial interventions with families or carers can be contemplated, they first have to be engaged with the services. In its own right, this may be one of the most important things we do. A supportive family (and most carers in mental health are families rather than friends or neighbours) can be the most powerful determinant of outcome for individuals with severe mental illness. Contrary to previous theories, which have implicated families in the genesis and exacerbation of psychoses (Chapter 14), the overwhelming evidence—both scientific and clinical—is that patients living with families do better than those without them. Of course this does not prove that families *cause* better outcomes. It is highly likely that less ill patients stay with families and more severely ill ones cannot tolerate the relationships (and sometimes the families cannot cope with them). On balance, however, despite the stresses and strains, it is better to have a family than not. As these family members are, therefore, actively engaged in trying to help and care for the patient it is essential that their efforts are taken seriously.

The need to recognize the carer burden (Harvey *et al.* 2001; Pai and Kapur 1981) is high on the health care agenda, alongside community care developments. Teams are expected to ensure that families are fully informed about treatment strategies, that their views on those treatments are taken into account, and that they are kept fully in the picture in terms of understanding the illness and the full range of possible treatments and care options. Put like that it sounds a tall order, but in practice it is usually rewarding and welcomed work.

Psychoeducation

Teaching patients and their families about the illness they have to contend with is generally referred to by the clumsy term 'psychoeducation'. At its most basic, it can comprise meeting the family and explaining what the diagnosis is, giving the best estimate of the prognosis, and explaining what the current treatment entails, with both its benefits and side-effects outlined. Providing carers with a copy of the care programme and talking it through with them can be a simple and efficient start to the process.

Psychoeducation can be significantly improved by using a more structured approach. The 'knowledge about schizophrenia' interview (KASI) (Barrowclough *et al.* 1987) provides a method of assessing the carer's prior knowledge about the illness. Specially prepared leaflets and information sheets, and even videos, are useful follow-ups. These allow the family member (and the patient) to read and reread the material—most of us know from personal experience how little we remember of the information our doctors' give us. Being able to take away a well-written information pack, tailored to the individual's needs, means they can study it at leisure. They can also ask about anything they are unclear of when they next meet their key worker or doctor. It is difficult to ascertain how effective psychoeducation is, because it is usually studied as part of a more comprehensive intervention (Hogarty *et al.* 1991; Leff *et al.* 1990).

Clinical experience confirms how essential explanations of illness and treatment are to any intervention that requires family members to work as part of the therapeutic team. It is vital not only to make sure we are all pulling in the same direction but also to dispel, as much as is possible, residual guilt and shame that are so common in parents of the mentally ill. Although we may have moved on from superficial theories blaming them for their offspring's illness (Chapter 14), they will certainly be regularly exposed to such prejudices in their daily life. They need to know that we do not share those views and psychoeducation is a very powerful means of emphasising this.

Behavioural family management

Work to understand why some patients with schizophrenia relapsed despite effective maintenance pharmacotherapy (Hirsch *et al.* 1973) led to studies of the family environment to which they were discharged. It was identified that patients from families who were emotionally intense and generally very involved were more likely to relapse. Work by Leff and colleagues further indicated that relapse was likely when the patient spent a lot of time with family members (the studies used 35 hours per week as the cut-off) and particularly so if the family members were critical of the patient. These families came to be referred to as 'high expressed emotion' ('high EE') families and a series of studies showed that family treatments to reduce high EE led to a reduction in relapse rates (Falloon *et al.* 1982; Leff *et al.* 1990; Linszen *et al.* 1996; Tarrier *et al.* 1989; Vaughan *et al.* 1992).

Most of these studies used an approach which comprised psychoeducation about schizophrenia (usually delivered jointly to patient and family members) followed by regular meetings (weekly or fortnightly) for several months to explore strategies to reduce or avoid critical comments towards the patient and to help the family disengage somewhat. Simple interventions are often remarkably welcome and effective. Pointing out to a concerned mother that her son may need to be left alone when he is aroused and disturbed is, in many ways, quite counter-intuitive (most of us want to comfort and care for distressed relatives). The education is about helping reduce the emotional charge which so many individuals with severe mental health problems (not just those with schizophrenia) find so difficult to handle.

Exploration of the family interactions often revealed common, repeated, and undramatic stresses (e.g. lying in bed all day, repetitive questioning, smoking in bed) that families struggle with. Helping find a form of words or action which modifies the behaviour without a row can be developed jointly by the therapist and family members, and they can be supported in practising it. Over time, families realize that this less confrontative and slightly more distanced style pays off and both they and the patient feel better. Family members really appreciate finding out that their problems are not unique, that it is not so much them as the problems the illness brings. Indeed, one study has shown better results by engaging in family problem-solving in a group session (McFarlane *et al.* 1995).

Behavioural family management is one of the evidence-based practices which is taught on Thorn courses. Being able to offer it to all families where there is clear evidence of high expressed emotion (there is no demonstrated benefit in 'low EE' families) ought to be a performance target for any dedicated assertive outreach team. In truth, even with small case loads, we find establishing such a provision very difficult. Firstly, it is very time consuming. In the initial series of studies, five courses of treatment were necessary to prevent one relapse and, in later studies (conducted perhaps with less committed families and less expert therapists), it required seven courses to prevent each relapse (Mari and Streiner 1994). Secondly, not only is the intervention difficult and time-consuming, but the results are not immediate. We should not underestimate how difficult it is to remain committed to a treatment which does not result in any direct improvement in well being but simply in a statistical reduction in risk. In one way we experience what the patient has to tolerate with maintenance medication—no immediate benefit but simply our reassurance that they are less likely to fall ill. Despite these difficulties, this is an effective treatment that can bring significant benefits to both patient and family, and teams need to develop strategies to encourage and support its provision.

We have found that making psychoeducation a top priority with the family means that we get to know them better. It gives us the basis for assessing whether or not they need interventions to reduce EE. We do not conduct long and detailed assessments of EE levels. Instead, we use a brief count of criticisms in a standard interview allied with clinical judgement. Even in its shortened form, the Camberwell Family Interview schedule (CFI) (Vaughn and Leff 1976) is long. The Relatives' Assessment Interview (RAI) (Barrowclough *et al.* 1998) is designed to look at relatives' experiences of caring and to identify areas of need rather than ratings of expressed emotion. For example, the RAI establishes levels of contact, household tension, and irritability, patient behaviours, and ability to contribute to household tasks, manage money, and interact socially. Very often tensions arise over patient underactivity or bizarre behaviour. In the close relationships developed through assertive outreach, it may be unnecessary to use such structured interviews, unless there is a desire to measure outcome more precisely.

Different cultures seem to have different levels of EE (Telles *et al.* 1995; Wig *et al.* 1987) and the Telles study suggested that the intervention can make things worse. We are, however, still deliberately lax about defining high EE. The result is that staff offer the intervention to most families. The common trap with such endeavours is to start with the most obvious and difficult cases. As confidence builds up with less extreme families one can attempt the really difficult ones.

There is some evidence that the success of behavioural family management is mediated through improved medication compliance, and so we offer medication management interventions concurrently.

Patient-focused interventions

Patients need the same, if not more, attention paid to engagement and explanation of their illnesses and treatments as do their families and carers. Like them, they need constant reassurance and repetition of the information if it is to be absorbed and psychoeducation is to be successful. What we are attempting to get over is complex, often distressingly ambiguous, and often lacking in the certainty that would fix it in the mind. Denial of the reality of their disorder is more common in patients than in families (although it is often very striking when it does occur in families and such shared denial is remarkably resistant to challenge or erosion). Patient education is generally easier to weave into ongoing treatment over a longer time. Unlike families, however, they are less likely to actively seek information. The team needs a mechanism to encourage and prompt it so that it becomes, like engagement, a constant strand in the approach.

In addition to these general approaches, there are three broad areas of psychosocial intervention aimed directly at the patient:

- CBT for delusions and hallucinations
- Motivational interviewing to improve compliance with prescribed medication and (hopefully) reduce the use of drugs and alcohol
- The development of early intervention strategies in relapse

CBT for delusions and hallucinations

CBT is a fast-developing area in mental health practice (Chapter 17) and there is real optimism about its potential in the treatment of delusions and hallucinations in schizophrenia. Two different theoretical approaches are identifiable (though in practice there is much overlap):

- Stress vulnerability model—emphasizes coping strategy enhancement
- Cognitive model—emphasizes similarity between normal and abnormal thinking

Both approaches draw heavily on the core principles of CBT :

- ◆ The central position of the patient as an active agent in the change process
- ◆ A collaborative rather than prescriptive exercise
- ◆ Scientific method (i.e. predicting consequences and testing those predictions)
- ◆ Focus on individual symptoms, not the disorder

The collaborative approach is probably the most important feature of all CBT approaches. Two key concepts often written about are 'collaborative empiricism' and the 'Socratic dialogue'. Collaborative empiricism describes the way the therapist and patient develop and test ideas together. They agree what would be the results of one view (the delusion) and what would happen if the delusion were not true, and then test out what actually does happen. Socratic dialogue refers to that Greek philosopher's habit of instructing his pupils by questioning them, so that eventually they came out with the answers themselves—they discovered what they already knew. In psychotic disorders it enables the inconsistency or inner doubts about delusions to be aired without a direct assault on them (which we have all learnt from bitter experience rarely works!).

Stress vulnerability model

This view accepts that the individual with a severe mental illness has some specific vulnerability to stress which manifests itself in the symptoms of the illness (Zubin and Spring 1977) and lies at the heart of much of assertive outreach practice described in this book. CBT techniques are aimed at reducing these stressors—whether they are the external stresses of family and friends or the stress of the symptoms themselves. In both cases it is understood that it is the patient's own 'appraisal' of the event which determines whether or not it is a stress, and if so, how severe.

Coping strategy enhancement

Tarrier and colleagues (Tarrier *et al.* 1998) consider that patients who have a wide range of coping strategies manage better with their psychotic experiences. They advise identifying empirically as many effective strategies as possible which reduce distress from the symptoms and encouraging the patient to use them. Such strategies can be *affective* (relaxation, sleep), *behavioural* (activity, seeking company), or *cognitive* (distraction, challenging). They are not concerned particularly with the content or meaning of the symptoms.

Falloon and Talbot (1981) take a similar approach to Tarrier but suggest that the consistent use of a single, well-trained strategy (rather than a range) is more likely to bring relief. Hogarty's highly structured personal therapy for schizophrenia (Hogarty *et al.* 1997) incorporates a similar approach to reducing 'affect dysregulation' (Chapter 14).

CBT to challenge delusions

Chadwick's approach (Chadwick *et al.* 1996) involves challenging delusions and assumptions about hallucinations based on the 'Socratic dialogue' outlined above. It explicitly draws on the evidence from normal psychology that most of us preferentially register information that strengthens our prejudices and ignore that which contradicts them. The approach is one of accessing the patient's inner doubts, often by working with the double awareness that is often so striking in psychotic patients (i.e. patients behave in ways that are totally at variance with their intensely held beliefs). Four components of this disputing approach are distinguished:

- Evidence for belief challenged (starting with less important issues first)
- Internal logic and plausibility challenged
- Reformulate as understandable response, seek meaningful alternative
- Assess alternative and delusion against available evidence

(Chadwick *et al.* 1996)

With hallucinations, the approach is probably less sucessful and the emphasis is often more on challenging the '*sense of omniscience*' attributed to the voices. This is done by demonstrating how the predicted consequences of the voices do not always happen. It is slow work. Helping the patient to recognize that they have some control over the voices (usually by getting them to deliberately bring them on in the interview and then to stop them for brief periods) can significantly reduce the fear they engender.

The research evidence for these approaches is growing, but it would be misleading to suggest that it is anywhere near as strong as that for medication or behavioural family management. Delusions seem to respond better than auditory hallucinations, and the main impact is on reduction of symptoms and associated distress and quicker recovery. There is no evidence for reducing relapse rates. Hogarty's work suggests that the approaches are probably better targeted on patients who do not live alone (Hogarty *et al.* 1997). Garety (Garety *et al.* 1997) considers it best to concentrate on patients who show a 'chink of insight'.

Motivational interviewing

Motivational interviewing was developed by Prochaska and Diclemente (1992) to help in the management of alcohol and drug abuse. In their 'stages of change' approach they emphasized the careful assessment of 'where the patient is at' in terms of confronting their addiction, and then tailoring treatment to that stage. The treatment takes the form of a series of interviews exploring the pros and cons of the current stage or of moving forward. (It is explained in greater detail in Chapters 11 and 18 which focus on medication compliance and substance abuse.)

The same observations apply to motivational interviewing as to other psychosocial interventions. It is an effective technique which is fairly easy to learn but equally easy to overlook in everyday practice. Systems within routine team functioning should ensure that once key workers have acquired the skills, they use them. Reporting back on them in reviews and planning and timetabling booster sessions at these reviews are ways of making sure that the skills are used. Given the strikingly positive effect of this intervention on drug compliance (Kemp *et al.* 1996), it is hard to explain why it is overlooked.

The results with substance abuse are probably not so well established—certainly not in patients with dual diagnosis of mental illness and substance abuse. It remains, however, one of the few approaches to harm minimization in these situations that can escape the sense of moral criticism or nagging that tends to be associated with simpler approaches to substance abuse.

Early intervention

Many patients have identifiable relapse signatures (i.e. a group of symptoms, experiences, or behaviours that herald an impending breakdown).

Common early warning signs

- Tensions, nervousness, irritability, sense of impending doom
- Difficulty sleeping and overactivity
- Social withdrawal; disengagement from services; self-neglect
- Increased positive symptoms—paranoia, thought disorder, auditory hallucinations

For some disorders there are well-recognized warnings that are specific to the disorder, rather than individual patients (e.g. poor sleep is very typical in incipient mania; being preoccupied and withdrawn is common in schizophrenia). All mental health workers learn to be alert for such indicators. It is the basis of much of our clinical training.

Early recognition of emerging patterns of breakdown, often before full-blown symptoms are obvious, comes with experience. Monitoring to assess mental state and functioning should take place (whether in depth or, more often, informally as part of another activity) as an integral part of any contact between a patient and a mental health professional. Using this monitoring as an opportunity to spot early signs of destabilization or breakdown is one of the primary purposes of any outreach service.

Relapse Signatures

As well as the more general early signs of relapse, there are some patients who have their own unique pattern which precedes breakdown. This is particularly so in bipolar disorder, and teaching patients (and their families) how to recognize such patterns, and what to do, can be an invaluable intervention. Agreeing what should be done and (most important) writing this agreement down as a contingency plan is increasingly routine practice. The procedures we use are outlined in the chapter on bipolar disorder (Chapter 15) and will not be repeated here.

Tarrier's work in this area (Perry *et al.* 1999) shows that the approach is of value for more patients than just those who have a strikingly obvious relapse signature. Most bipolar patients and their families can be helped to identify the early stages of relapse and encouraged and taught what to do. We have been using a similar approach in our CBT with schizophrenia, but have not found making a distinction between 'relapse signatures' and responding to periods of increased stress that valuable. With our schizophrenia patients we focus on identifying indicators of stress and worry and strategies to use should the need arise, rather than conceptualizing it as relapse prevention.

As with psychosocial interventions generally, early intervention has the added benefits of empowerment and reducing the sense of hopelessness for both patient and family.

Understanding and support

At the beginning of this chapter and at other places in this book we have warned against the possible downside of being excessively evidence-based in approach. Yes, we do need to make sure that most of our time and efforts go into providing treatments that are known to work—whether these are broadly psychological, social, or medical. On the other hand, we must not forget that this work is about people and relationships. Patients and their families need understanding and support, though not as an alternative to effective psychosocial interventions. They may need them even more when they are receiving such psychosocial interventions because these treatments are demanding and can (despite our best efforts) be quite stressful.

Time needs to be devoted to simply being nice to patients and their families. If we cannot learn to respect and like them, and them us, then we are unlikely to be able to help them even with the most sophisticated treatments. Expressing sympathy and support, paying attention to the broader canvas of patients' lives, are necessary foundations for collaborative work. It is not wasted time or a case of 'avoiding the issue'. It is one of the great advantages of having a capped case load that key workers can be more welcoming and generous with their patients. In a health service with unlimited demand and limited resources, staff do not actively seek work. Adopting a rather business-like tone has traditionally been one way of managing the pressures. With the severely mentally ill this approach is probably inefficient in the long term. A welcoming and genuinely supportive approach, which leads to problem solving earlier on, will save time in the long run.

Older counselling approaches (whether non-directive or Rogerian or psychodynamic) have a role to play in outreach work. Tragic and difficult events are far from uncommon for our patients, who need the opportunity to talk them through, make sense of them, and come to terms with them. Most mental health workers appreciate the value of such approaches. The trick is to avoid dogma. There is no set number of sessions or length of session that must be followed. What is important is that the sessions are safe, respectful, and supportive.

Received wisdom is that psychodynamic approaches with individuals with severe mental illnesses do more harm than good. Where this means attempting to interpret and uncover unconscious material in an individual who has difficulty distinguishing the inner world from the outer at the best of times, we would agree. However, concepts like 'denial', 'unconscious worrying', 'transference', having a 'complex' about something are all useful ways of understanding experience. The language is intuitive and now easily understood by all involved and can help make otherwise confusing experiences more understandable.

While we would not encourage psychoanalytical therapy for our patients, we see no harm in using many of the terms and ideas that derive from it. These terms are generally regarded as more respectful and equal than the technical terms we use in formal therapies (e.g. 'automatic thoughts'). Psychodynamic language is that which patients hear on the television (e.g. 'you're just repressing it') and that they know we use about each other—it is no longer associated with illness. It is also a robust conceptual framework which makes some sort of sense of difficult experiences in ways that help us, as therapists, to keep sight of the patient's essential humanity.

Conclusions

In the broad, holistic approach used in outreach work, patients and their families are seen as complete individuals, in all their complexity. The work ranges from the narrowly prescriptive aspects of medication, to social and personal support, through dramatic life crises. The rather vague concept of 'psychosocial interventions' straddles this range. It consists of a group of disparate treatments with proven efficacy, and which are based on using understanding (and the collaborative relationship that develops from it) to achieve quite specific behavioural changes. They are both effective and conceptually attractive to outreach workers.

Such interventions are, however, often unhelpfully presented as being easy. *Learning* to do them, and to do them well, is reasonably easy. They are well described and operationalized. Most of our staff have been able to gain a working ability with the main three or four interventions in a one-year day-release course. But *applying* them, and applying them consistently, is not easy (see Chapter 26)—that requires effort, sensitivity, and persistence. Time for them needs to be protected in the midst of crises, admissions, etc. Their results are very real but not immediately obvious, and their success requires continued attention to detail. None of this is easy, and we should not pretend it is.

Research and developments in this area are frenetic; improvements are happening all the time. The real challenge is not to keep at the cutting edge but to ensure that established and effective psychosocial interventions are made available to those who can benefit from them. In no other field is there such a pressing need to monitor and audit to ensure that we deliver what we know works (rather than simply search for newer and more effective treatments).

Part III

Structural issues

Chapter 26

Managing the team

Introduction

Assertive outreach is an effective method of delivering intensive and comprehensive packages of care to severely mentally ill individuals. It relies on co-ordination, communication, and a clearly understood policy framework at a team level. It is a labour-intensive activity and deals with complex issues. Assertive outreach teams need a clinical team leader who is a mental health professional and capable of combining team case work with operational management, in order that the team functions effectively on all these levels.

In the NHS, the consultant psychiatrist has a complementary leadership role and ultimate clinical accountability. This chapter sets out the relative roles and tasks, and presents a model for organizing the team's resources day to day. For the many staff who graduate from clinical to managerial roles, basic management concepts are covered along with the contemporary policy framework. Throughout, key issues are raised for managers responsible for assertive outreach services.

Role of the team leader

Below are the main tasks that make up the role of the team leader. Assertive outreach presents us with the demands of an extended key-worker role in our work with patients. For the team leader this is compounded by the demands of co-ordinating a busy team, day to day, often over seven days or even with 24-hour cover. The role calls for a generalist with clinical experience, sound judgement, and the ability to plan and prioritize the many varied tasks into a week's work. It's like juggling a number of balls at the same time—and some of those balls can cause damage if they are dropped!

Key tasks of the team leader

- Clinical work with own case load of patients, plus team patients
- Co-ordinating the handovers and meeting schedule
- Management supervision of team members
- Co-ordinating clinical supervision
- Staff recruitment and selection/retention

> **Key tasks of the team leader (*Continued*)**
>
> - Co-ordinating induction and training
> - Managing the budget
> - Implementing and protecting the model and policies
> - Dealing with problems—clinical and operational (e.g. complaints, untoward incidents)
> - Delivering and managing processes and strategies for change
> - Representing the team externally
> - Linking and negotiating with external agencies
> - Overseeing the team's case load size, mix, and priorities
> - Monitoring and evaluation of the service; regular audit
> - Decision making in conjunction with the consultant

This is clearly not a job that suits everyone and the following are some important characteristics to include in the person specification:

> - Clear communicator
> - Good interpersonal skills
> - Able to work under pressure
> - Able to make key decisions for both day-to-day problem solving and strategy
> - Able to lead by example in clinical work
> - Good presentational skills
> - Able to work as part of a team
> - Able to delegate tasks and responsibilities
> - Able to involve and motivate the team

Role of the consultant psychiatrist

Standards for assertive outreach indicate the importance of medical staff being fully integrated (Allness and Knoedler 1998; Burns *et al*. 2001*a*; Teague *et al*. 1998). A single consultant for the team provides direction and a consistent approach to patient care, and simplifies care programme and Mental Health Act procedures and accountability. Teams that use external CMHT medical resources experience different levels of consultant commitment, delays, disputes, and communications which can dilute the application of the model.

The consultant and junior medical staff should feel part of the team, even though they do not key work because of the multiple calls on their time. The tasks that make up the consultant's role are:

- Directing team vision, model, and priorities
- Responsible medical officer for the purposes of the Mental Health Act (Department of Health 1999*b*)
- Primary clinical decision maker
- Clinical work across entire team case load
- Medical input to clinical reviews
- Representing the team externally
- Line managing medical staff

Structuring a week in assertive outreach

A flexible team needs a predictable timetable. The timetable shown in Fig. 26.1 is the one used by our team and is one way of co-ordinating team activity over a seven-day period with limited weekend cover. Teams that operate a shift system or are on call may have a handover at the beginning and end of each shift. Our model represents a compromise between a team that operates in normal office hours and one that is on call 24 hours a day, seven days a week. The majority of time is unstructured for patient contact and activity. This activity is not predictable and key workers need to allow time in their diaries for the unexpected.

Monday morning's handover is important for planning the week ahead. Sharing of case loads with a modified whole-team approach (Chapter 5) means that individual visits and tasks can be allocated throughout the week. Different weekdays may have a specific focus—collecting clozapine blood samples on one particular day, conducting a ward round on another, planning weekend activity on a Friday, etc.

Such a weekly schedule accommodates many factors such as consultant availability, postgraduate training, and in-patient unit schedules and shifts. Meetings should be just long enough for co-ordination, cover, communication, and support, allowing the majority of time for patient contact. A 'tight' meeting will limit expansive and overly detailed backgrounds and discussion. A strategy in our team is to bring drifting discussion into line by asking for the 'headline' first, followed by any relevant facts. For example, the headline may be 'Patrick wants to negotiate a reduction in his medication', and the facts might be that there are relevant side-effects and mental state assessment shows absence of positive symptoms, drug history indicates relapse often occurs following negotiation down to subclinical doses. Brief multidisciplinary discussion can then occur and a plan agreed.

	MONDAY	TUESDAY	WEDNESDAY	THURSDAY	FRIDAY	SATURDAY	SUNDAY
MORNING	09.30 –10.00 HANDOVER To include team approach planning of visits for week 10.00 –11.00 CLINICAL SUPERVISION (alternate weeks) 10.00 –11.00 DEVELOPMENT MEETING (monthly)	09.00 –11.00 COMMUNITY REVIEW MEETING	09.30 –10.00 HANDOVER	09.30 –10.00 HANDOVER	09.30 –10.00 HANDOVER	09.00 –17.00 ROUTINE VISITS (with capacity for emergency cover)	09.00 –17.00 ROUTINE VISITS (with capacity for emergency cover)
AFTERNOON		11.00 –12.00 BUSINESS MEETING (monthly) 15.30 –17.00 IN-PATIENT WARD ROUND		16.00 –17.00 MINI WARD ROUND			

Fig. 26.1   A weekly timetable for an assertive outreach team

Handover/briefing

'Handover' is a nursing term for relaying information from shift to shift. Many American and Australian assertive outreach teams operate shifts. Not all UK teams have adopted this pattern despite the literature promoting extended hours and 24-hour cover (see Chapter 6). With shared case loads, effective transmission of verbal and written information is essential on a daily basis.

Most assertive outreach teams in the UK use a key-worker system (Department of Health 1990), strengthened with a team approach for patients needing daily visits or with specific difficulties. The CPA currently only applies to England and not the whole of the UK. Where key workers are identified and shift work is not operating, the 'handover' is more of a morning briefing session.

Format for handover/briefing

- Takes place first thing in the morning (or beginning and end of the day when using a shift system).
- 15–30 minutes depending on case-load size.
- Chairperson to mention each patient by name (alphabetical order or by key worker).
- Discussion only occurs if there has been a change, development, or concern, or advice is needed, or where visit allocation or cover is needed.
- Chairperson to curtail lengthy discussion or refer to clinical supervision or weekly review meeting.
- Junior doctor present.
- Monday handover may be more involved with allocation of work for the week e.g. which patients to be visited each day, tasks for the support worker.
- Friday handover may include time for planning support over the weekend if cover is limited.

Functions of handover/briefing

- Structured exchange of information on every patient, in a time-efficient forum.
- Allocation of tasks and visits.
- Organization of cover for staff on leave, training, or away sick.
- Organization of joint visits either for safety or specific input.
- Group support and multidisciplinary problem solving.
- Prioritization of resources for the day.

Functions of handover/briefing (*Continued*)

♦ Regular access to a doctor for advice, prescriptions, medicine titration, or changes.

♦ Reinforces 'teamness' through face-to-face planning and discussion.

Weekly review meeting

Patients with complex needs, such as those cared for by assertive outreach teams, require a regular review of their treatment and care. Regular reviews are required for all patients on enhanced CPA incorporating health and social care elements. We review in depth every six months. The high level of needs of assertive outreach patients does not mean that this in-depth process should necessarily occur more often: our patients are routinely assessed frequently. Exceptions may be patients subject to aftercare under supervision ('supervised discharge') and those considered high risk and where the care plan does not adequately resolve concerns. For example, a patient who remains out of contact despite intensive attempts to engage, and for whom risks are apparent, may need full multidisciplinary review every few months.

Wherever possible, all those involved with the care and welfare of the patient are invited to the meeting. This may include the patient, carers, and voluntary sector and day/residential care workers. A balance has to be struck, however, between such inclusiveness and the efficient use of team time. We routinely review five patients each week, allocating 20 minutes to each review.

Functions of CPA review meeting

♦ Forum for involving users, carers, and other agencies in care planning and review process.

♦ Opportunity for extended discussion with full multidisciplinary team and all revelant parties to current and long-term management.

♦ Statutory requirement (Care Programme Approach—Department of Health 1990).

♦ Agreement and completion of full documentation—CPA, care plan, risk and contingency plans, treatment plan, review of aftercare under supervision, etc.

By providing such practical assistance as transport, reminders, and reassurance it is possible to facilitate the presence of the patient and their carers routinely at the review. Sometimes patients do not want to be present to hear all their history and prefer to come into the review for input to the discussion of the care plan. The following format is one we evolved in our team. Some staff members need training and support in developing the skills of concise and effective review presentations.

Preparations for CPA review

- Put reviews in your diary.
- Arrange joint visit with SHO.
- Repeat BPRS, side-effects, or any other relevant structured assessment scales e.g. Beck inventory.
- Invite the patient and carer or relevant others. Book a time slot and arrange transport if necessary.
- Prepare the patient well; explain the purpose and procedure. Explain the time limitations. Agree whether they wish to hear all their history or only wish to attend care planning.
- Plan what you and your patient each need to get out of the review.

If the patient is attending, it will be necessary to adjust the style and content of the review to allow for, sensitivity to potential embarrassment, denial, and third-party information received. With this caveat, the following information should be covered:

Content of review

- Name and age
- Length of time with team
- Diagnosis
- Summary of relevant family/social history
- Summary of psychiatric history:
  —number and frequency of admissions
  —relapse signature
  —untoward events
  —risks associated with relapse
  —treatment responses
  —medication summary
- Social circumstances
- Medical history
- Current situation/problems:
  —current BPRS and mental health
  —current medication

Content of review (*Continued*)

> —side-effect assessment
>
> —Mental Health Act status: supervision register/supervised discharge/Section 17 leave
>
> —prioritize other problems from physical health, housing, finance, occupation, daily living skills
>
> —risks
>
> ◆ Discussion
>
> ◆ Presentation of new care plan
>
> ◆ Presentation of risk documentation
>
> ◆ Review contingency plan

There is currently such emphasis on completing paperwork in reviews that it is easy to forget that their main purpose is to plan treatment. Key workers need to schedule in 'post-review' time (and energy) to make sure the paperwork is completed that day. Leaving it for a day or so risks confusion and the possibility of forgetting important issues.

During this post-review time, the care plan, contingency plan, and risk documentation should be completed *fully* and filed in the correct section of the notes with copies to the GP and other agencies as necessary and agreed.

Business meetings, team days, and development meetings

Business meetings

A rolling programme of business and development meetings ensures regularity and helps team members to organize their time. Business meetings provide a structured space for senior staff to inform of changes affecting the team or external agencies (e.g. information on new community groups, changes in arrangements for accessing meals on wheels, pharmacy opening times over bank holidays, forthcoming conferences, deadlines for returning monitoring information). Consultation on strategic changes and discussion on operational policies can take place. Generation of new working practices or ideas is encouraged from individual team members. A single team leader cannot resolve and contain all aspects of team dynamics, individual anxieties, organizational change, or team direction and adaptation. Nor should they attempt to. All teams have a wealth of professional and personal experience. Solutions are usually readily found through collective effort.

Team days

Business meetings should be backed up by regular team days (once or twice a year) which can focus on major, non-clinical decision making. Team days are generally best arranged away from the base. They provide additional 'thinking time' and need an agenda that will allow both brainstorming and detailed constructive problem solving. A typical agenda might include a mix of specific topics that have filtered through from business meetings, re-organization, and specific incidents, as well as issues from clinical supervision and unstructured time.

Team days can be stressful when conflicts are confronted so it is good to finish with some team building. The vogue for masculine activity sports is over as team members pick up potential industrial injuries or feel pressurised to participate for the sake of the team! Stick to relatively safe fun, like ten-pin bowling or a trip to the greyhound races.

Facilitators

The decision to have a professional outside facilitator is best decided by the team as a whole. Structured, business parts of the day will not generally require an outside facilitator, but the team may choose to have one for that part of the programme which is more personal and more to do with team dynamics.

Development meetings

Development meetings are part of the team training and audit cycle (Chapter 27). Team members can take it in turns to facilitate or present a training topic, or external speakers can be invited. Group training in the use of agreed structured assessment tools (e.g. BPRS—Overall and Gorham 1962; EDOS—Chaplin *et al.* 1999; and HoNOS—Wing *et al.* 1999) generates greater inter-rater reliability and team understanding, plus it reinforces a common language used to discuss change. Specific topics can be introduced in development sessions by external speakers. A relevant new publication or research paper can be presented. In this way the development meeting becomes a learning aid, helping staff to keep up to date and encouraging evidence-based practice.

Development meetings can also generate audit ideas or standards, or even be used to conduct an audit. For example, to audit risk assessment documentation each team member can scan 10 sets of notes in the meetings and the whole process can be completed in a single meeting. Team members also get to understand how and why audits are performed.

Operational policy

The team's culture, purpose, and objectives should be defined in an operational policy. This should include local criteria for accepting referrals, for discharge, and team structure. Operational policies can also include specific team-level priorities and targets on measurable and achievable activities such as frequency of contact or interventions offered. Assertive outreach is fortunate in that it has a relatively clear, evidence-based model to provide the framework. An assertive outreach worker, when asked what they believe is their core purpose and objectives, is likely to provide a clearer answer than many in the mental health field. Operational policies give a concise overview of the functions and structure of the team to new and existing staff, other clinical colleagues, and to managers and commissioners.

Key areas for operational policy

- Model and philosophy of teams
- Team aims and objectives
- Target patient group
- Referral criteria
- Discharge criteria
- Team-level priorities and targets
- Relationships with other parts of the service
- Team staffing, composition, and accountability
- Operating hours and cover arrangements
- Training and staff support
- Research and outcome measures

Using the operational policy to set team priorities, goals, and targets allows for management by objectives. Drucker (1993) described a model whereby staff can measure their own activity against agreed organizational objectives which in turn focus, guide, and help their individual work. Drucker's model can be applied to assertive outreach teams. For example, the organization's mission statement may be: 'To provide the best mental health services for people in the locality'. This lacks any specific information on how to achieve or measure it. At the team level, targets must be more realistic. For assertive outreach workers with small case loads our team aims to: 'Provide an intensive service for those most in need'. This is equally vague. An objective to 'provide an average of two visits per week per patient' informs the individual worker of their target. The worker and their manager can measure this activity, and it is realistic. With a staff to patient ratio of 1:10, the objective becomes 20 visits per week per worker.

Management approaches

Team-based management is the accepted model for assertive outreach teams large enough to be self- sufficient (i.e. multidisciplinary, with designated medical input and upwards of five staff and fifty patients). The leadership style should be that of an accessible and supportive facilitator rather than a remote and supervisory manager. Leadership implies inspiring a group of people towards a common set of objectives rather than simply getting things done through instructing them.

Autocratic leadership may evolve where an experienced and confident senior clinician leads an inexperienced team with a number of unqualified support workers. The advantages are that leadership is clear and decisions made quickly, maximizing time available for patients. The disadvantages include concentration of responsibility around one person leading to inhibition of learning, growth, and ownership within the group. The team may function poorly in the absence of the leader and he or she is bombarded with requests from staff to sanction each decision they make.

The style generally favoured for effective team functioning is more democratic. The advantages are that commitment and responsibility is fostered in all team members. The potential disadvantages are delay, or even paralysis, of decision making. This can slow down the flexible, rapid response to both patient need and organizational change. Meetings become larger and less efficient, delegation becomes diffuse, and difficulties achieving goals or time pressures cause frustrations.

In practice, consultation and involvement of all staff as a cohesive, but multidisciplinary, team is essential. Style will not be fixed and a shift to a more autocratic style is common when there are crises or the workload is excessive.

Accountability and responsibility

An individual team member has responsibilities to patients and their families, to other team members, and to the team as a whole. They are also accountable to their line manager, to their professional body, and, under the law, to society The cycle of responsibility is shown in Fig. 26.2.

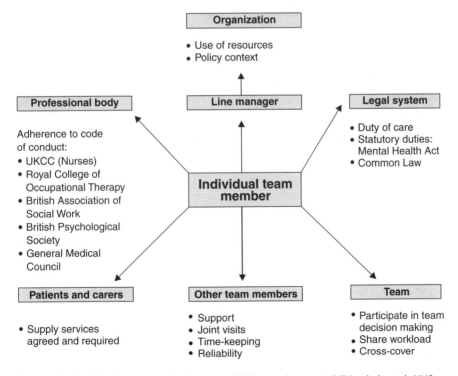

Fig. 26.2 An individual team member's responsibilities and accountabilities (adapted, NHS Training Authority 1990)

Management supervision

Management supervision is one of the key tasks referred to at the beginning of this chapter. Most team leaders from a clinical background find managing staff the hardest new skill to master. Regular, structured, one-to-one supervision with team members, together with handovers and team meetings, are the mechanisms to shape and lead staff members.

Management supervision provides 'a hierarchical system of monitoring individual staff performances, standards, and development'.

Management supervision creates a formal time in which staff can raise specific questions and requests with their line manager relating to their employment.

Content of management supervision

- Provide feedback and check performance of individual staff
- Encourage, recognize, and develop strengths of staff
- Help identify and problem solve weaknesses
- Individual performance review (annual)
- Monitor activity and documentation standards
- Monitor sickness and annual leave
- Help identify training needs and delivery of training
- Negotiate and agree goals and targets with staff member
- Allocate and delegate tasks, projects, and case load

Documentation

The content of management supervision sessions needs to be recorded in a suitable format in order to provide continuity and for appraisal. The form should outline the date, areas covered, action agreed, and time-scale for implementation. Sometimes forms require signing by the line manager and the supervisee to agree content and outcomes. Should changes fail to take place and disciplinary action is indicated, these records provide the necessary evidence. Documents should be stored safely and securely.

The frequency of management supervision does not need to be set in the operational policy. New staff and staff experiencing difficulties will need management supervision every few weeks. Experienced and more autonomous staff may require only periodic supervision every few months. Frequency needs to be negotiated with each individual and not assumed.

Personal issues

One-to-one management supervision will inevitably deal with personal and inter-personal matters that have a bearing on a person's ability to do their job. Domestic problems and family commitments will impact periodically, for example, on time-keeping, concentration, and motivation. Being able to discuss these reduces the stress on the staff member and the level of frustration on the part of the manager at under-performance. It is the manager's responsibility, however, to deal with such feelings and circumstances without the process slipping into a counselling session.

Cross-disciplinary supervision

Cross-disciplinary supervision requires an understanding and acceptance of the different styles of working that create a dynamic multidisciplinary team. For the same objective of helping a patient find work, the social worker may use the language of 'discrimination'; an occupational therapist, 'activity analysis'; and a psychologist, 'graded exposure'. Varied styles should not be at the expense of the common purpose defined by the model and operational policy.

Difficulties can arise with supervision arrangements because of the multidisciplinary nature of the team. The position of social workers remains anomalous—integrated into teams but still often separately managed. Separate legal frameworks and budgets can mean delays for patients. The merging of NHS and local authority responsibilities for all health and social care under single management, envisaged in *The NHS Plan* (Department of Health 2000), should simplify the position of social workers in assertive outreach teams. Many parts of the UK already have long-standing arrangements for close working.

Single management and budgets fit into the philosophy of assertive outreach by reducing the fragmentation of services to the benefit of the service user. Single management for staff also emphasizes the generic role of the clinical case managers/outreach workers over and above their original professional background.

Clinical supervision

How does clinical supervision differ from management supervision? Is it appropriate for a line manager to also give clinical supervision to their staff? These are difficult questions and it is worth making a clear distinction between the two activities.

Clinical supervision is a system which 'brings practitioners and skilled supervisors together to reflect on practice. Supervision aims to identify solutions to problems, improve clinical practice and increase understanding of professional issues.' Supervision in the case of nurses is not a statutory requirement, neither is it hierarchical or a management control system.

(UKCC 1996)

A good use of clinical supervision in assertive outreach is to support staff in the clinical use of the skills they have learnt. For example, staff sent on training courses such as the Thorn course (Gournay and Birley 1998), required for psychosocial interventions, have often failed to employ these interventions with patients where there is no post-course supervision.

Content of clinical supervision

- Reflection on complex or difficult cases
- Evaluation to improve clinical practice
- Support of developing skills such as the use of sophisticated psychosocial interventions
- Consideration of professional issues
- Sharing of new ideas and practice

Practice varies as to whether it is the role of the team leader to provide clinical supervision as well as management supervision for each case manager. Doing both can develop the relationship between the key worker and manager through a two-way process of feedback. Clinical supervision is focused on individual patients and is more likely to result in the development of skills such as behavioural family management. Combining the two functions can, however, carry risks. The clinical supervisor's other role as line manager may inhibit the supervisee from expressing concerns. Confidentiality and trust may be more difficult to maintain in the supervisory relationship (King's Fund 1994). Conflicts of interest may also arise, such as where a team leader is involved in disciplinary action against a staff member.

One model is to set up regular group clinical supervision with the assertive outreach workers, perhaps for one hour every two weeks. This session has a facilitator who may be a senior, experienced member of the team—but is not the team leader . The role of the facilitator is to avoid the development of cosy peer supervision, which can lack the rigour to confront poor practice. Staff in assertive outreach subscribe to a common model and purpose which makes group clinical supervision a good option. It is arguably a more effective use of time than one-to-one supervision because of the generic approach to patient care. A drawback of the team leader's absence from group clinical supervision is that it can insulate him or her from the real anxieties and concerns of their staff. Group clinical supervision needs to retain confidentiality within the group to allow free expression. Feedback by the facilitator to the team leader is not an option, unless sanctioned by the group.

Burn out and supervision

The combination of management and clinical supervision aims to produce a competent and confident practitioner who feels well supported and understood by the system in which he or she works (Nursing Times 2000). Developing flexibility and a degree of role blurring requires the confidence to step out of the safety of traditional professional roles and to take positive risks. This will not happen if the team member is not secure in their role or within the organization.

High levels of burn out are often claimed for assertive outreach—usually by those not working in the field. Our own team's seven-year experience has consistently shown staff turnover rates of 10% per year. This compares with average turnover rates for the NHS of 15%, the public sector in general in the UK of 13.9%, and the private sector of 14.3% (Noakes and Johnson 1999). Retention is enhanced by well-resourced and well-remunerated teams, as well as opportunities to be involved in research, training, and project work. A clear model, or vision, which incorporates role flexibility, and the relative autonomy associated with community working keeps staff motivated.

Proponents of the team approach argue that shared case loads help to reduce burn out (Bond 1991). There is no evidence of this. In a survey of multidisciplinary team members in 57 UK CMHTs, Onyett *et al.* (1997) found that burn out was not associated with case-load size or composition, or the frequency with which patients were seen.

Nevertheless, assertive outreach produces some unique pressures on staff. Patients are referred precisely because they are hard to engage, yet the model requires strenuous efforts to engage them. Patients may be less than grateful, even hostile, for your hard work. The extended key worker role places enormous responsibility on staff. Some staff find shopping and practical assistance tasks do not best reflect their professional expertise and may choose to work in more traditional areas. Extended hours and on-call working also take their toll. An effective system of management and clinical support is time well spent in the development and retention of expensive and experienced staff.

Recruitment and selection of staff

The practice of assertive outreach in the UK is relatively new. It is rare to be able to recruit an experienced practitioner familiar with what is, by definition, an expanded role that crosses traditional professional barriers. In addition to the skills and competencies outlined in the job description, personal characteristics are highly relevant to assertive outreach.

Desirable personal characteristics

- Flexible
- Pragmatic
- Practical problem-solving ability
- Patient needs-led approach
- Nurturing and supportive style
- Gentle firmness
- Non-judgemental
- A 'can do' attitude

Patients are often very demoralized and pessimistic, having failed so often in the past. The assertive outreach worker has to be able to contribute his or her optimism to the joint effort. There are always a million reasons why something may not be possible. What is needed from the assertive outreach worker is a desire to make it happen, perhaps in very small steps. A 'can do' attitude is an essential care quality.

Undesirable personal characteristics

- Over controlling
- 'Macho'
- Needing to do for others
- Pessimistic approach to patients' motives and behaviours; 'seen it all' attitude
- Protective of professional boundaries
- Unwilling to use self-disclosure as part of engagement process

Some staff apply to work in assertive outreach teams expecting to be a mobile agent of control, safeguarding society from its most troublesome members. This may come from in-patient experiences of our patients when they are at their most unwell. Our experience has shown that attempts to work with patients in their own homes draws on collaboration and nurturing. 'Macho' attempts to control do not generally provide long-term solutions. Patients also quickly understand staff and their underlying motives and values. Staff who harbour negative stereotypes of patients, or who have over-rigid ideas of what is, and is not, appropriate, will not be able to establish an 'authentic' therapeutic relationship.

Specific interview questions and scenarios can elicit the types of responses that might indicate desirable or undesirable characteristics and attributes. For example: 'During the course of building up a relationship with a patient they ask if you are married and how many children you have. How would you respond?'

The traditional person specification summarizes skills and personal qualities into essential and desirable. Communication skills and the ability to cope with pressure sit alongside more formally acquired knowledge and qualifications. In our mental health trust 'personal experience of mental health problems' is entered into all clinical person specifications as desirable (unless specific exemptions are agreed by the Chief Executive). US experience has shown us that 'consumer workers' are a valuable resource in assertive outreach, particularly in relation to engagement. In recent years, UK 'service users' have become fully-paid employees in many aspects of mental health services including assertive outreach teams.

There is currently no unemployment among occupational therapists, nurses, psychologists, or social workers in the UK. Assertive outreach is labour-intensive, with skilled labour making up the majority of the team's budget. The ability to develop a long-term, therapeutic relationship with difficult patients is vital to the success of the undertaking. For all these reasons, and more, the investment of time and energy in recruitment and selection will pay dividends in the longer term. Short-term approaches to filling vacancies with relocated internal staff and secondees, who do not go through full selection procedures and filters, can be a costly mistake.

Conclusions

In this chapter we have tried to set out basic operational management activities and applied them to a typical week in assertive outreach. More generic tasks like managing budgets, strategic planning, managing change, service review, have been omitted as they are dealt with in more general publications (Reynolds and Thornicroft 1999; Wood and Carr 1998). Chapters 28 and 29 of this book also examine service planning and service evaluation.

The central resource is people. Successful teams rely on the skills and commitment of individual staff members. The managerial role is to harness these skills in a clear, meaningful, and effective operational framework. In the NHS we are used to management activities that divert clinicians from patient care. Such external forces are usually about servicing the organization. A team-based manager is in a position to have a dual perspective, in which promoting patient care remains dominant.

Chapter 27

Training

Introduction

> Not all mental health service staff, even those trained relatively recently, have the skills and com-
> petencies to deliver modern mental health services. For example, psychological interventions,
> such as cognitive behaviour therapy, and complex medication management.
>
> (Department of Health 1999*b*)

Professional training and education has not kept up with the development of assertive
outreach as a specialism. Unless exposed to assertive outreach on a placement during
training, staff are unlikely to have had any theoretical or practical exposure to this way
of working. The comprehensive and generalist approach to the care of the severely
mentally ill enshrined in the model means that it utilizes wide-ranging skills and
knowledge. This chapter sets out the competencies that inform the scope of training
from induction and conceptual model, practical skills and knowledge, through to
sophisticated assessment and treatments. Much applies equally to unqualified support
workers.

Two aspects of basic level professional training should be considered. Firstly, common gaps in knowledge can be anticipated from a new team member's professional
background. For example, assessing side-effects of medication is likely to be a new skill
for an occupational therapist, and detailed knowledge of the welfare benefits system a
challenge for a nurse. Secondly, mental health nurses now receive 18 months of generic
nurse training before specializing under Project 2000 (English National Board 1996).
Therefore they qualify with significantly less mental health learning and experience
than previously. This common foundation programme may soon be shortened, allowing more time for specific mental health training (Sainsbury Centre for Mental Health
1997). Social worker training involves even less mental health practice.

Pre-qualification training is too often a preparation for independent practice rather
than a preparation for working with agencies and co-ordinating comprehensive care in
partnership with other professions (Muijen 1997).

Changing needs and roles

The Sainsbury Centre for Mental Health's review, *Pulling together* (Sainsbury Centre
for Mental Health 1997), examines the future roles and training of mental health staff
working with the severely mentally ill in the UK. The review recognizes that the
transition from largely hospital-based to community-based services, increasing patient

and carer involvement and choice, and the blurring of roles across health and social care boundaries have all affected practice:

- Rigid professional demarcations increasingly fail to reflect current workload requirements and current practice.
- Professional staff roles overlap considerably between the various disciplines and with support staff.
- The demands of purchasers of services and of training consortia are forcing a reconsideration of the skill mix required in mental health services.
- There is increasing emphasis on competent performance of role rather than qualification and status.

(Sainsbury Centre for Mental Health 1997)

In addition, new interventions are evolving in the treatment of psychotic illnesses. Increasingly, patients and professionals are finding the advantages of novel antipsychotic medications with more tolerable side-effect profiles. Psychosocial interventions have become integral components in the management of schizophrenia rather than just worthy extras (Burns 1997a). Each step forward increases knowledge and carries training implications.

Establishing core competencies for assertive outreach

Competence combines the general attributes of knowledge, skill, and attitudes, but also incorporates professional or personal judgement. A competence describes what is important for the workforce and provides performance anchor points. Most person specifications for professional jobs in assertive outreach will ask for at least two years' post-qualification experience and experience of work in the community.

There is a tendency to adapt or copy job descriptions from other teams without a great deal of thought for specific core competencies. Competencies for unqualified support workers are perhaps more important. The inquiry into the killing of Jonathan Newby by a mentally ill resident in a care home in which he worked identified the importance of training for staff not from a professional mental health background (Davies 1995). This inquiry led to the establishment of the 'Newby competencies', which are incorporated into the Mental Health Foundation Certificate in Community Mental Health (Mental Health Foundation 1997).

The first of 20 recommendations of *Pulling together* is that core competencies be established for mental health workers across specialisms (Sainsbury Centre for Mental Health 1997). *Capable Practitioner*, was produced by The Sainsbury Centre for Mental Health (2001) as a report for the National Service Framework workforce action team.

The report outlines a framework of generic capabilities for the key professional disciplines working in mental health, and is intended as the foundation for a national set of competencies. The following list is adapted for assertive outreach from the competencies found in *Capable Practitioner*, *Pulling together*, and the 'Newby competencies'. It highlights basic competences applicable to all clinical staff, including non-professional support workers.

Basic competencies for all clinical staff

- An understanding of the signs and symptoms of major mental illness and the ways in which people with a mental health problem may feel and experience the world. A non-judgemental attitude to mental illness.
- Interpersonal skills including the ability to communicate with patients, professionals, and colleagues in a multi-agency environment. Awareness of the need to work in partnership with carers and social networks.
- Knowledge of the priority group of people with severe and enduring mental health problems.
- An ability to observe and monitor the well-being of someone with a mental illness and to recognize when to call for expert assistance.
- An ability to establish, sustain, disengage, and re-establish working relationships with a patient.
- An understanding of the most commonly used medical and psychological treatments and their likely effects.
- An ability to assess and provide a flexible range of approaches for the patient's practical and social needs including housing, finance, occupation, and problem solving.
- Supporting patients and their carers in presenting their own needs and interests, ensuring access to an independent advocate when required.
- An understanding of the systems for arranging and managing care, including assertive outreach, the care programme approach, and the Mental Health Act.
- Knowledge and skill in risk assessment and the prevention and management of behaviour which is dangerous to self or others.
- An understanding of substance abuse, its effects, and how to recognize, monitor, and manage it.
- Accurate, appropriate, sensitive, and accountable record-keeping.
- Safe and ethical practice. Conforming to organizational policies and procedures related to confidentiality, equal opportunities, etc.

Additional competencies for professionally trained key workers

- Ability to plan, manage, and evaluate care in conjunction with the multidisciplinary team.
- Ability to guide and manage support in the delivery of packages of care.
- Up-to-date skills and understanding of medical and psychological treatment approaches to psychotic disorders e.g. novel antipsychotics and clozapine therapy, schizophrenia family work, CBT, compliance therapy, vocational rehabilitation.
- Effective liaison with all levels of the organization and other agencies.
- Ability to write clear and relevant reports.
- Knowledge of policy and legislation in relation to modern mental health care.
- Capable of educating patients and carers on aspects of illness, treatments, and mental health services.
- Capable of facilitating the participation of patients and carers in the development, delivery, and evaluation of individual care plans.
- Capable of developing and promoting the use of evidence-based practice within the team.

Induction and conceptual model

There are many conceptual issues to take on board when starting work in an assertive outreach team. On the one hand, assertive outreach seems like commonsense; on the other, it seems complex and overwhelming. Achieving an understanding of all the components and a perspective which puts assertive outreach in the context of the whole care system takes a long time. At the same time, you have all the research to digest. Just when you begin to feel you have an overview, practice and legislation moves on! This sort of knowledge cannot be assimilated in an intensive course. It requires time, practice, reflection, and the opportunity to compare with other localities and teams. What the team can, and should, provide for new staff is a clear and unambiguous model, an operational policy, a system of supervision and mentorship, and an induction programme.

Staff entering a team where there are disputes over elements of the model between individuals or professions, or where the model is ill-defined, will find it harder to settle in. What are the aims of the team? What is expected of me? What standards and targets apply? (See Chapter 26.) For new teams setting up there is often more time for comprehensive induction as case loads are built up over several months. There is also scope for the team, collectively, to develop their operational policy. Members of the team from different professional backgrounds can 'cross-train' each other. This makes for a more dynamic induction process and strengthens team integration. Sessions from an occupational therapist on daily living skills' training, from medical staff on psychopharmacology, and a social worker on housing are some obvious examples.

External trainers and visits make up the rest of the induction package. A speaker from the local social security office gave us some excellent tips on completing disability living allowance forms. Familiarization visits to local drop-in centres, work schemes, and hostels are well worth scheduling in the induction phase, as time will be scarce when you have a full case load.

It is important to get to know each part of the whole care and social system. A great deal of activity occurs in the voluntary sector including work activities, social clubs, hostels, and befriending schemes. The church plays a part in many communities. With its emphasis on mainstreaming, assertive outreach also requires a working knowledge of everyday resources that might be available in the locality, such as adult education courses.

Both qualified and unqualified staff must be aware of certain basics before they enter a patient's home alone. Our first-day induction checklist requires completion to show that the new member of staff has read and discussed the policy on dealing with violence, aggression, and risk. This includes communication procedures for home visits, such as daily diaries, to ensure that the team knows where staff are and how to contact them. Reporting in safe at the end of the day is essential.

Assessment skills

There is a plethora of structured assessment tools, some of which are designed for research and some for routine practice in mental health. Previously, such tools were only used by psychiatrists, psychologists, or specialized therapists. We would strongly advocate the use of a limited number of assessment tools by the whole team in routine practice. Consideration needs to be given to the need to collect the information, what will be done with it, and whether this will improve service delivery and outcomes in routine clinical practice. If satisfactory rationales are not obvious, then valuable time would be better employed in delivering interventions. Table 27.1 summarizes some commonly used structured assessment tools and the rationales for their use. Each can be used with all team members.

Training the whole team, together, in the use of structured assessment tools, helps to build a shared language and structure around which to discuss patient care and progress at team meetings. Team members will then struggle less to describe in what ways they believe an individual patient has improved or deteriorated. The frequent contact with a patient means that it is quite difficult to perceive gradual improvements or deteriorations in mental state without structured assessments. Comparing assessment scores at six-month intervals can often highlight such insidious changes.

Table 27.1   Common structured assessments

Training	Source of training	Rationale
Beck depression inventory (Beck *et al.* 1961)	Within team	Self-assessment of depressive symptoms and suicidality
Brief psychiatric rating scale (Overall and Gorham 1962)	Within team or as part of psychosocial intervention course	Brief, structured assessment of psychiatric symptoms; informs intervention and evaluation of the interventions when repeated
Camberwell assessment of need scale (CANS) (Slade *et al.* 1999)	Within team or as part of psychosocial intervention course	Structured assessment of needs including housing, finance, and occupation
Drug attitude inventory (Hogan *et al.* 1983)	Within team or as part of psychosocial intervention course	Helps to guide compliance negotiation and management
HoNOS (Wing *et al.* 1999)	Within team	Structured assessment of symptoms, behaviour, and social environment
Risk assessment (local format)	Within team or organization	Detection and management of risks to the patient and others
Side-effect rating scales e.g. EDOS (Chaplin *et al.* 1999; Simpson and Angus 1970), akathisia scale (Barnes 1989)	Within team or as part of psychosocial intervention course	Structured assessment of medication side-effects; informs compliance, prescribing, and titration

Improvements in inter-rater reliability derive from training together as a team to achieve common understandings of terminology and anchor points used in each of the scales. Training to use these scales is brief and can be easily accommodated within the team's induction and development time.

Other assessment skills (e.g. the Approved Social Worker, a doctor's Mental Health Act assessment, an occupational therapist's functional or vocational assessment) are part of routine professional training and practice and need no special mention here.

Intervention skills

Training to deliver interventions to patients should be fundamental to assertive outreach. Theories and models help with knowledge but skills such as engagement skills, compliance skills, managing substance abuse, daily living skills' training, employment strategies, and filling in benefit forms are our core activities. In assertive outreach, however, practical skills can often be more appreciated by the patient. How good are we at helping them fix that door lock or assembling flat-pack furniture?

Thorn courses

An important development in the last decade has been the setting up of the Thorn training initiative (Gournay and Birley 1998). This training programme was established in response to the policy shift towards severe and enduring mental illness and the appearance of effective psychosocial treatments for schizophrenia. Initially designed to equip CPNs with new skills, the course has embraced multidisciplinary education. Dissemination of the programme by training teachers has led to the expansion of the programme across the country, beyond the original London and Manchester sites. Furthermore, local 'Thorn-like' courses have been set up and accredited using a similar format.

The core components of the Thorn and other psychosocial interventions courses are modules in case management or assertive outreach for the severely mentally ill, schizophrenia family work, and psychological interventions such as CBT. The course demonstrates a commitment to evidence-based practice and is the most obvious 'off-the-peg' diploma-level course for those working in assertive outreach from mental health professional backgrounds. Courses run on a day-release basis, over an academic year, with 40–50 study days. There are practice as well as theory assessments and supervision is built into the course. Practice involves the conducting and writing up of interventions with patients in the student's workplace. For example, the student is expected to conduct a formal programme of schizophrenia family work with a suitable family, including assessments, delivery, and evaluation. The theoretical assignment might be to write an essay reviewing the evidence base for family interventions.

The increasing use of novel antipsychotics has had implications for our team training. As we have succeeded in increasing access and the number of patients on clozapine, it has been necessary to train team members to take blood from patients in their homes. Venepuncture clinics and clozapine clinics are not an option for some of our more disabled patients. The ability to have their blood taken at home by their key worker or a member of the team has reduced the fragmentation of services and increased our ability to maintain people on this treatment. So far we have only trained nurses and support workers to perform this activity. The prospect of training a social worker or occupational therapist to take blood presents obstacles from their professional regulators more than from the staff concerned.

Medication compliance therapy techniques (Kemp *et al.* 1997) represent a focused and effective area for training, particularly in assertive outreach. More basic approaches to compliance enhancement such as the use of concordance aids (dosette boxes), telephone reminders to patients, and supervision of oral medication in the patient's home are skills that team members can pass on to each other.

Operational training

Operational training describes the skills and knowledge required to enable a team to function safely, sensitively, and efficiently as a unit. For example, when discussing new staff induction we stressed the importance of early exposure to team policies and procedures on safety, communication, and managing risk. Table 27.2 outlines some of these brief courses. In many ways, parts of the case management module of the psychosocial intervention course constitute operational training since case management and assertive outreach are not treatments in themselves but methods of delivery. Some other examples are outlined in Table 27.2.

Risk assessment and breakaway technique are concerned with the safe operation and outcome of the service. Staff working in the community are not trained in control and restraint techniques like their in-patient colleagues, as usually they are working one to one in the patient's home. It is much better to make a safe exit, or to breakaway from any assault or hold, than to attempt to restrain a patient in such situations.

Table 27.2   Operational training courses

Training	Source	Rationale
Breakaway technique	Internal Trust	Assist in prevention and management of violence and aggression; staff safety
Cultural awareness	Internal Trust	Improve cultural sensitivity of service
Fire safety	Internal Trust	Health and safety at work
Note-keeping	Internal, Trust or team	Effective communication and treatment planning; legal documents
Organizational policies and procedures	Within team	Safe and ethical practice e.g. confidentiality, patient access to notes, administration of medicines
Risk assessment	Within team or organization	Detection and management of risks to the organization; assessment training where rationale is to detect and manage risks to the patient and others

Keeping accurate patient notes is a skill and cannot be assumed. There are standards and legal consequences of note-keeping. Co-ordination and communication in the team also rely on notes being accurate and complete. It is annoying (not to say unsafe) to spend time and energy trying to raise the occupant of house number 23 when the address on the front sheet of the notes should have read 23a.

Monitoring training needs, outcomes, and competencies

It is good practice to keep a 'live list' of the training received by each member of staff in the team. This record enables the team leader to identify staff who have missed out on training or still need to be recommended. Management supervision and appraisal is the mechanism for identifying training needs with individuals. Appraisal is also an opportunity to ensure that skills learnt on training courses are being incorporated into practice. Further training needs for the whole team are often led by changes such as the introduction of new risk assessment protocols or in response to critical incidents.

Outcomes of training are often overlooked. What matters is if the training translates to practice and influences patient outcomes. Staff training and supervision positively influence the likely success of psychosocial interventions (Brooker *et al.* 1994). Barriers often exist to the use of those skills, and there is considerable inertia in the system, with staff allowing their acquired skills to lie dormant on return to routine clinical practice. Fadden (1997) surveyed 86 trainees in the UK who had completed a behavioural family therapy course for work with patients with schizophrenia. Nine months to three-and-a-half years after training, 70% reported that they had been able to use the approach with families. However, this use was modest—equating to 1.7 families seen per therapist and 8% of the therapists accounting for 40% of the interventions. A significant number of staff from all disciplines had simply not been implementing their new skills. This is not an isolated finding. With small case loads this neglect is unacceptable.

Local audits provide useful information to quantify the effect of training on practice. How many patients in your current service have been assessed using the BPRS, or assessed for side-effects? We would suggest a standard of more than 90% for such an audit, if the routine use of such measures is agreed in the team. We audited the number of our patients who had significant contact with a carer. A surprisingly low figure of 27% demonstrated the degree of isolation experienced by many of our patients. We then audited how many of those carers demonstrated high expressed emotion and how many had received family intervention. The majority had received intervention to at least the psychoeducation stage, demonstrating utilization of learning, but few had been engaged in extended problem-solving sessions.

Conclusion

Throughout this book there is a recurring theme of investing in people, in what is a low-tech but demanding, skilled, labour-intensive activity. The team contains individual and multidisciplinary knowledge, skills, and experience in abundance. Organizing the team so that these can be passed on through clinical supervision, handover meetings, review meetings, and development meetings is as important as the provision of formal training and induction.

Assertive outreach provides an excellent system of care through which to deliver up-to-date pharmacological and psychosocial treatment packages. Diploma-level psychosocial intervention courses are best for developing the more sophisticated knowledge and skills. These courses require a large investment of time and resources. The team must facilitate and audit the routine implementation of these skills to justify that investment. A focus on competencies provides a framework for unqualified support staff and trained professionals against which to judge training needs and performance.

Chapter 28

Service planning

Introduction

By April 2001, the UK government's *NHS plan* had seen 170 assertive outreach teams established, with a further 50 teams expected by 2004. These teams should serve all 20 000 people with severe and enduring mental health problems estimated to be hard to engage and in need of intensive support in the community (Department of Health 2000). This is an ambitious commitment and reflects the degree of centralized service planning in this country. By contrast, the North American experience has seen assertive outreach develop through a 'franchising' process (Bond 1991). Model assertive outreach programmes have been copied by other parts of the country over a relatively long time period. Using a particularly American metaphor, Bond suggests that service planners may be able to learn something from the fast food industry in its successful transmission of standards to new locations!

The expansion of assertive outreach in the UK is not only driven from central policy. Below are listed the main drivers for expansion—some are valid, others are more questionable.

- Government policies: *Modernizing Mental Health Services* (Department of Health 1998a), *A National Service Framework* (Department of Health 1999a), *The NHS Plan* (Department of Health 2000), *The mental health policy implementation guide* (Department of Health 2001).
- Shift in emphasis towards meeting the complex needs associated with severe and enduring mental illness.
- Research evidence for efficacy of assertive outreach (Hoult *et al.* 1983; Marshall and Lockwood 1998; Stein and Test 1980).
- Improvements in evidence-based treatments (Kane and McGlashan 1995).
- Government response to well-publicized homicides by mentally ill people (Department of Health 1999c; Ritchie 1994).
- Desire to provide 'added value' through comprehensive, high-quality services.

This chapter aims to guide practitioners and managers in setting up assertive outreach services from a non-technical service-planning perspective. The truth behind some of these drivers and their relevance and applicability to different types of locality in the UK needs examination. Examples of different service configurations will be discussed with their relative merits and drawbacks. Issues of model fidelity that are important for the outcomes of the service are discussed in detail in Chapter 4. Evaluation of services is covered in the chapter on research and development (Chapter 29).

Fundamental questions

Despite the UK government having specified the types of services they expect from a modern mental health service (Department of Health 2001), we still need to ask ourselves fundamental questions when considering setting up and when reviewing assertive outreach services. Chapter 3 of this book deals in detail with the first and second most important questions:

1. *What do we hope to achieve by having an assertive outreach service?* What is assertive outreach for? What evidence-based treatments and care packages can we provide with assertive outreach that we are not providing consistently now?
2. *How many individuals are there in our locality who require assertive outreach?* Who is it for? What are the defining characteristics of the target population?

The staffing and size of the team will, in the main, be determined by these two questions. The skills mix should be determined by the range of interventions to be provided. Prioritizing sophisticated psychosocial interventions may lead to the employment of trained staff with this specialist training and the inclusion of a psychologist in the team. Prioritizing symptom management through improved medication compliance and access to novel antipsychotics will require a minimum quota of trained nurses. Engaging and working with patients from ethnic minorities will necessitate ethnic diversity in the prospective workforce.

A third question perhaps needs also to be asked:

3. *What might we not achieve by having an assertive outreach team?*

This question relates to the scepticism suggested earlier about some of the drivers for assertive outreach. There has been a tendency in the UK, as in the US, for assertive outreach to become entwined with the ongoing debate over risk and the severely mentally ill. Both the government and service planners wish, understandably, to find solutions when criticized after well-publicised 'failures' in community care. Planners who see assertive outreach teams as a final solution to risk and untoward events are probably under a misapprehension.

The role of assertive outreach in reducing risk to the general public is overplayed. Teams work best when they engage patients collaboratively, rather than attempting to control them (Chapter 8). They certainly can help with managing risk in patients where such behaviour is associated with psychosis. Improved medication compliance and treatment can reduce the risk. Patients who offend irrespective of their mental state, due to delinquency or other personality traits, however, present a very different problem. The most striking studies of failure of ACT to impact on outcome have been with offender patients (Solomon and Draine 1995*b*). We have experience of patients who offend only when they are well. Indeed you need a modicum of social skills and contacts to manage a significant drug habit or to exploit others!

Assertive outreach can provide better co-ordination of services and frequent contact with vulnerable or moderately dangerous individuals. If in-patient units, which provide 24-hour care for vulnerable patients, can experience untoward incidents, then so can assertive outreach services. We advise against becoming a hostage to fortune by marketing services primarily as a method of removing risk.

Neither can assertive outreach be commissioned any longer on the basis that it will reduce costs by reducing hospital admission or duration (Tyrer 1998; UK700 Group: Byford *et al.* 2000). Randomized controlled trials in Europe and, latterly, in North America (Chapter 29) do not bear out these assumptions (Mueser *et al.* 1998). A more modest, and honest, rationale lies in a desire to provide a better service (added value) to this patient group through comprehensive, intensive services, delivering effective treatments and care.

How does assertive outreach fit into the whole system?

The *NHS plan* (Department of Health 2000) correctly views assertive outreach as only one part of a whole system of modern mental health services necessary to meet the needs of patients. The cornerstones of mental health service provision are GPs and CMHTs. Unless these parts of the system are supported, endorsed, and enhanced (in the way assertive outreach currently is), then not even the best assertive outreach teams can deliver.

Our assertive outreach team operates in support of the CMHTs. It is currently unclear, in the UK, whether or not this will remain the case with implementation of the *NHS plan*. This seems to suggest a non-hierarchical relationship between a series of functional teams (assertive outreach, crisis, early onset, CMHT). Awareness of, and sensitivity to, evolution of the whole system of care is essential for effective functioning of an assertive outreach team.

Keys to engagement (Sainsbury Centre for Mental Health 1998) describes those essential services required to support hard-to-engage people who need intensive services. They are outlined in Table 28.1.

In this context we can see assertive outreach as a small but necessary part of a modern mental health service. The team is reliant on other parts of the mental health system being present and effective but, equally importantly, retains functional autonomy in that it does not make referrals to other services lightly. The team avoids fragmentation of care between providers where possible but cannot compensate for fundamental gaps or failures in other parts of the system.

Table 28.1 Required local services for those with severe mental health problems*

Community support	24-hour care, residential and housing	Day care and activities	Financial support
Primary care	Ordinary housing	Ordinary employment	Welfare advice service
Generic CMHTs	Low-, medium-, and high-support hostels	Supported employment	
Community-based alternatives to acute care	Residential homes	Adult education	
Assertive outreach	24-hour nursed accommodation	Clubhouse	
Crisis intervention	Acute in-patient care; low-, medium-, and high-security provision	Day centres; drop-in centres	

* Keys to engagement (Sainsbury Centre for Mental Health 1998)

Problems occur in the wider system when there are boundary confusions or disputes between specialist services in their response to particular patients with challenging needs. The generic CMHT accepts referrals from GPs for people with mental health problems with few explicit exclusions. Tertiary services, such as forensic, assertive outreach, and rehabilitation, have explicit criteria which can protect their services as well as focus treatment and support on their target groups.

Case study

A CMHT has been struggling with a psychotic patient who is poorly compliant with medication and abuses 'crack' cocaine regularly. His offending behaviour is escalating and he has a forensic history of dangerous behaviour.

The CMHT knows that the local forensic service only takes people with very serious index offences—usually those who have been through the courts. They are not sure how such seriousness is measured. Will their patient be taken on by the community forensic team or will they only offer an opinion? The local drug and alcohol service has difficulty engaging psychotic patients who are poorly motivated to change their drug-taking behaviour.

Finally, they consider a referral to assertive outreach but know that the local team has a waiting list and may be concerned about the severity of the forensic history. How are the current needs of the patient to be met?

Further boundary issues occur between assertive outreach and rehabilitation or continuing care services since both concentrate on severe and enduring mental health problems. In the UK, assertive outreach services have evolved both within rehabilitation services and adult CMHT services. Our local protocol is that patients who need intensive support and who are living in independent accommodation are referred to the assertive outreach team. Those patients who require staffed residential accommodation and intensive support should be referred to the rehabilitation service which has a specific outreach service for them. The assertive outreach team provides for people who are hard to engage and require a high level of input due to unstable mental state and frequent relapses. The continuing care team is for those patients who have established stable mental states but require continuing support. In North Birmingham, the assertive outreach team and the continuing care team have the same manager. This single management arrangement means that patients can move easily and flexibly between the two services according to need.

The planning process

We have emphasized the dimension of the local whole-care system in identifying needs and priorities for this patient group. Vested interests of professional groups impinge on and complicate the process. It is not as simple as just planning an assertive outreach team based on estimates of numbers of patients and resources available. In many areas, teams are being set up using joint funding from social service and health money. This creates further complications as priorities and organizational cultures differ. The establishment of single-care agencies under the *NHS plan* (Department of Health 2000) may simplify organizational change of this type.

The diversity of stakeholders and the need for consultation requires (in most cases) a cumbersome, but ultimately effective, planning process based on the framework described below.

Steering group

The steering group is responsible for leading the change process, prioritizing the resources, defining the broad policy framework, and setting the values and principles of the proposed service. The steering group includes senior members of the major professions, senior managers who will be responsible for the service, and representatives from the major agencies of health and social care. The North American franchising process (described above) demonstrates the value of co-opting an expert with experience of assertive outreach who can clarify and cut through unnecessary debate. Local politics will determine the profile of user and carer representatives, primary care input, and perspectives from local minority groups or voluntary agencies.

Stakeholder conference or focus groups

A large stakeholder conference may be more appropriate for wholesale changes in the provision of community services. Focus groups are an alternative way of defining needs and demands across a range of perspectives. With either approach, the advantages of two-way exchange of information and enhanced validity for the planning process are derived. These strategies influence assessment of local needs rather than decisions on service configurations.

Local needs profile

Estimating population needs is a complex and potentially bottomless task. Data exists at national level and from local health authorities and social service departments. For assertive outreach, a case register of potential referrals can be derived from surveying referring CMHTs with reference to the agreed referral criteria. How many patients do you have with more than two admissions in the last two years? Of these patients how many would also qualify as hard to engage, poorly compliant with treatment, dual diagnosis, risks associated with relapse, living in independent accommodation? Converting data to something manageable that can inform decision making is a job for a small project group. This should be set up by, or from within, the steering group.

Reynolds and Thornicroft (1999) describe epidemiological, service utilization, service provision and deprivation weighted-index approaches to assessing needs. Certainly these are valid exercises for planning entire services but may be unnecessarily cumbersome where establishing an assertive outreach team is the only change proposed. The authors suggest that:

> A more pragmatic managerial approach is to assess local needs for services by interpreting the incomplete mosaic of data that is to hand.

Writing the service proposal

The next step will be for the steering group to agree a model, priorities, and resources, and for the chair or clinical expert to write the service proposal. The proposal can be used to secure the funding and as a consultation document for feedback. The service proposal will contain a timescale for implementation and feedback.

Service configuration

Assertive outreach is traditionally delivered by discrete, multidisciplinary teams operating alongside local mental health services. The team is the primary provider of services to its case load and is responsible for admission and discharge to its own in-patient beds. The team provides continuity of care and care givers across functional areas and across time (Test 1992). This summary describes the orthodox view of service configuration and many argue that without these components outcomes for patients are compromised. Despite these reservations, local adaptations abound and are determined by local needs, resources, and circumstances.

American assertive outreach teams vary immensely despite the orthodox view often portrayed in the literature. Bond (1991) describes a number of variations. In Chicago, the original orthodox Bridge programme was adapted for different patient populations including the homeless and those with hearing impairments. In contrast to the continuity of care described earlier by Test, one Chicago programme experimented with short-term outreach intervention aimed at stabilizing patients before handing them back to less intensive services (half the patients stayed with the short-term programme longer than was planned).

Model fidelity

The Department of Health and organizations such as The Sainsbury Centre for Mental Health caution against major adaptations of the basic PACT model described by Stein and Test (1980). They do so on the grounds of preserving the model on which the evidence base rests, though little scientific work has been done to test which model ingredients are critical to successful outcomes.

The mental health policy implementation guide (Department of Health 2001) states that assertive outreach teams are best provided by a discrete team whose members' sole responsibility is assertive outreach. It suggests a team case load of approximately 90 patients with a ratio of no more than 12:1 between patients and care co-ordinators. Although geography and demographics will play a large part, each team is likely to serve a population of around 250 000.

Integrated assertive outreach workers

A common adaptation, however, is the so-called 'integrated model' where one or two CPNs are 'bolted on' to existing CMHTs and asked to provide an assertive outreach function to a small case load of CMHT patients. The assertive outreach workers are well integrated into the CMHTs but too often dislocated from like-minded colleagues and a consistent model. To achieve the critical mass for a stand-alone team at least five workers and 50 potential patients are required. Below this number the team cannot safely and effectively provide cross cover and multidisciplinary input for itself. Some services, particularly in more rural areas, have adopted this 'bolt on' worker solution described to overcome this problem of few prospective patients or patients spread over a wide rural area.

Table 28.2, adapted from Kent and Burns (1996), outlines the two sides to this debate. The 'bolt on' approach is not supported by the Department of Health in the UK except in remote regions where only a few individuals might meet the criteria for assertive outreach.

Assertive outreach appears to work best (just like CMHTs) when a team has clinical responsibility for all aspects of patient care both as an in-patients and within the community. The daily living programme (Marks *et al.* 1994) was one example of a UK assertive outreach team that had hospitalization outcomes compromised when it lost control over admission and discharge. This arrangement leads to divided consultant responsibility and sometimes divisive negotiating with consultants less familiar or less committed to assertive outreach priorities. For example, discharging a patient home early on the understanding that they remain on long leave and are visited daily with supervised medication may not require much consideration when you have consultant responsibility for your own beds. When that bed (and therefore the leave) is the responsibility of another consultant the potential for disagreement is considerable.

We have no evidence from our local experience that the establishment of assertive outreach diminished the CMHT focus on the severely mentally ill. Through taking on

Table 28.2 Integrating ACT key workers into existing CMHTs*

Potential advantages	Potential disadvantages
Full multidisciplinary support where the alternative would be a small unrepresentative team	Loss of programme fidelity
Vertical and horizontal service integration	Secondment of key workers to other (non-ACT) tasks
Avoids fragmentation of sectorized community mental health services	Inefficient use of time (e.g. multiple meetings)
Retains CMHT focus on severely mentally ill	Professional isolation
Skill sharing	Changes of consultant responsibility for ACT patients and in-patient treatment where more than one CMHT involved in the ACT service

* Adapted from Kent and Burns 1996

10–15 of the most complex or unstable patients from each CMHT, the balance of patients with longer-term psychotic disorders and the whole range of other disorders referred by GPs was not significantly altered. Still over half of the case loads of local CMHTs are patients with severe and enduring mental health problems.

We have had experience of assertive outreach workers integrated into CMHTs as part of a network. The resulting problems soon led us to move on towards a stand-alone team. Simple audits and comparisons showed up how some CMHTs expected their assertive outreach workers to participate in duty systems or referral meetings which took them away from intensive and frequent patient contact and had little or no relevance to their targeted role. We evolved through the stages of increasing model fidelity shown in Fig. 28.1, using our own experience of the drawbacks of less faithful service configurations.

Service examples

In Wandsworth, the assertive outreach team is one of a handful of targeted tertiary level specialist teams. The sectorized CMHTs provide the foundation of services and are the access point for all referrals to these specialist services. CMHTs can make referrals to forensic services, assertive outreach, or rehabilitation services according to agreed referral criteria. Each of these three specialist teams has access to their own in-patient beds.

North Birmingham Mental Health NHS Trust, on the other hand (Wood and Carr 1998), carried out a thorough review and reorganization of its adult services coinciding with a merger of three mental health units in 1994. The CMHTs were renamed 'primary care liaison teams' and were the access point for all non-emergency referrals not requiring home treatment or in-patient admission. Emergency activity and access to

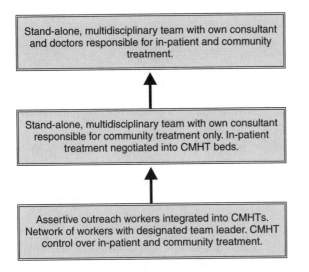

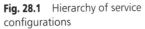

Fig. 28.1 Hierarchy of service configurations

in-patient beds became the responsibility of 24-hour home-treatment teams. Both home-treatment teams and the primary care liaison service can refer to assertive outreach and continuing care teams which have separate access to their own rehabilitation and continuing care beds.

External resistance

Lack of commitment, perceived threats to status, and narrow professional interests all conspire to undermine the change process, and in our experience should not be underestimated. Recent government endorsement of assertive outreach has helped to overcome this somewhat. One must be prepared, however, for colleagues who insist that they have been practicing assertive outreach all along but have called it 'rehabilitation' or 'forensic community psychiatric nursing' or such like.

Seeking clarification of the model and operational policies of this 'prodromal' assertive outreach service will often meet with vague responses. The clarity of definitions of assertive outreach is unusual in mental health services and can be perceived by colleagues as implied criticism of the imprecision that is traditionally accepted (Kent and Burns 1996). Despite the frustration that resistance to change may generate, it is worth reminding ourselves that resistance is inevitable and normal.

> It is important to keep in mind that those placing obstacles in the path of change are doing so for heartfelt and legitimate reasons. It is too easy to become overly cynical, imputing the worst motives.
>
> (Onyett 1992)

Conclusions

Service planning and evaluation is a continuous process. By careful attention to model, fidelity service configuration in relation to the whole system, and a local needs analysis, many mistakes can be avoided. It will not, however, be possible to establish an effective, smooth running team immediately from scratch. Fine tuning and problem solving needed, and teams evolve towards their optimum. Lessons can be learnt from visits and assistance from demonstration sites, and from the literature.

The official line is not to adapt the basic PACT model overly for fear of losing beneficial outcomes. Compromises inevitably happen and local needs analysis may make it difficult to establish a centralized stand-alone team (e.g. in rural populations). In practice, patients who fit assertive outreach criteria are heavily concentrated in the towns.

Pitfalls exist if other parts of the mental health service are not sufficiently developed, or not flexible enough to respond to changing patient needs. If an assertive outreach team is occupied with inappropriate patients whose problems are not centrally related to unstable psychotic illness because there are gaps in the local system, it will compromise outcomes.

External resistance undoubtedly occurs and must be dealt with sensitively. Assertive outreach is currently enjoying favour and funding from central government. It is at the service planning level that the foundation is laid for ensuring that it does fulfil its promise and result in improvements for patients.

Chapter 29

Research and development

Introduction

This is a handbook primarily for practitioners and not for academics or researchers. However, assertive outreach has been promoted and introduced as one of the models, par excellence, of evidence-based practice (Chapters 1 and 4). Its practice has been healthily associated with an enhanced concern with a more critical approach to mental health care—not doing things in a set way simply 'because they have always been done that way'. As the range of possible interventions has increased within finite resources, we must make sure we use our time in the most effective way. This is an ethical as much as an economic issue—we owe it to our patients to ensure that they get the best out of what is available. These concerns are heightened in assertive outreach as many teams are established with time-limited funding, with continuation often dependent on 'an evaluation'.

A number of separate evaluative activities tend to get bundled together under the rubric of 'doing research'. These can be disentangled into four, three of which should be carried out by all teams and one (research) only embarked upon after considerable thought.

Mental health service evaluative activities

- **Monitoring:** routine or special collection of data e.g. case-load demographics, occupied bed days, referrals, untoward incidents.
- **Clinical audit:** the systematic analysis of the quality of clinical care assessed against a known quality standard.
- **Service development:** the considered and reflective introduction of changes in practice.
- **Formal research:** using controlled comparison groups to test a hypothesis, often related to innovation.

Each of these methodologies can be used to explore and measure three aspects of mental health provision: outcomes, processes, and inputs.

Outcomes

The most commonly reported outcomes for assertive outreach at a patient level traditionally include symptom severity, hospitalization, and loss to follow-up. Framing such measures as positive targets is more constructive and we can convert these traditional outcomes to symptom reduction, community tenure, and engagement. It is important to remember, however, that patients and their families would not necessarily view these as that important and stress social and vocational outcomes more (e.g. Chapter 23).

Aggregated outcomes provide the information at a service level that can be compared against a standard for an audit or against a control group in the case of focused research.

Processes

Thornicroft and Tansella (1999) define process as 'those activities which take place to deliver mental health services'.

An audit of the frequency of contact with patients is an evaluation of process. Monitoring case load or the use of clozapine or 'aftercare under supervision' are also measuring processes. Process evaluation relates to our fundamental questions about why we want to set up an assertive outreach team. What do we hope to achieve by having an assertive outreach service? What will we do differently? What evidence-based treatments and care can we provide with assertive outreach that we cannot provide without it? It is with these processes that we hope to achieve positive outcomes for patients.

Inputs

Inputs are the resources that are put into mental health services. Individual treatments with cost implications, like novel antipsychotic medication, are inputs but also have process and outcome implications. At the service level, the obvious inputs are staffing, training, hospital beds, equipment, and buildings. The level of investment to train a member of staff to diploma level in the use of psychosocial interventions for psychosis is considerable. Comparing inputs and outcomes is how the efficiency of a service is judged. Stein and Test's study (1980) was so influential because it demonstrated efficacy with reduced costs.

Routine monitoring of care

All professionals have to keep records. The most important records are the patients' clinical case notes and, in any legal process, it is these which will be examined. We have learnt over the last decades just how important it is to keep up-to-date, high-quality notes. For assertive outreach work, the recording of 'failed visits' (visits where the patient was not in or we were unable to make contact with them) is of particular importance. The legal profession assumes that if nothing is recorded then nothing happened. We have stressed these issues throughout, but good-quality notes are also essential for audit (see below).

In addition to clinical case notes, we are also required to return 'statistics' on our work. For the most part this is simply a record of the number of contacts with patients and (depending on the sophistication of the local IT) the time spent. In many countries, the content of that contact—its purpose and activities involved—is also recorded. This is especially so in insurance-based systems where the payment for different activities will differ. For instance, in one US state case managers cannot 'bill' time spent picking up groceries provided free for mentally ill individuals if they do it alone, whereas if the patient comes along in the car then it becomes 'billable time'.

Regular inputting of contact data is generally considered one of the less enjoyable parts of the job. Whilst a core, it is, however, an essential part of the job if we are to be taken seriously in an increasingly hard-nosed and accountable health care system. In this area the UK clearly lags behind current practice, and visits to other systems (often with much more paperwork) demonstrate just how routine and simple monitoring can be.

Making routine monitoring more acceptable

Part of the resistance to routine monitoring is that it often appears to be imposed from without and to have no clinical relevance. However, it is not going to go away. So it is worth considering how it can be used to serve the team's purposes and, consequently, seem more worthwhile. Using this data to monitor and review current practice is one way to do this.

1. Emphasize the 'professionalism' of data returns.
2. Use routine data for individual supervision.
3. Use routine data for monitoring model fidelity.

Emphasize the 'professionalism' of data returns

If the work we do is worthwhile, then it is worth recording. The increased insistence that nursing and community activity is recorded is evidence that it is taken seriously. Instead of focusing on the 'big brother' aspect of being checked up on, focus on the importance that the activity is being accorded. This emphasis can be strengthened by taking seriously the activity of making returns and setting time aside for it. We encourage all our team members to timetable in an hour or so a week for doing their returns. This means they have some chance of being done accurately—not rushed at the end of a month when the computer unit is demanding them and memory has faded. In a team like ours, which aims for about 20–25 contacts a week, an hour should be more than enough. We emphasize also that it is 'thinking time'. Inevitably, when entering data, there is stimulus to think about where one is going with a specific patient. A scheduled session in the office once a week (when statistics can be done, notes reviewed, and some paperwork completed) should be part of any outreach worker's routine.

Use routine data for individual supervision

Routine data can often highlight patterns of practice for individuals that need attention. We aim for 20–25 contacts a week but this inevitably includes considerable variation. Depending on their needs, some patients will require frequent short visits (e.g. daily meds) and some, fewer, more extensive visits (e.g. a well-established patient who now needs complex negotiations to help him get a flat or job). If an individual case manager's contact frequency is very different from his or her peers, however, this may indicate problems that need to be taken up in supervision. It can be just as problematic if the rate is too high as if it is too low.

Case study

Anne is a new case manager who has wanted to join the team for a long time. She contributes extensively in review meetings and is optimistic and enthusiastic for her patients. Six months into the job her statistics still average out at 35 + visits a week and she is seeing four of her patients on a daily basis, five days a week. In supervision her enthusiasm is recognized and praised. The high visit frequency is used as a way into discussing her anxiety levels about her new patients and the need to let herself trust them more.

Robert's contact frequency falls from a steady 20 + per week to a month when it is routinely 12–15 visits a week (and with more failed visits than usual). In supervision he has not commented on any difficulties. When the downturn is highlighted it becomes clear that the start of this occurred after an unfounded accusation from a female patient, when he had felt unsupported by the organization. He had hardly been aware of the impact himself until his change in visit pattern was discussed.

Obviously, this use of statistical returns needs to be sensitive and collaborative. It has an enormous potential to seem persecutory and to mediate against good data collection.

Use routine data for monitoring model fidelity

Just as routine monitoring data can be used for individual supervision, so can it be used for team supervision. This is often referred to as monitoring fidelity to the agreed model of care and is covered in detail in Chapter 4. It is remarkably easy, for even the most committed team, to 'drift' in its practice. Getting an overview of how well the team is meeting its target of two visits per patient per week can be accurately picked up from such data, along with an understanding of how these visits vary between different patient groups and different case managers. Comparing clinical impression against routinely collected data can be a sobering experience! It is remarkable how different reality and rhetoric can become without anyone noticing.

This monitoring of model fidelity is a form of audit to be dealt with below. More sophisticated team assessments will require more detailed recording of contacts. In the course of a research study involving several case management teams (UK700 Group:

Creed *et al.* 1999), a set of simple categories for each contact was developed (Burns *et al.* 2000) and used to compare practice against PACT standards. Each contact or 'event' was recorded according to the main focus of activity or intervention. While such detailed recording would be hard to justify for routine practice it may be necessary for individual audits.

Event record categories for assertive outreach

- Housing
- Occupation and leisure
- Finance
- Daily living skills
- Criminal justice system
- Carers and significant others
- Engagement
- Physical health
- Specific mental health intervention/assessment
- Medication
- Case conference

Audit

Audit does not involve finding out new knowledge about how to provide care, but examining how well proven methods of care are being applied locally. It consists of a cycle of setting standards of care that one expects to provide and then testing whether these are being met. If they are not, then efforts have to be made to do so and the audit repeated after an appropriate time. If they are being met, then a decision can be made whether or not the achieved standards should be raised for a further cycle or whether one is happy with that level and a different target is chosen for audit. The audit cycle is well described (Firth–Cozens 1993) and clinical audit is a requirement for services in the UK (Department of Health 1998*b*). As with routine data collection, one can either suffer audit as a necessary evil or embrace it as an opportunity to reflect on, improve, and celebrate good practice. We would encourage the latter!

Although most organisations provide extensive help with audit, the real value is in doing it oneself. Increasingly, the centrally driven audit agenda is about routine monitoring of bureaucracy, such as compliance with the care programme approach or discharge procedures. To avoid bad feeling, it is worth spending time together as a team to understand the benefits of such non-negotiable activities. Where there are requirements for a set number of internal audits, and there is discretion on the topics, then it is equally important that the team discusses the rationale for them and is interested in the answers. We have conducted audits on out-of-hours contacts and the proportion of family contacts, and a series of paper-based audits on the content of individual care plans. We have been surprised by some of our results (e.g. the low level of contact with relatives despite consistent efforts) and heartened by others (e.g. the extremely low rate of out-of-hours emergency contacts with services).

Audits gets increasingly sophisticated as teams get more settled and teething problems are resolved. They may influence the way data is recorded, either temporarily or permanently. No matter how skilful or sophisticated, however, it will be a waste if the topic is not 'owned' by the team. To sustain ownership we ensure that there is team discussion about the standard to be audited and the mechanism chosen to do it. We prioritize audits where the complete team can be involved in the whole process (e.g. auditing 10 sets of notes each to identify frequency of vocational activity recorded). Where possible, we do this all in the room together and make 'an event' of it. If this approach is not possible, we aim for a rapid turn-round so that the results are available fairly soon after the question has been set. Usually one member of the team takes responsibility for ensuring that the audit is conducted and for timetabling it in. This person is responsible for 'seeing it happens'—not for doing it.

Service development

It is not just hospital services that can become rigid and inward-looking.Community teams and assertive outreach teams can become institutionalized too. Paradoxically, assertive outreach services may be more at risk of it than other mental health services precisely because they are often set up with an explicit model and a commitment to model fidelity. While we have regularly stressed the value of an explicit model for a service, it does carry with it a risk of 'fossilization' and a focus on structure rather than content and quality of care. Service development is an essential, ongoing aspect of service planning.

CMHTs need to have a mechanism for overviewing their practice and making sure that it adapts to changes around them. This may be as basic as responding to an influx of refugees to the area or reorganizing liaison meetings with primary care following a restructure. Developments may, however, have to be more substantial to reflect new techniques or treatments. For instance, our team has reorganized considerably to accommodate an increased use of clozapine in our resistant schizophrenia patients (Chapter 15). This was one of the major drivers for a move to a seven-day a week service, but it has also had knock-on effects because of the increased volume of daily supervised medicines. Two examples of service developments from this have been the purchase of a motor scooter to speed up the drug rounds through late-afternoon rush-hour traffic and the training of all staff in venepuncture.

Service developments should be thought through carefully at events such as team away days (Chapter 26) and we would strongly advise that a review date should be set for any innovation. The current zeitgeist is that virtually all innovation is good. Indeed 'innovative' is routinely used as a term of approval of services and taken to imply 'improvement'. Not all changes are improvements. Innovations need to be reviewed with at least three questions in mind:

1. Is the change sustainable?
2. Does it bring demonstrable benefits?
3. What price is paid to achieve it?

The value of introducing any major change in practice on a 'pilot' basis is that it is then impossible to neglect these questions. It is no use introducing a change that only lasts as long as it has novelty value. A good test is how much support it receives from those who have to provide the input over sustained periods. The enthusiast who comes up with the idea is not the one to judge it. We have had a series of safety-reporting systems that have all seemed brilliant when first launched (e.g. detailed diaries for each member with complex ringing-in obligations), but none has persisted, apart from a simple, efficient notification of risky visits. A preordained review is vital in such circumstances because it avoids complacency and the assumption that a system is in place when it has, in fact, fallen into disuse.

That an idea seems good does not necessarily mean that it makes any real difference. Providing an out-of-hours service both reflected received wisdom for assertive outreach and has an impelling logic. After several years of providing only flexible evening work we undertook to introduce extended-hours availability on a routine basis. Although there were no complaints from the staff about it, a review of the use of the provision showed that it simply was not used (Chapter 6). On the other hand, the review of our extension to seven days a week showed that the contact frequency was high, targeted, and effective in improving medication compliance. That innovation continues.

Even if an innovation is effective, careful thought must be given to its 'cost-effectiveness'. Its benefits should be weighed against the alternative activities that could be provided in the staff time devoted to it. The economic concept of 'opportunity cost' examines alternative use of those inputs within the whole system. For every use of resources, there is an alternative lost opportunity. We faced this dilemma at our inception. Do we use finite health money to establish a new assertive outreach service or to enhance our existing CMHTs? This is a much trickier question than deciding whether or not an innovation is effective. There are methods of estimating added health value for different treatments (e.g. QUALYs—quality-adjusted life years) (Smith 1987). The use of these is complex and very time-consuming and rarely feasible outside of highly-resourced research projects. There is currently no simple, convincing mechanism for comparing the value of a mental health treatment in one area with another, and personal professional judgement will have to suffice.

Being open to innovation is, despite these caveats, an essential virtue in community mental health practice. Not only does it allow teams to adopt new and more effective treatments more quickly, but it also keeps our perspective fresh. Even the most evidence-based interventions will be of limited effect if they are delivered in a stale, mechanistic manner. A culture of enquiry and flexibility is an asset in its own right.

Research

Research is a process by which new knowledge is acquired. It is not the only way. New knowledge can be obtained by careful clinical observation and even by pure chance. What is special about scientific research is that it uses well-tested and tried methods to resolve difficult questions. Most typically such research uses an *experiment* to test which of two or more outcomes is associated with an intervention. There are a number of experimental (and so-called 'quasi-experimental') approaches to answering difficult questions.

Research is distinguished from audit by its aim to derive new knowledge about its subject matter rather than test how well current knowledge is being used locally. It is distinguished from local surveys and needs assessments by the 'generalizability' of its findings. Research questions are usually framed in such a manner that their answers should be as independent as possible of local conditions and, therefore, applicable in a wide range of settings. For instance, demonstrating the successful outcome of an operation simply by examining the results obtained by an outstandingly good surgeon does not tell us how successful that operation is. It tells us how successful that surgeon is with the patients referred to him. To research the success of the operation we would need to have it applied by a fairly representative group of surgeons and ensure that the patients receiving it are also a relevant cross-section. We easily recognize these issues in other fields of endeavour. For example, good exam results in a school are not automatically evidence of the superiority of its teaching methods—we need to think about what sort of pupils it gets and the quality of its teachers, etc.

Why are research methods important?

Why do academics seem to spend so much time arguing about methodology? Are research methods that important in mental health? Surely it is often quite obvious when a treatment works? Sometimes it is and there is no need for careful research studies. The first heart transplants are a good example—all the patients would have died without a transplant, and many of them lived for a long time with their transplants. However, as transplants became more common, the point at which the clinical decision to undertake one advanced. No longer is immediate death the inevitable alternative and, also, there are differing techniques for undertaking the procedure. Individual surgeons are unlikely to be able to make careful and convincing comparisons; they will stick to the method they know best and feel safest with. At this point more careful scientific research needs to be designed to answer these questions.

Attention to detail is particularly essential to resolve long-running controversies where, despite extensive experience, experts continue to disagree. How can trained people continue to have strongly held differences of opinion despite accumulating evidence? The reasons for this are basically twofold. Firstly, there is enthusiasm and the natural tendency we all share to be optimistic for the treatments we use and the approaches we adopt. This is not surprising—we use them because they have worked in the past and also because they resonate with our view of the task. Thus, enthusiasts for family work will persist longer with a difficult family and are more likely to judge the outcome successful than a sceptic. Similarly, an enthusiast for aggressive psychopharmacology would persist longer with the same patient with various drug changes and be more likely to attribute any natural improvements to that intervention.

Few responses by individual patients in mental health practice are a simple 'either/or', so there is inevitably scope for interpretation of results. In psychotherapy research, professionals consistently rate more change in their patients than either the patients or external observers would. The healthy optimism that therapists need to make a success of their treatments makes interpreting the outcome difficult.

Bias in research

The second difficulty is bias. Most research structures are aimed at reducing bias. Bias refers to all those extraneous factors (other than the intervention whose effect is to be judged) which can affect the outcome. We have already mentioned the therapist's bias. This is not wilful or deliberate but normal human behaviour ('giving people the benefit of the doubt', 'hoping for the best for them'). For this reason one of the commonest aspects of research is that 'independent' researchers, rather than the clinicians, collect the outcome data.

Bias can also come from a number of other sources.

Sampling bias

How the patients are recruited may exert a powerful influence on outcome. Two examples of this are particularly relevant to assertive outreach. If patients are recruited into the experimental service at the point where they would otherwise have entered hospital (e.g. Muijen *et al.* 1992; Stein and Test 1980), then there is an in-built bias in favour of these so called 'diversion studies'. You cannot increase the admission rate in the experimental group as the control groups are all going in! Easier to overlook is the influence of when, in the natural history of the disorder, one selects patients. If we select patients for assertive outreach because they have been very ill and in hospital often recently, it is the natural pattern of these illnesses that they will be comparatively better in the next couple of years. These are fluctuating disorders and so there is a natural 'regression to the mean' if we select people at their worst. For this reason, pre-post studies (i.e. comparing hospital usage for the same patients for a period before and after the introduction of a new service) can be very misleading. Such studies should be interpreted very cautiously, as there is often a significant improvement in the control patients in RCTs!

If a clinic can choose its patients, then it may attract either less ill or possibly more ill patients. This is one reason why outcome in specialist clinics may be much worse than in routine ones. For instance, modern research into the outcome in anorexia nervosa arose because psychiatrists (who saw the difficult cases) thought it was a very serious disease, whereas physicians (who treated first-episode and easier cases) thought it was a brief, mild disorder (Beck and Brochner–Mortensen 1954).

Another form of sampling bias in clinical practice is to base opinions on follow-up patients and forget to account for those who do not come back for follow-up. Most of us have a much gloomier view of the long-term prognosis for schizophrenia than the evidence suggests (Ciompi 1988; Harding *et al.* 1987) because we work long term with those who do not get better.

Hawthorne effect

One of the most important sources of bias in mental health research is the Hawthorne effect (Grufferman 1999). This describes the improvement in outcome in behavioural studies that are a result of the extra attention that the study generates. It is generally recognized that patients do better in research trials than in routine practice, and there are a lot of reasons for this (sampling, better adherence by both patient and doctor to proper procedures, etc).

The Hawthorne effect is the overall sense of well-being that comes from all that extra attention. After all, patients with long-term disorders may be fairly demoralized and the sense that 'something new is being done' can boost morale both for them and staff and produce a direct effect in outcome. The most famous example of this in mental health practice was the continued use of modified insulin coma therapy, which persisted despite serious doubts and with no coherent theoretical basis. A very careful trial demonstrated that equally improved outcome was achieved by transfer to a specialist unit and the increased nursing care required for the insulin therapy, even when the insulin was not given. It was the extra attention and hope that made the difference. Clinical observation could not have made this distinction, but a careful clinical research trial has saved a generation of patients from a potentially risky procedure.

All of us involved in new and exciting service developments need to be aware of the potential for bias in interpreting our success. We may select easier patients (or have them selected for us) or may attribute to the way of working, benefits that come from having more motivated, enthusiastic, or better-trained staff. Research increasingly attempts to control for these factors. In themselves they are not bad things—a team that can foster and attract such staff may have a real story to tell about improving care. What careful research aims to achieve is clarity about exactly what is influencing what.

The hierarchy of research methods

This is not the book to discuss individual study methods and research structures in great detail. As will be obvious from the above, it is more important for clinicians to understand the purpose of having such tightly defined methodologies in research so that conclusions can be drawn with confidence and be generalizable. If one agrees to become involved in research it will have an impact on one's work. No matter what approach is used—even pragmatic trials (see below)—it will inevitably involve more careful recording of activity and data collection. It does not, however, necessarily mean that there will have to be a randomized controlled trial (RCT).

The randomized controlled trial (RCT)

The RCT has come to dominate research practice since its development over 40 years ago. It is often referred to as the 'gold standard' in research and is certainly the most powerful format to test a question. It reduces bias at the start of the trial by randomly allocating patients to either the experimental arm (in which they receive the treatment under scrutiny) or the control arm (in which they receive either no treatment (i.e. a placebo controlled trial) or another standard, accepted treatment). Neither patient nor therapist has any say in which treatment is given.

This is the only trial design which can really answer questions about causality— whether or not the experimental treatment is responsible for the outcome. To do so it needs to be designed with a single variable differentiating the experimental and control arms. This is not easy to do in community psychiatry studies where the interventions are often complex. Where it is done (e.g. the UK700 study) (UK700 Group: Burns *et al*. 1999*b*), it may be criticized for being too narrow or for distorting practice. Other designs can only tell us about association (i.e. that an intervention is associated or correlated with a type of outcome).

Blinding

Because of rater bias and patient expectations, the usual aim is to make RCTs 'double blind'. This means that neither the patient nor the research or clinical staff know if the patient is receiving the experimental treatment or the control. Thereby, their expectations are not allowed to affect outcome. For instance, in antidepressant trials both patients and staff would expect those getting the drug to do better and would rate them so. Surprisingly however, large numbers of patients in such trials complain of side-effects from placebo!

It is rarely possible to achieve blinding in studies of complex mental health interventions such as assertive outreach. The alternative approach is to try and make the measures as concrete as possible, reducing the scope for bias by defining outcomes very carefully and training and retraining the raters.

Statistics

Results of such trials are generally interpreted 'probabilistically'. This means that statistics are used to estimate the likelihood of any difference found being due to chance. Results are often presented as 'statistically significant', but it is important to remember that this is not a statement of absolute fact but of the likelihood that the study results represent reality. Given that people vary and few results are black and white, most studies have to compare the range of outcomes in the experimental group with that in the control group. To be able to draw conclusions from this difference requires a calculation (*before the study is started*) about whether the sample is big enough to draw such conclusions. This is called a 'power calculation'.

It is also important to bear in mind that a result can be highly statistically significant but not be at all *clinically significant*. This is especially so in very large studies where, say, a reduction in blood pressure by 2 mm/Hg can be firmly demonstrated for a new drug. But is a reduction of 2 mm/Hg clinically worthwhile?

Power

If there is a lot of natural variation and the expected treatment differences are modest, then studies need to be large. This is the case for community mental health research. However, we persist with a tradition of conducting 'under–powered' studies. This is a serious failing in our discipline (Coid 1994; Burns 2000*b*) and needs to be resolved. It is particularly important for assertive outreach workers because of the likelihood of being asked to take part in local evaluations that drift into research projects. It is very unlikely indeed that a study of 50–100 patients can sustain scientific interpretation unless the questions are asked in an extraordinarily careful manner. Certainly the question of testing whether a team with such a patient sample reduces bed usage is not possible for all the reasons outlined above. And yet such studies are still being conducted, soaking up time and energy to produce questionable results. A multi-centre study of the same question but employing several teams will, however, achieve that power. It will also reduce local Hawthorne effects and probably cover a more representative patient sample.

Non-experimental studies

An RCT, with its attendant costs and disruption, is really only indicated if an important question cannot be resolved by simpler research methods. The following list outlines the commonest research designs, ranked according to their rigour (i.e. the degree to which we can place confidence in their results).

Cohort studies consist of following up a defined group of individuals or patients (a 'cohort') over a defined period and recording their outcomes. By having detailed descriptions of them at baseline we can draw conclusions about outcomes in different groups. Long-term follow-up studies in schizophrenia are an example of this. There is no experimental intervention but, at the end we may know more about the predictors of outcome, such as the influence of gender or family history, if this had been recorded (Ciompi 1988; Harding *et al.* 1987).

Common research designs

Experimental studies

- RCT—double-blind; single-blind; open
- Case control

Non-experimental studies

- Cohort study
- Case series
- Individual case history

Exposure to treatment may be one of the characteristics and in some cases (where the exposure or non-exposure has been in a relatively consistent manner) this can be called a 'quasi-experimental' study. Although the patients have not been randomly allocated to two treatments, such allocations have arisen in the form of a 'natural experiment'. Examples of this are when a service is available in one area but not in another and the outcomes are then compared (Dean *et al*. 1993; Thornicroft *et al*. 1998*a*). There are real risks in how such studies are interpreted and causality is often attributed where it cannot really be defended. How carefully the study is conducted can make up for these limitations.

Case control studies are a type of cohort study where for each subject followed up there is a control patient, matching as closely as possible on all measures apart from the one under examination. Thus, the control patient is usually about the same age and same gender, and perhaps has other similarities. Very careful matching in case control trials (Thornicroft *et al*. 1998*a*) can bring them close to RCTs in explanatory power, but remain open to much greater risks of bias.

Case series and individual case histories are often dismissed in research but are essential for very rare conditions. They can be very helpful in relatively neglected areas (such as bipolar disorder in assertive outreach) (Hackman *et al*. 1999) or for reporting new variations in treatment patterns (e.g. our experience with establishing patients on clozapine at home) (O'Brien and Firn 2002).

Pragmatic trials, clinical effectiveness, and meta-analyses

The complexity and cost of RCTs has led to concerns that simpler, yet important questions are often overlooked in research and that results are poorly transferable to 'the real world' of day-to-day clinical practice (Thornley and Adams 1998). In particular, the contrast is drawn between 'therapeutic efficacy', which tells us how well a treatment works under optimal conditions, and 'clinical effectiveness' (Thornicroft *et al*. 1998*b*), which indicates what we can expect under normal clinical conditions where patients sometimes forget to take their drugs and miss appointments.

Pragmatic trials are an attempt to address this. These trials are designed to be easy to conduct in routine clinical practice, with no onerous data collection (Thornley and Adams 1998). They can be RCTs, but have few exclusion criteria and have simple randomization procedures with tightly defined and unequivocal outcome measures. To allow for the extensive variation within them, they need enormous samples—typically several thousand patients. The establishment of organizations such as the Commission for Health Improvement in the UK (which requires evidence of clinical effectiveness data for new treatments) is likely to redress the current, possibly excessive, attention paid to RCTs.

Systematic reviews, such as those published by the Cochrane database (Marshall and Lockwood 1998), involve bringing together the results of all the RCTs in the relevant area. These are graded for quality of work (including how well randomization was conducted, how complete the follow-up was, etc.) and then subject to meta-analysis. This involves subjecting all the studies to the same analysis against a single outcome measure. It also involves re-analysing all the data together so that a total effect can be deduced. This is certainly a major research advance, but there remain significant challenges in applying it in mental health research where the interventions are often complex and poorly defined and where the study context and control conditions can exert a powerful effect that cannot be estimated.

Qualitative research

This chapter has concentrated on research designs based on measuring processes and outcomes as accurately as possible, and then subjecting these results to statistical analysis. This is often referred to as 'quantitative' research to emphasize the counting aspect of it. Quantitative research is usually employed to test hypotheses (beliefs about the nature of the subject) which are stated as precisely as possible right at the beginning. Where do these hypotheses come from? For the most part they come from clinical impressions. We work with a group of patients over time and gradually the idea emerges that, say, 'men benefit more from daily supervised meds'. If we want to be certain whether this is the truth or not (we doubt it!), then we propose it as a hypothesis and design a study to test it.

Sometimes qualitative research is used to generate hypotheses. Qualitative research is an emerging branch of science with increasing credibility. It arises more from social sciences, where it is much more difficult to conduct controlled experiments. Qualitative methods draw on a number of techniques from both social sciences and anthropology to refine the process of understanding what is going on in a situation. It encompasses a whole range of approaches from focus groups to participant observation.

There is an ongoing debate about whether qualitative work is purely 'hypothesis generating' or whether it can give definitive answers in its own right. The argument is muddied by an unfortunate practice of sometimes calling poorly thought-out or under-powered research, qualitative. It is clear that high-quality qualitative research requires as much (if not more) rigour than quantitative. It is beyond our competence to advise on it other than to point out that it should not be undertaken without highly skilled supervision.

Conclusions

Assertive outreach has come to prominence at the same time as a rising interest in evidence-based practice. It is also an unusually well-defined form of care, and earlier examples were subjected to research studies that produced remarkable results which became internationally famous. Not surprisingly then, assertive outreach staff have been involved in much more clinical research than most mental health teams (Mueser *et al.* 1998). All of us are likely to be increasingly involved in audit, research, and development. The benefits of this in keeping us critical and reflective in our thinking are enormous if we take it seriously and do not simply collect data.

We owe it to ourselves to make sure that research in this area is conducted ethically and sensibly. Questions have to mean something and clinicians, patients, and carers have much to contribute in both the setting of the questions and the design and conduct of the research. Only if there is a rich dialogue between all stakeholders will it deliver the results we really need. We can also ensure that time and energy are not wasted on small-scale, under-powered studies whose results will not advance our understanding. There is a whole range of new questions (Burns *et al.* 2001*b*) to ask (not just effects on hospital use) and who better to raise them than the people who receive or work in the services?

References

Al–Kubaisky, T., Marks, I.M., Logsdail, S., and Marks, M.P. (1992) Role of exposure homework in phobia reduction: a controlled study, *Behaviour Therapy*, **23**, 599–621.

Allness, D. and Knoedler, W. (1998) *The PACT model of community based treatment for persons with severe and persistent mental illness: a manual for PACT start-up*, National Alliance for the Mentally Ill Anti-Stigma Campaign, Arlington VA.

Altshuler, L.L., Post, R.M., Leverich, G.S., Mikalauskas, K., Rosoff, A., and Ackerman, L. (1995) Antidepressant-induced mania and cycle acceleration: a controversy revisited, *American Journal of Psychiatry*, **152:8**, 1130–8.

American Psychiatric Association (1980) *Diagnostic and statistical manual of mental disorders* (3rd edn), American Psychiatric Association, Washington DC.

American Psychiatric Association (1994) *Diagnostic and statistical manual of mental disorders* (4th edn), American Psychiatric Association, Washington DC.

Angermeyer, M.C., Loffler, W., Muller, P., Schulze, B., and Priebe, S. (2001) Patients' and relatives' assessment of clozapine treatment, *Psychological Medicine*, **31:3**, 509–17.

Appleby, L., Shaw, J., Amos, T., McDonnell, R., Kiernan, K., and Davies, S. (1999) *Safer services. Report of the National Confidential Inquiry into Suicide and Homicide by people with mental illness*, HMSO, London.

Appleby, L., Morriss, R., Gask, L., Roland, M., Perry, B., Lewis, A., *et al.* (2000) An educational intervention for front-line health professionals in the assessment and management of suicidal patients (the STORM Project), *Psychological Medicine*, **30:4**, 805–12.

Audit Commission (1994) *Finding a place: a review of mental health services for adults*, HMSO, London.

Barnes, T.R. (1989) A rating scale for drug-induced akathisia, *British Journal of Psychiatry*, **154**, 672–6.

Barnes, T.R., Hutton, S.B., Chapman, M.J., Mutsatsa, S., Puri, B.K., and Joyce, E.M. (2000) West London first-episode study of schizophrenia: clinical correlates of duration of untreated psychosis, *British Journal of Psychiatry*, **177**, 207–11.

Barrowclough, C., Tarrier, N., Watts, S., Vaughn, C., Bamrah, J.S., and Freeman, H.L. (1987) Assessing the functional value of relatives' knowledge about schizophrenia: a preliminary report, *British Journal of Psychiatry*, **151**, 1–8.

Barrowclough, C., Marshall, M., Lockwood, A., Quinn, J., and Sellwood, W. (1998) Assessing relatives' needs for psychosocial interventions in schizophrenia: a relatives' version of the Cardinal Needs Schedule (RCNS), *Psychological Medicine*, **28:3**, 531–42.

Bartels, S.J., Drake, R.E., and McHugo, G.J. (1992) Alcohol abuse, depression, and suicidal behavior in schizophrenia, *American Journal of Psychiatry*, **149:3**, 394–5.

Bartels, S.J., Teague, G.B., and Drake, R.E. (1993) Service utilisation and costs associated with substance use disorder among severely mentall ill patients, *Journal of Nervous & Mental Disease*, **177**, 400–7.

Barton, R. (1959) *Institutional neurosis*, John Wright, Bristol.

Bateson, G., Jackson, D., Haley, J., and Weakland, J. (1956) Towards a theory of schizophrenia, *Behavioral Science*, 1, 251–64.

Beard, J.H., Malamud, T.J., and Rossman, E. (1978) Psychiatric rehabilitation and long-term rehospitalization rates: the findings of two research studies, *Schizophrenia Bulletin*, 4:4, 622–35.

Beard, J.H., Propst, R.N., and Malamud, T.J. (1982) The Fountain House model of rehabilitation, *Psychosocial Rehabilitation Journal*, 5:1, 47–53.

Bech, P., Allerup, P., Gram, L.F., Reisby, N., Rosenberg, R., Jacobsen, O., *et al.* (1981) The Hamilton depression scale. Evaluation of objectivity using logistic models, *Acta Psychiatrica Scandinavica*, 63: 3, 290–9.

Beck, A.T., Ward, C.H., Mendelson, M., Mock, J.E., and Erbaugh, J.K. (1961) An inventory for measuring depression, *Archives of General Psychiatry*, 4, 561–71.

Beck, A.T., Hollon, S.D., Young, J.E., Bedrosian, R.C., and Budenz, D. (1985) Treatment of depression with cognitive therapy and amitriptyline, *Archives of General Psychiatry*, 42: 2, 142–8.

Beck, J.C. and Brochner–Mortensen, K. (1954) Observations on the prognosis in anorexia nervosa, *Acta Medica Scandinavica*, 149, 409–30.

Beeforth, M., Conlan, E., and Grayley, R. (1994) *Have we got views for you: user evaluation of case management*, Sainsbury Centre for Mental Health, London.

Bhugra, D. and Bhui, K. (2001) *Cross cultural psychiatry: a practical guide*, Edward Arnold, London.

Bhugra, D., Desai, M., and Baldwin, D.S. (1999) Attempted suicide in west London. I: rates across ethnic communities, *Psychological Medicine*, 29:5, 1125–30.

Bindman, J., Beck, A., Thornicroft, G., Knapp, M., and Szmukler, G. (2000) Psychiatric patients at greatest risk and in greatest need. Impact of the supervision register policy, *British Journal of Psychiatry*, 177, 33–7.

Bines, W. (1994) *The health of single homeless people*, Centre of Housing Policy, York University, York.

Birchwood, M. and Iqbal, Z. (1998) Depression and suicide thinking in psychosis: a cognitive approach. In *Outcome and innovation in psychological management of schizophrenia*, (ed. T. Wykes, N. Tarrier, and S. Lewis), Wiley, Chichester, 81–100.

Birchwood, M., Smith, J., Cochrane, R., Wetton, S., and Copestake, S. (1990) The social functioning scale. The development and validation of a new scale of social adjustment for use in family intervention programmes with schizophrenic patients, *British Journal of Psychiatry*, 157, 853–9.

Birchwood, M., Smith, J., Drury, V., Healy, J., MacMillan, F., and Slade, M. (1994) A self-report insight scale for psychosis: reliability, validity and sensitivity to change, *Acta Psychiatrica Scandinavica*, 89:1, 62–7.

Birchwood, M., McGorry, P., and Jackson, H. (1997) Early intervention in schizophrenia, *British Journal of Psychiatry*, 170, 2–5.

Bleuler, E. (1950) *Dementia praecox or the group of schizophrenias* (translated by J. Zinkin), International Universities Press, New York.

Bond, G.R. (1991) Variations in an assertive outreach model, *New Directions for Mental Health Services*, 52, 65–80.

Bond, G.R. (1992) Vocational rehabilitation. In *Handbook of psychiatric rehabilitation* (ed. R.P. Liberman), Macmillan, New York.

Bond, G.R. and Dincin, J. (1986) Accelerating entry into transitional employment in a psychosocial agency, *Rehabilitation Psychology*, 31, 135–45.

Bond, G.R., Witheridge, T.F., Dincin, J., Wasmer, D., de Webb, J., and Graaf–Kaser, R. (1990) Assertive community treatment for frequent users of psychiatric hospitals in a large city: a controlled study, *American Journal of Community Psychology*, 18:6, 865–91.

Bond, G.R., McGrew, J.H., and Fekete, D.M. (1995) Assertive outreach for frequent users of psychiatric hospitals: a meta-analysis, *Journal of Mental Health Administration*, **22:1**, 4–16.

Bond, G.R., Drake, R.E., Mueser, K.T., and Becker, D.R. (1997) An update on supported employment for people with severe mental illness, *Psychiatric Services*, **48:3**, 335–46.

Bowden, C.L., Brugger, A.M., Swann, A.C., Calabrese, J.R., Janicak, P.G., Petty, F., *et al.* (1994) Efficacy of divalproex vs lithium and placebo in the treatment of mania. The Depakote Mania Study Group, *JAMA*, **271:12**, 918–24.

Bowlby, J. (1961) Process of mourning, *International Journal of Psychoanalysis*, **42**, 317–40.

Braun, P., Kochansky, G., Shapiro, R., Greenberg, S., Gudeman, J.E., Johnson, S., *et al.* (1981) Overview: deinstitutionalization of psychiatric patients, a critical review of outcome studies, *American Journal of Psychiatry*, **138:6**, 736–49.

Brayne, H.A. and Martin, G. (1990) *Law for social workers*, Blackstone Press Limited, London.

Brooker, C., Falloon, I., Butterworth, A., Goldberg, D., Graham–Hole, V., and Hillier, V. (1994) The outcome of training community psychiatric nurses to deliver psychosocial intervention, *British Journal of Psychiatry*, **165:2**, 222–30.

Brown, G.W., Birley, J.L., and Wing, J.K. (1972) Influence of family life on the course of schizophrenic disorders: a replication, *British Journal of Psychiatry*, **121:562**, 241–58.

Burns, T. (1986) Use of the term 'borderline patient' by Swedish psychiatrists, *International Journal of Social Psychiatry*, **32:4**, 32–9.

Burns, T. (1994) Mrs Bottomley's Ten Point Plan, *Psychiatric Bulletin*, **18:129**, 130.

Burns, T. (1997*a*) Psychosocial interventions, *Current Opinion in Psychiatry*, **10**, 36–9.

Burns, T. (1997*b*) Case management, care management and care programming, *British Journal of Psychiatry*, **170**, 393–5.

Burns, T. (2000*a*) Maxwell Jones lecture: the legacy of therapeutic community practice in modern community mental health services, *Therapeutic Communities*, **21:3**, 165–74.

Burns, T. (2000*b*) Psychiatric home treatment. Vigorous, well designed trials are needed, *BMJ*, **321:7254**, 177.

Burns, T. (2000*c*) Supervised discharge orders, *Psychiatric Bulletin*, **24:401**, 402.

Burns, T. (2001) Balancing the service elements. In *Textbook of community psychiatry* (ed. G. Thornicroft and G. Szmukler), Oxford University Press, Oxford.

Burns, T. and Bale, R. (1997) Establishing a mental health liaison attachment with primary care, *Advances in Psychiatric Treatment*, **3**, 219–24.

Burns, T. and Cohen, A. (1998) Item-of-service payments for general practitioner care of severely mentally ill persons: does the money matter?, *British Journal of General Practice*, **48**, 1415–16.

Burns, T. and Kendrick, T. (1997) The primary care of patients with schizophrenia: a search for good practice, *British Journal of General Practice*, **47:421**, 515–20.

Burns, T. and Priebe, S. (1996) Mental health care systems and their characteristics: a proposal, *Acta Psychiatrica Scandinavica*, **94:6**, 381–5.

Burns, T., Beadsmoore, A., Bhat, A.V., Oliver, A., and Mathers, C. (1993*a*) A controlled trial of home-based acute psychiatric services. I: clinical and social outcome, *British Journal of Psychiatry*, **163**, 49–54.

Burns, T., Raftery, J., Beadsmoore, A., McGuigan, S., and Dickson, M. (1993*b*) A controlled trial of home-based acute psychiatric services. II: treatment patterns and costs, *British Journal of Psychiatry*, **163**, 55–61.

Burns, T., Fiander, M., Kent, A., Ukoumunne, O.C., Byford, S., Fahy, T., *et al.* (2000) Effects of case load size on the process of care of patients with severe psychotic illness, *British Journal of Psychiatry*, **177:427**, 433.

Burns, T., Knapp, M., Catty, J., Healey, A., Henderson, J., Watt, H., *et al.* (2001*a*) Home treatment for mental health problems: a systematic review, *Health Technology Assessment*, **5**:15.

Burns, T., Fioritti, A., Holloway, F., Malm, U., and Rossler, W. (2001*b*) Case management and assertive community treatment in Europe, *Psychiatric Services*, **52**: 5, 631–6.

Butler, R. (1975) *Report of the Committee on Mentally Abnormal Offenders*, HMSO, London.

Byrne, D.L., Asmussen, T., and Freeman. Descriptive terms for women attending antenatal clinics: mother knows best? In *British Journal of Obstetrics and Gynaecology*, **107**, 1233–1236.

Caplan, G. (1964) *Principles of preventive psychiatry*, Basic Books, New York.

Carey, K.B. (1995) Treatment of substance use disorders and schizophrenia. In *Double jeopardy: chronic mental illness and substance abuse* (ed. A.F. Lehman and L.B. Dixon), Harwood Academic Publishers, Baltimore.

Catty, J., Burns, T., Knapp, M., Watt, H., Wright, C., Henderson, J., *et al.* (in press) Home treatment for mental health problems: a systematic review, *Psychological Medicine*.

Chadwick, P.D., Birchwood, M., and Grower, P. (1996) *Cognitive therapy for delusions, voices and paranoia*, John Wiley, Chichester.

Chaplin, R. and Kent, A. (1998) Informing patients about tardive dyskinesia. Controlled trial of patient education, *British Journal of Psychiatry*, **172**, 78–81.

Chaplin, R., Gordon, J., and Burns, T. (1999) Early detection of antipsychotic side-effects, *Psychiatric Bulletin*, **23**, 657–60.

Charlton, J., Kelly, S., Dunnell, K., Evans, B., and Jenkins, R. (1994) Suicide deaths in England and Wales: trends in factors associated with suicide deaths. In *The prevention of suicide* (ed. R. Jenkins *et al.*), HMSO, London.

Chaulk, C.P. and Pope, D.S. (1997) The Baltimore City Health Department program of directly observed therapy for tuberculosis, *Clinics in Chest Medicine*, **18**:1, 149–54.

Ciompi, L. (1988) Learning from outcome studies toward a comprehensive biological-psychosocial understanding of schizophrenia, *Schizophrenia Research*, 1, 373–84.

Coid, J.W.(1994) Failure in community care: psychiatry's dilemma, *BMJ*, **308**:6932, 805–6.

Coid, J.W. (1996) Dangerous patients with mental illness: increased risks warrant new policies, adequate resources, and appropriate legislation, *BMJ*, **312**:7036, 965–6.

Committee of Inquiry (1969) *Report of the Committee of Inquiry into allegations of ill-treatment of patients and other irregularities at the Ely Hospital, Cardiff, presented to Parliament by the Secretary of State of the Department of Health and Social Security*, HMSO, London.

Cookson, J. (1997) Lithium: balancing risks and benefits, *British Journal of Psychiatry*, 171, 120–4.

Cooper, J.E. (1979) Crisis admission units and emergency psychiatric services. In *Public health in Europe, No. 2*, WHO, Copenhagen.

Craig, T. and Timms, P.W. (1992) Out of the wards and onto the streets? Deinstitutionalization and homelessness in Britain, *Journal of Mental Health*, 1, 265–75.

Crow, T.J. (1980) Molecular pathology of schizophrenia: more than one disease process?, *BMJ*, **280**:6207, 66–8.

Crow, T.J., MacMillan, J.F., Johnson, A.L., and Johnstone, E.C. (1986) A randomised controlled trial of prophylactic neuroleptic treatment, *British Journal of Psychiatry*, 148, 120–7.

Crowther, R.E., Marshall, M., Bond, G.R., and Huxley, P. (2001) Helping people with severe mental illness to obtain work: systematic review, *BMJ*, 322, 204–8.

Cunningham–Owens, D.G. (1999) *A guide to the extrapyramidal side effects of antipsychotic drugs*, Cambridge University Press, Cambridge.

Curson, D.A., Barnes, T.R., Bamber, R.W., Platt, S.D., Hirsch, S.R., and Duffy, J.C. (1985) Long-term depot maintenance of chronic schizophrenic out-patients: the seven-year follow-up of the Medical Research Council fluphenazine:placebo trial. III. Relapse postponement or relapse prevention? The implications for long-term outcome, *British Journal of Psychiatry*, 146, 474–80.

Curtis, J.L., Millman, E.J., Struening, E., and D'Ercole, A. (1992) Effect of case management on rehospitalization and utilization of ambulatory care services, *Hospital & Community Psychiatry*, 43:9, 895–9.

David, A.S. (1990) Insight and psychosis, *British Journal of Psychiatry*, 156, 798–808.

David, A., Buchanan, A., Reed, A., and Almeida, O. (1992) The assessment of insight in psychosis, *British Journal of Psychiatry*, 161, 599–602.

Davies, W. and Frude, N. (1993) *Preventing face-to-face violence: the T-PIP programme*, The Association of Psychological Therapies, Leicester, England.

Dean, C., Phillips, J., Gadd, E.M., Joseph, M., and England, S. (1993) Comparison of community based service with hospital based service for people with acute, severe psychiatric illness, *BMJ*, 307:6902, 473–6.

Degen, K., Cole, N., Tamayo, L., and Dzerovych, G. (1990) Intensive case management for the seriously ill, *Administration and Policy in Mental Health*, 17:4, 265–69.

Denicoff, K.D., Smith–Jackson, E.E., Disney, E.R., Ali, S.O., Leverich, G.S.,and Post, R.M. (1997) Comparative prophylactic efficacy of lithium, carbamazepine, and the combination in bipolar disorder, *Journal of Clinical Psychiatry*, 58:11, 470–78.

Department of Health (1959) *The Mental Health Act: England and Wales*, Department of Health, London.

Department of Health (1990) *The Care Programme Approach for people with a mental illness referred to the Special Psychiatric Services*, Joint Health/Social Services Circular HC (90) 23/LASS (90) 11, Department of Health, London,.

Department of Health (1992) *The Health of the Nation: A strategy for health in England*, HMSO, London.

Department of Health (1995) *Patients in the Community Mental Health Act 1995*, HMSO, London.

Department of Health (1998a) *Modernising Mental Health Services, Safe, Sound and Supportive*, HSC 1998/233/LAC(98)25, Department of Health, London,

Department of Health (1998b) Key components of the clinical governance framework In *A first class service – quality in the new NHS*, HMSO, London, pp. 35–8.

Department of Health (1999a) *Modern Standards and Service Models: National Service Framework for Mental Health*, Department of Health, London.

Department of Health (1999b) *Code of practice: Mental Health Act 1983*, HMSO, London.

Department of Health (1999c) *Safer services: national confidential inquiry into suicide and homicide by people with mental illness*, Department of Health, London.

Department of Health (2000) *The NHS plan—a plan for investment, a plan for reform*, Department of Health, London.

Department of Health (2001) *The mental health policy implementation guide*, Department of Health, London.

Deren, S., Stephens, R., Davis, W.R., Feucht, T.E., and Tortu, S. (1994) The impact of providing incentives for attendance at AIDS prevention sessions, *Public Health Report*, 109:4, 548–54.

Dincin, J. and Witheridge, T.F. (1982) Psychiatric rehabilitation as a deterrent to recidivism, *Hospital and Community Psychiatry*, 33:8, 645–50.

Drake, R.E. and Becker, D.R. (1996) The individual placement and support (IPS) model of supported employment, *Psychiatric Services*, 47:5, 473–5.

Drake, R.E. and Mercer–McFadden, C. (1995) Assessment of substance use among persons with chronic mental illnesses. In *Double jeopardy: chronic mental illness and substance abuse* (ed. A.F. Lehman and L.B. Dixon), Harwood Academic Publishers, Baltimore.

Drake, R.E. and Wallach, M.A. (1993) Moderate drinking among people with severe mental illness, *Hospital and Community Psychiatry*, **44:8**, 780–2.

Drake, R.E., Osher, F.C., and Wallach, M.A. (1989) Alcohol use and abuse in schizophrenia. A prospective community study, *Journal of Nervous & Mental Disease*, **177:7**, 408–14.

Drake, R.E., McHugo, G.J., and Noordsy, D.L. (1993) Treatment of alcoholism among schizophrenic outpatients: 4-year outcomes, *American Journal of Psychiatry*, **150:2**, 328–9.

Drake, R.E., Noordsy, D.L., and Ackerson, T. (1995) Integrating mental health and substance abuse treatments for persons with chronic mental disorders: a model. In *Double jeopardy: chronic mental illness and substance abuse* (ed. A.F. Lehman and L.B. Dixon), Harwood Academic Publishers, Baltimore.

Drake, R.E., Yovetich, N.A., Bebout, R.R., Harris, M., and McHugo, G.J. (1997) Integrated treatment for dually diagnosed homeless adults, *Journal of Nervous & Mental Disease*, **185:5**, 298–305.

Drake, R.E., McHugo, G.J., Clark, R.E., Teague, G.B., Xie, H., Miles, K., *et al.* (1998) Assertive community treatment for patients with co-occurring severe mental illness and substance use disorder: a clinical trial, *American Journal of Orthopsychiatry*, **68:2**, 201–15.

Drake, R.E., McHugo, G.J., Bebout, R.R., Becker, D.R., Harris, M., Bond, G.R., *et al.* (1999*a*) A randomized clinical trial of supported employment for inner-city patients with severe mental disorders, *Archives of General Psychiatry*, **56:7**, 627–33.

Drake, R.E., Becker, D.R., Clark, R.E., and Mueser, K.T. (1999*b*) Research on the individual placement and support model of supported employment, *Psychiatric Quarterly*, **70:4**, 289–301.

Drucker, P.F. (1993) *Management: tasks, responsibilities and practice*, Harper Business, New York.

English National Board (1996) *Working in partnership: a collaborative approach to care. Report of the mental health nursing review team. Progress two years on*, English National Board, London.

Fadden, G. (1997) Implementation of family interventions in routine clinical practice following staff training programs: a major cause for concern, *Journal of Mental Health*, **6:6**, 599–612.

Falloon, I.R. and Talbot, R.E. (1981) Persistent auditory hallucinations: coping mechanisms and implications for management, *Psychological Medicine*, **11:2**, 329–39.

Falloon, I.R., Boyd, J.L., McGill, C.W., Razani, J., Moss, H.B., and Gilderman, A.M. (1982) Family management in the prevention of exacerbations of schizophrenia: a controlled study, *New England Journal of Medicine*, **306:24**, 1437–40.

Falret, J. (1854) Memoire sur la folie circulaire, *Bulletin de la Acadamie Imperiale de Medicin, Paris*, 19, 382–400.

Fatemi, S.H., Rapport, D.J., Calabrese, J.R., and Thuras, P. (1997) Lamotrigine in rapid-cycling bipolar disorder, *Journal of Clinical Psychiatry*, **58:12**, 522–7.

Firth–Cozens, J. (1993) *Audit in mental health services*, Lawrence Erlbaum, Hove, East Sussex.

Fleischhacker, W.W., Roth, S.D., and Kane, J.M. (1990) The pharmacologic treatment of neuroleptic-induced akathisia, *Journal of Clinical Psychopharmacology*, **10:1**, 12–21.

Ford, R. and Repper, J. (1994) Taking responsibility for care, *Nursing Times*, **90:31**, 54–6.

Frank, A.F. and Gunderson, J.G. (1990) The role of the therapeutic alliance in the treatment of schizophrenia. Relationship to course and outcome, *Archives of General Psychiatry*, **47:3**, 228–36.

Franklin, J.L., Solovitz, B., Mason, M., Clemons, J.R., and Miller, G.E. (1987) An evaluation of case management, *American Journal of Public Health*, **77:6**, 674–8.

Freeman, M. and Stoll, A. (1998) Mood stabilizer combinations: a review of safety and efficacy, *American Journal of Psychiatry*, **155**, 12–21.

Fromm–Reichmann, F. (1948) Notes on the development of treatment of schizophrenics by psycho-analytic psychotherapy, *Psychiatry*, 11, 263–70.

Fujiwara, P.I., Larkin, C., and Frieden, T.R. (1997) Directly observed therapy in New York City. History, implementation, results, and challenges, *Clinics in Chest Medicine*, 18:1, 135–48.

Garety, P., Fowler, D., Kuipers, E., Freeman, D., Dunn, G., Bebbington, P., *et al.* (1997) London-East Anglia randomised controlled trial of cognitive-behavioural therapy for psychosis. II: predictors of outcome, *British Journal of Psychiatry*, 171, 420–6.

Geddes, J., Freemantle, N., Harrison, P., and Bebbington, P. (2000) Atypical antipsychotics in the treatment of schizophrenia: systematic overview and meta-regression analysis, *BMJ*, 321:7273, 1371–6.

Giuffrida, A. and Torgerson, D.J. (1997) Should we pay the patient? Review of financial incentives to enhance patient compliance, *BMJ*, 315:7110, 703–7.

Goffman, I. (1960) *Asylums: essays on the social situation of mental patients and other inmates.* Penguin Books, Harmondsworth, Middlesex.

Goldstein, R.B., Black, D.W., Nasrallah, A., and Winokur, G. (1991) The prediction of suicide. Sensitivity, specificity, and predictive value of a multivariate model applied to suicide among 1906 patients with affective disorders, *Archives of General Psychiatry*, 48:5, 418–22.

Goodwin, F.K. and Jamison, K.R. (1990) *Manic-depressive illness*, Oxford University Press, New York.

Gournay, K. and Birley, J. (1998) Thorn: a new approach to mental health training, *Nursing Times*, 94:49, 54–5.

Green, M.F. (1996) What are the functional consequences of neurocognitive deficits in schizophrenia?, *American Journal of Psychiatry*, 153:3, 321–30.

Greenwood, N., Hussain, F., Burns, T., and Raphael, F. (2000) Asian in-patient and carer views of mental health care. Asian views of mental health care, *Journal of Mental Health*, 9:4, 397–408.

Grove, B. (1999) Mental health and employment: shaping a new agenda, *Journal of Mental Health*, 8, 131–40.

Grove, B. (2000) *Work and employment*, Health Advisory Service, London.

Grufferman, S. (1999) Complexity and the Hawthorne effect in community trials, *Epidemiology*, 10:3, 209–10.

Gunnell, D. (1991) *The potential for preventing suicide. A review of the literature on the effectiveness of interventions aimed at preventing suicide*, Health Care Evaluation Unit, University of Bristol, Department of Epidemiology and Public Health Medicine.

Hackman, A.L., Ram, R.N., and Dixon, L.B. (1999) Psychosocial treatment of bipolar disorder in the public sector: program for assertive community treatment model. In *Bipolar disorders. Clinical course and outcome* (ed. J.F. Goldberg and M. Harrow), American Psychiatric Press, Washington DC, pp. 259–74.

Hallström, R.V. (1985) *Judgement of Mr Justice McCullough in the High Court of Justice, Queen's Bench Division*, Royal Court of Justice.

Harding, C.M., Brooks, G.W., Ashikaga, T., Strauss, J.S., and Breier, A. (1987) The Vermont longitudinal study of persons with severe mental illness. II: long-term outcome of subjects who retrospectively met DSM-III criteria for schizophrenia, *American Journal of Psychiatry*, 144:6, 727–35.

Harris, E.C. and Barraclough, B. (1998) Excess mortality of mental disorder, *British Journal of Psychiatry*, 173, 11–53.

Harrison, G., Glazebrook, C., Brewin, J., Cantwell, R., Dalkin, T., Fox, R., *et al.* (1997) Increased incidence of psychotic disorders in migrants from the Caribbean to the United Kingdom, *Psychological Medicine*, 27:4, 799–806.

Harvey, K., Burns, T., Sedgwick, P., Higgitt, A., Creed, F., and Fahy, T. (2001) Relatives of patients with severe psychotic disorders: factors that influence contact frequency. Report from the UK700 trial, *British Journal of Psychiatry*, 178, 248–54.

Herinckx, H.A., Kinney, R.F., Clarke, G.N., and Paulson, R.I. (1997) Assertive community treatment versus usual care in engaging and retaining clients with severe mental illness, *Psychiatric Services*, **48**:10, 1297–1306.

Hinton, J. (1967) *Dying*, Penguin Books Ltd, Middlesex, England.

Hirsch, S. (1988) *Psychiatric beds and resources: factors influencing bed use and service planning*, Gaskell Press (Royal College of Psychiatrists), London.

Hirsch, S.R., Gaind, R., Rohde, P.D., Stevens, B.C., and Wing, J.K. (1973) Outpatient maintenance of chronic schizophrenic patients with long-acting fluphenazine: double-blind placebo trial. Report to the Medical Research Council Committee on clinical trials in psychiatry, *BMJ*, **1**:854, 633–7.

Hogan, T.P., Awad, A.G., and Eastwood, R. (1983) A self-report scale predictive of drug compliance in schizophrenics: reliability and discriminative validity, *Psychological Medicine*, **13**:1, 177–83.

Hogarty, G.E., Anderson, C.M., Reiss, D.J., Kornblith, S.J., Greenwald, D.P., Ulrich, R.F., *et al.* (1991) Family psychoeducation, social skills training, and maintenance chemotherapy in the aftercare treatment of schizophrenia. II. Two-year effects of a controlled study on relapse and adjustment. Environmental–Personal Indicators in the Course of Schizophrenia (EPICS) Research Group, *Archives of General Psychiatry*, **48**:4, 340–7.

Hogarty, G.E., Kornblith, S.J., Greenwald, D., DiBarry, A.L., Cooley, S., Flesher, S., *et al.* (1995) Personal therapy: a disorder-relevant psychotherapy for schizophrenia, *Schizophrenia Bulletin*, **21**:3, 379–93.

Hogarty, G.E., Kornblith, S.J., Greenwald, D., DiBarry, A L., Cooley, S., Ulrich, R.F., *et al.* (1997) Three-year trials of personal therapy among schizophrenic patients living with or independent of family. I: description of study and effects on relapse rates, *American Journal of Psychiatry*, **154**:11, 1504–13.

Holloway, F. (1988) Prescribing for the long-term mentally ill. A study of treatment practices, *British Journal of Psychiatry*, **152**, 511–15.

Holloway, F. and Carson, J. (1998) Intensive case management for the severely mentally ill: controlled trial, *British Journal of Psychiatry*, **172**, 19–22.

Holloway, F., Oliver, N., Collins, E., and Carson, J. (1995) Case management: a critical review of the outcome literature, *European Psychiatry*, **10**, 113–28.

Hoult, J. (1986) Community care of the acutely mentally ill, *British Journal of Psychiatry*, **149**, 137–44.

Hoult, J., Reynolds, I., Charbonneau–Powis, M., Weekes, P., and Briggs, J. (1983) Psychiatric hospital versus community treatment: the results of a randomised trial, *Australian & New Zealand Journal of Psychiatry*, **17**:2, 160–7.

Hoult, J., Rosen, A., and Reynolds, I. (1984) Community orientated treatment compared to psychiatric hospital orientated treatment, *Social Science & Medicine*, **18**:11, 1005–10.

Hsu, L.K., Meltzer, E.S., and Crisp, A.H. (1981) Schizophrenia and anorexia nervosa, *Journal of Nervous & Mental Disorders*, **169**:5, 273–6.

Ingham, C. (2000) *Panic attacks*, Thorsons, London.

Intagliata, J. (1982) Improving the quality of community care for the chronically mentally disabled: the role of case management, *Schizophrenia Bulletin*, **8**:4, 655–74.

Jackson, H., McGorry, P., Edwards, J., Hulbert, C., Henry, L., Francey, S., *et al.* (1998) Cognitively-oriented psychotherapy for early psychosis (COPE). Preliminary results, *British Journal of Psychiatry Supplement*, **172**:33, 93–100.

Johannessen, J.O. (1998) Early intervention and prevention in schizophrenia: experiences from a study in Stavanger, Norway, *Seishin Shinkeigaku Zasshi*, **100**:8, 511–22.

Johnson, M.J., Williams, M., and Marshall, E.S. (1999) Adherent and non-adherent medication—taking in elderly hypertensive patients, *Clinical Nursing Research*, **8**:4, 318–35.

Johnson, S. and Thornicroft, G. (1993) The sectorisation of psychiatric services in England and Wales, *Social Psychiatry & Psychiatric Epidemiology*, **28:1**, 45–7.

Johnson, S. and Thornicroft, G. (1995) Service models in emergency psychiatry: an international review. In *Emergency mental health services in the community* (ed. M. Phelan, G. Strathdee, and G. Thornicroft), Cambridge University Press, Cambridge.

Jones, D. (1982) The Borders mental health service, *British Journal of Clinical & Social Psychiatry*, **2**, 8–12.

Jones, M. (1952) *Social Psychiatry: a study of therapeutic communities*, Tavistock, London.

Jorm, A.F., Korten, A.E., Jacomb, P.A., Rodgers, B., Pollitt, P., Christensen, H., *et al.* (1997) Helpfulness of interventions for mental disorders: beliefs of health professionals compared with the general public, *British Journal of Psychiatry*, **171**, 233–7.

Juniper, D. (2000) *Overcoming depression*, How-to Books, Oxford.

Kane, J., Honigfeld, G., Singer, J., and Meltzer, H. (1988) Clozapine for the treatment-resistant schizophrenic. A double-blind comparison with chlorpromazine, *Archives of General Psychiatry*, **45:9**, 789–96.

Kane, J.M. and McGlashan, T.H. (1995) Treatment of schizophrenia, *Lancet*, **346:8978**, 820–5.

Kemp, R., Hayward, P., Applewhaite, G., Everitt, B., and David, A. (1996) Compliance therapy in psychotic patients: randomised controlled trial, *BMJ*, **312:7027**, 345–9.

Kemp, R., Hayward, P., and David, A. (1997) *Compliance therapy manual*, King's College School of Medicine and Dentistry and Institute of Psychiatry, London.

Kemp, R., Kirov, G., Everitt, B., Hayward, P., and David, A. (1998) Randomised controlled trial of compliance therapy. 18-month follow-up, *British Journal of Psychiatry*, **172:5**, 413–19.

Kendler, K.S., Kessler, R.C., Walters, E.E., MacLean, C., Neale, M.C., Heath, A.C., *et al.* (1995) Stressful life events, genetic liability, and onset of an episode of major depression in women, *American Journal of Psychiatry*, **152:6**, 833–42.

Kendrick, T. (1996) Cardiovascular and respiratory risk factors and symptoms among general practice patients with long-term mental illness, *British Journal of Psychiatry*, **169:6**, 733–9.

Kendrick, T., Burns, T., Freeling, P., and Sibbald, B. (1994) Provision of care to general practice patients with disabling long-term mental illness: a survey in 16 practices, *British Journal of General Practice*, **44:384**, 301–5.

Kendrick, T., Millar, E., Burns, T., and Ross, F. (1998) Practice nurse involvement in giving depot neuroleptic injections: development of a patient assessment and monitoring checklist, *Primary Care Psychiatry*, **4**, 149–54.

Kendrick, T., Burns, T., Garland, C., Greenwood, N., and Smith, P. (2000) Are specialist mental health services being targeted on the most needy patients? The effects of setting up special services in general practice, *British Journal of General Practice*, **50**, 121–6.

Kennerley, H. (1997) *Overcoming anxiety*, Robinson, London.

Kent, A. and Burns, T. (1996) Setting up an assertive community treatment service, *Advances in Psychiatric Treatment*, **2:4**, 143–50.

Kernberg, O.F. (1984) *Severe personality disorders: psychotherapeutic strategies*, Yale University Press, New Haven, CT.

Khan, D., Ross, R., and Rush, A. (1996) Expert consensus treatment guidelines for bipolar disorder, *Journal of Clinical Psychiatry*, **57**, 1–8.

Kielhofner, G., Mallinson, T., Crawford, C., Nowak, M., Rigby, M., Henry, A., *et al.* (1998) *A users nanual for the occupational performance history interview (version 2.0) OPHI-II*, University of Illinois, Chicago.

Kingdon, D.G. and Turkington, D. (1994) *Cognitive-behavioural therapy for schizophrenia*, Guildford Press, New York.

King's Fund (1994) *Clinical supervision in practice*, King's Fund, London.

Kinzel, A.F. (1970) Body-buffer zone in violent prisoners, *American Journal of Psychiatry*, 127:1, 59–64.

Kissling, W., Kane, J.M., Barnes, T.R.E., Dencker, S J., Fleischhacker, W.W., Goldstein, M.J., *et al.* (1991) Guidelines for neuroleptic relapse prevention in schizophrenia: towards a consensus view. In *Guidelines for neuroleptic relapse prevention in schizophrenia* (ed.W. Kissling), Springer–Verlag, Berlin, pp. 155–63.

Kleinman, A. (1980) *Patients and healers in the context of culture*, California Press, California.

Koffman, J. and Fulop, N.J. (1999) Homelessness and the use of acute psychiatric beds: findings from a one-day survey of adult acute and low-level secure psychiatric patients in North and South Thames regions, *Health & Social Care in the Community*, 7:2, 140–7.

Kosky, N. and Burns, T. (1995) Patient access to psychiatric records: experience in an in-patient unit, *Psychiatric Bulletin*, 19, 87–90.

Kovess, V., Boisguerin, B., Antoine, D., and Reynauld, M. (1995) Has the sectorization of psychiatric services in France really been effective?, *Social Psychiatry & Psychiatric Epidemiology*, 30:3, 132–8.

Kraepelin, E. (1919) *Dementia praecox and paraphrenia* (translated by R.M. Barclay), facsimile edn (1971), Kreiger, New York.

Kuipers, E., Garety, P., Fowler, D., Dunn, G., Bebbington, P., Freeman, D., *et al.* (1997) London-East Anglia randomised controlled trial of cognitive-behavioural therapy for psychosis. I: effects of the treatment phase, *British Journal of Psychiatry*, 171, 319–27.

La Grenade, J. (1999) The National Health Service and ethnicity: services for black patients. In *Ethnicity: an agenda for mental health* (ed. D. Bhugra and K. Bahl), Gaskell, London.

Laing, R.D. (1960) *The divided self*, Tavistock, London.

Lancet (editorial) (1995) Care-management: a disastrous mistake, *Lancet*, 345, 399–401.

Laugharne, R. (1999) Evidence-based medicine, user involvement and the post-modern paradigm, *Psychiatric Bulletin*, 23, 641–3.

Lees, J., Manning, N., and Rawlings, B. (1999) *Therapeutic community effectiveness. A systematic international review of therapeutic community treatment for people with personality disorders and mentally disordered offenders.* CRD Report 17 NHS, Centre for Reviews and Dissemination, University of York, York.

Leff, J. (1993) All the homeless people—where do they all come from?, *BMJ*, 306:6879, 669–70.

Leff, J. and Vaughn, C. (1981) The role of maintenance therapy and relatives' expressed emotion in relapse of schizophrenia: a two-year follow-up, *British Journal of Psychiatry*, 139, 102–4.

Leff, J., Berkowitz, R., Shavit, N., Strachan, A., Glass, I., and Vaughn, C. (1990) A trial of family therapy versus a relatives' group for schizophrenia. Two-year follow-up, *British Journal of Psychiatry*, 157, 571–7.

Lehman, A.F. and Dixon, L.B. (1995) *Double jeopardy: chronic mental illness and substance abuse*, Harwood Academic Publishers, Baltimore.

Lehman, A.F., Myers, C.P., Thompson, J.W., and Corty, E. (1993) Implications of mental and substance use disorders. A comparison of single and dual diagnosis patients, *Journal of Nervous & Mental Disease*, 181:6, 365–70.

Lehman, A.F., Dixon, L.B., Kernan, E., DeForge, B.R., and Postrado, L.T. (1997) A randomized trial of assertive community treatment for homeless persons with severe mental illness, *Archives of General Psychiatry*, 54:11, 1038–43.

Lehman, A.F., Dixon, L., Hoch, J.S., Deforge, B., Kernan, E., and Frank, R. (1999) Cost-effectiveness of assertive community treatment for homeless persons with severe mental illness, *British Journal of Psychiatry*, 174, 346–52.

Letts, P. (1998) *Managing other people's money*, Age Concern, London.

Liberman, R.P., Wallace, C.J., Blackwell, G., Kopelowicz, A., Vaccaro, J.V., and Mintz, J. (1998) Skills training versus psychosocial occupational therapy for persons with persistent schizophrenia, *American Journal of Psychiatry*, 155:8, 1087–91.

Lidz, R.W. and Lidz, T. (1949) The family environment of schizophrenic patients, *American Journal of Psychiatry*, 106, 332–45.

Linehan, M.M., Armstrong, H.E., Suarez, A., Allmon, D., and Heard, H.L. (1991) Cognitive-behavioral treatment of chronically parasuicidal borderline patients, *Archives of General Psychiatry*, 48:12, 1060–4.

Linszen, D., Dingemans, P., Van der Does, J.W., Nugter, A., Scholte, P., Lenior, R., *et al..* (1996) Treatment, expressed emotion and relapse in recent onset schizophrenic disorders, *Psychological Medicine*, 26:2, 333–42.

Littlewood, R. and Lipsedge, M. (1997) *Aliens and alienists: ethnic minorities and psychiatry*, Routledge, London.

Mandel, M.R., Severe, J.B., Schooler, N.R., Gelenberg, A.J., and Mieske, M. (1982) Development and prediction of postpsychotic depression in neuroleptic-treated schizophrenics, *Archives of General Psychiatry*, 39:2, 197–203.

Mari, J.J. and Streiner, D.L. (1994) An overview of family interventions and relapse on schizophrenia: meta- analysis of research findings, *Psychological Medicine*, 24:3, 565–78.

Marks, I.M., Connolly, J., Muijen, M., Audini, B., McNamee, G., and Lawrence, R.E. (1994) Home-based versus hospital-based care for people with serious mental illness, *British Journal of Psychiatry*, 165, 179–94.

Marshall, M. (1996) Case management: a dubious practice, *BMJ*, 312:7030, 523–4.

Marshall, M. and Lockwood, A. (1998) *Assertive community treatment for people with severe mental disorders (Cochrane Review)*, The Cochrane Library [3].

Marshall, M., Lockwood, A., and Gath, D. (1995) Social services case-management for long-term mental disorders: a randomised controlled trial, *Lancet*, 345:8947, 409–12.

Marshall, M., Bond, G., Stein, L.I., Shepherd, G., McGrew, J., Hoult, J., *et al.* (1999) PRISM psychosis study: Design limitations, questionable conclusions, *British Journal of Psychiatry*, 175, 501–3.

Maslow, A.H. (1954) *Motivation and personality*, Harper and Row, New York.

Mayfield, D., McLeod, G., and Hall, P. (1974) The CAGE questionnaire: validation of a new alcoholism screening instrument, *American Journal of Psychiatry*, 131:10, 1121–3.

Mayou, R.A., Ehlers, A., and Hobbs, M. (2000) Psychological debriefing for road traffic accident victims. Three-year follow-up of a randomised controlled trial, *British Journal of Psychiatry*, 176, 589–93.

McCrone, P., Menezes, P.R., Johnson, S., Scott, H., Thornicroft, G., Marshall, J., *et al.* (2000) Service use and costs of people with dual diagnosis in South London, *Acta Psychiatrica Scandinavica*, 101:6, 464–72.

McFarlane, W.R., Lukens, E., Link, B., Dushay, R., Deakins, S.A., Newmark, M., *et al.* (1995) Multiple-family groups and psychoeducation in the treatment of schizophrenia, *Archives of General Psychiatry*, 52:8, 679–87.

McFarlane, W.R., Dushay, R.A., Deakins, S.M., Stasny, P., Lukens, E.P., and Toran, J. (2000) Employment outcomes in family-aided assertive community treatment, *American Journal of Orthopsychiatry*, 70:2, 203–14.

McGlashan, T.H. (1998) Early detection and intervention of schizophrenia: rationale and research, *British Journal of Psychiatry Supplement*, 172:33, 3–6.

McGrew, J.H. and Bond, G.R. (1995) Critical ingredients of assertive community treatment: judgments of the experts, *Journal of Mental Health Administration*, 22:2, 113–25.

McGrew, J.H., Bond, G.R., Dietzen, L., and Salyers, M. (1994) Measuring the fidelity of implementation of a mental health program model., *Journal of Consulting & Clinical Psychology*, **62:4**, 670–8.

McGrew, J.H., Bond, G.R., Dietzen, L., McKasson, M., and Miller, L.D. (1995) A multisite study of client outcomes in assertive community treatment, *Psychiatric Services*, **46:7**, 696–701.

McHugo, G.J., Drake, R.E., Teague, G.B., and Xie, H. (1999) Fidelity to assertive community treatment and client outcomes in the New Hampshire dual disorders study, *Psychiatric Services*, **50:6**, 818–24.

Meissen, G., Powell, T.J., Wituk, S.A., Girrens, K., and Arteaga, S. (1999) Attitudes of AA contact persons toward group participation by persons with a mental illness, *Psychiatric Services*, **50:8**, 1079–81.

Menezes, P., Johnson, S., Thornicroft, G., Marshall, J., Prosser, D., Bebbington, P., *et al.* (1996) Drug and alcohol problems among individuals with severe mental illness in South London, *British Journal of Psychiatry*, **168**, 612–19.

Mental Health Foundation (1996) *MHF briefing no. 3. Mental health and housing*, Mental Health Foundation, London.

Mental Health Foundation (1997) *MHF briefing no. 9. Community mental health training: Core knowledge, skills and attitudes for community mental health care*, Mental Health Foundation, London.

Menzies, R., Rocher, I., and Vissandjee, B. (1993) Factors associated with compliance in treatment of tuberculosis, *Tubercle & Lung Disease*, **74:1**, 32–7.

Merson, S., Tyrer, P., Duke, P., and Henderson, F. (1994) Interrater reliability of ICD-10 guidelines for the diagnosis of personality disorders, *Journal of Personality Disorders*, **8**, 89–95.

Milgram, S. (1963) Behavioural study of obedience, *Journal of Abnormal & Social Psychology*, **67**, 371–8.

Miller, W.R. and Rollinick, S. (1991) *Motivational interviewing: Preparing people to change addictive behavior*, Guildford Press, New York.

Minghella, E., Ford, R., Freeman, T., Hoult, J., McGlynn, P., and O'Halloran, P. (1998) *Open all hours: 24 hour response for people with mental health emergencies*, Sainsbury Centre for Mental Health, London.

Moncrieff, J. (1997) Lithium: evidence reconsidered, *British Journal of Psychiatry*, **171**, 113–19.

Moore, S. (1961) A psychiatric out-patient nursing service, *Mental Health*, **20**, 51–55.

Morgan, G. (1994) Assessment of risk. In *The prevention of suicide* (ed. R. Jenkins *et al.*), Department of Health, HMSO, London.

Morgan, S. (1993) *Community mental health: practical approaches to long term problems*, Chapman Hall, London.

Mueser, K.T., Bennett, M., and Kushner, M.G. (1995) Epidemiology of substance abuse disorders among persons with chronic mental illness. In *Double jeopardy: chronic mental illness and substance abuse* (ed. A.F. Lehman and L.B. Dixon), Harwood Academic Publishers, Baltimore.

Mueser, K.T., Bond, G.R., Drake, R.E., and Resnick, S.G. (1998) Models of community care for severe mental illness: a review of research on case management, *Schizophrenia Bulletin*, **24:1**, 37–74.

Muijen, M. (1997) The future of training, *Journal of Mental Health*, **6:6**, 535–8.

Muijen, M., Marks, I.M., Connolly, J., Audini, B., and McNamee, G. (1992) The daily living programme. Preliminary comparison of community versus hospital-based treatment for the seriously mentally ill facing emergency admission, *British Journal of Psychiatry*, **160**, 379–84.

Muijen, M., Cooney, M., Strathdee, G., Bell, R., Hudson, A., (1994) Community psychiatric nurse teams: intensive support versus genetic case. *British Journal of Psychiatry*, **165**: 211–217.

Munro, E. and Rumgay, J. (2000) Role of risk assessment in reducing homicides by people with mental illness, *British Journal of Psychiatry*, **176**, 116–20.

National Services Framework (1999) *Better act now! NSF's views on the Mental Health Act Review*, NSF, London.

NHS Training Authority (1990) *Effective team working in the community*, MacMillan Intek Ltd, Hove.

Nicol, M.M., Robertson, L., and Connaughton, J.A. (2000) *Life skills programmes for chronic mental illness*, The Cochrane Library, Issue 1.

Nicola Davies (1995) *The report of the inquiry into the circumstances leading to the death of Jonathan Newby*, Oxfordshire Health, Oxford.

Noakes, B. and Johnson, N. (1999) Primary care. Don't leave me this way, *Health Service Journal*, 109:5645, 20–2.

Noffsinger, S.G. and Resnick, P.J. (1999) Violence and mental illness, *Current Opinion in Psychiatry*, 12:6, 683–7.

Nursing Times (2000) Open learning: clinical supervision: make your experience work: cross-disciplinary supervision. In *Nursing Times*, 96(7), 47–50, Feb 17–23.

O'Brien, A. and Firn, M. (in press) Clozapine initiation in the community, *Psychiatric Bulletin*.

O'Donnell, I. and Farmer, R. (1995) The limitations of official suicide statistics, *British Journal of Psychiatry*, 166:4, 458–61.

Onyett, S. (1992) *Case management in mental health*, Chapman Hall, London.

Onyett, S., Pillinger, T., and Muijen, M. (1997) Job satisfaction and burnout among members of community mental health teams, *Journal of Mental Health*, 6:1, 55–66.

Osher, F.C. and Kofoed, L.L. (1989) Treatment of patients with psychiatric and psychoactive substance abuse disorders, *Hospital & Community Psychiatry*, 40:10, 1025–30.

Overall, J.E. and Gorham, D.L. (1962) The brief psychiatric rating scale, *Psychological Reports*, 10, 799–812.

Owen, R.R., Fischer, E.P., Booth, B.M., and Cuffel, B.J. (1996) Medication noncompliance and substance abuse among patients with schizophrenia, *Psychiatric Services*, 47:8, 853–8.

Owens, D.G. (1996) Adverse effects of antipsychotic agents. Do newer agents offer advantages? *Drugs*, 51:6, 895–930.

Pai, S. and Kapur, R.L. (1981) The burden on the family of a psychiatric patient: development of an interview schedule, *British Journal of Psychiatry*, 138, 332–35.

Pasamanick, B., Scarpitti, F.R., and Leyton, M. (1964) Home versus hospital care for schizophrenics, *Journal of the American Medical Association*, 187, 177–81.

Paykel, E.S. (1978) Contribution of life events to causation of psychiatric illness, *Psychological Medicine*, 8:2, 245–53.

Paykel, E.S., Myers, J.K., Lindenthal, J.J., and Tanner, J. (1974) Suicidal feelings in the general population: a prevalence study, *British Journal of Psychiatry*, 124, 460–9.

Pelosi, A.J. and Jackson, G.A. (2000) Home treatment—enigmas and fantasies, *BMJ*, 320:7230, 308–9.

Perkins, R. and Burns, T. (2001) Home treatment, *International Journal of Social Psychiatry*, 47:3, 55–66.

Perkins, R., Evanson, E.A., and Davidson, B. (2000) *The Pathfinder user employment programme*, South West London and St George's Mental Health NHS Trust, London.

Perris, C. 1969, The separation of biplor (manic-depressive) from unipolar recurrent depressive psychoses, *Behavioural Neuropsychiatry*, 1: 8, 17–24.

Perry, A., Tarrier, N., Morriss, R., McCarthy, E., and Limb, K. 1999, Randomised controlled trial of efficacy of teaching patients with bipolar disorder to identify early symptoms of relapse and obtain treatment., *BMJ*, 318, 149–153.

Powell, E. (1961) *Opening speech, annual conference*, National Association for Mental Health, London.

Prance, N. (1993) Travelling companions, *Nursing Times*, 89:5, 28–30.

Priebe, S. and Gruyters, T. (1995) Patients' assessment of treatment predicting outcome, *Schizophrenia Bulletin*, 21:1, 87–94.

Priebe, S., Broker, M., and Gunkel, S. (1998) Involuntary admission and posttraumatic stress disorder symptoms in schizophrenia patients, *Comprehensive Psychiatry*, **39:4**, 220–4.

Prochaska, J.O. and Diclemente, C.C. (1992) Stages of change in the modification of problem behaviors, *Progress in Behaviour Modification*, **28**, 183–218.

Querido, A. (1968) *The development of socio-medical care in the Netherlands*, Routledge and Kegan Paul, London.

Rapp, C.A. (1992) The strengths perspective of case management with persons suffering from severe mental illness. In *The strength model of social work: power in the people* (ed. D. Saleebey), Longman, New York.

Rapp, C.A. (1998) The active ingredients of effective case management: a research synthesis, *Community Mental Health Journal*, **34:4**, 363–80.

Rapp, C.A. and Wintersteen, R. (1989) The strengths model of case management: results from 12 demonstrations, *Psychosocial Rehabilitation Journal*, **13:1**, 23–32.

Razali, M.S. and Yahya, H. (1995) Compliance with treatment in schizophrenia: a drug intervention program in a developing country, *Acta Psychiatrica Scandinavica*, **91**, 331–5.

Reed, J.L. (1992) *Review of health and social services for mentally disordered offenders and others requiring similar services—final summary report*, Department of Health, London.

Reed, P.G. and Leonard, V.E. (1989) An analysis of the concept of self-neglect, *Advances in Nursing Science*, **12:1**, 39–53.

Regier, D.A., Farmer, M.E., Rae, D.S., Locke, B.Z., Keith, S.J., Judd, L.L., *et al.* (1990) Comorbidity of mental disorders with alcohol and other drug abuse. Results from the Epidemiologic Catchment Area (ECA) Study, *Journal of the American Medical Association*, **264:19**, 2511–18.

Reynolds, A. and Thornicroft, G. (1999) *Managing mental health services*, Open University Press, Buckingham, Philadelphia.

Rinaldi, M. and Hill, R. (2000) *Insufficient concern*, Merton Mind, London.

Ritchie, C.W., Hayes, D., and Ames, D.J. (2000) Patient or client? The opinion of people attending a psychiatric clinic, *Bulletin*, **24**, 447–450.

Ritchie, J.H. (1994) *The report of the inquiry into the care and treatment of Christopher Clunis presented to the Chairman of the North East Thames and South East Thames Regional Health Authorities*, HMSO, London.

Rollinick, S., Heather, N., and Bell, A. (1992) Negotiating behaviour change in medical settings: the development of brief motivational interviewing, *Journal of Mental Health*, **1**, 25–37.

Rorstad, P. and Checinski, K. (1996) *Dual diagnosis: facing the challenge*, Wynne House Publishing, Guildford.

Rosen, A., Hadzi–Pavlovic, D., and Parker, G. (1989) The life skills profile: a measure assessing function and disability in schizophrenia, *Schizophrenia Bulletin*, **15:2**, 325–37.

Rosenthal, D., Wender, P.H., Kety, S.S., Welner, J., and Schulsinger, F. (1971) The adopted-away offspring of schizophrenics, *American Journal of Psychiatry*, **128:3**, 307–11.

Rounsaville, B.J., O'Malley, S., Foley, S., and Weissman, M.M. (1988) Role of manual-guided training in the conduct and efficacy of interpersonal psychotherapy for depression, *Journal of Consulting & Clinical Psychology*, **56:5**, 681–8.

Royal College of Psychiatrists (1993) *Community supervision orders*, Report to Council, Royal College of Psychiatrists, London.

Ryle, A. (1997) The structure and development of borderline personality disorder: a proposed model, *British Journal of Psychiatry*, **170**, 82–7.

Sachs, G.S., Printz, D.J., Kahn, D.A., Carpenter, D., and Docherty, J.P. (2000) The expert consensus guideline series: medication treatment of bipolar disorder, *Postgraduate Medicine, Special Report*, 1–104.

Sackett, D.L., Straus, S.E., Richardson, W.S., Rosenberg, W., and Haynes, R.B. (1997) *Evidence based medicine—how to practice and teach EBM*, Churchill Livingstone, Harcourt Publishers Ltd, London.

Sainsbury Centre for Mental Health (1997) *Pulling together: the future roles and training of mental health staff*, Sainsbury Centre for Mental Health, London.

Sainsbury Centre for Mental Health (1998) *Keys to engagement: a review of care for people with serious mental illness who are hard to engage with services*, Sainsbury Centre for Mental Health, London.

Sainsbury Centre for Mental Health (2001) *Capable practitioner: a framework and list of practitioner capabilities required to implement the National Service Framework for mental health,* Sainsbury Centre for Mental Health, London.

Schneider, K. (1923) *Die psychopathischen personalichkeiten*, Springer, Berlin.

Schneider, K. (1959) *Clinical psychopathology* (translated by M.W. Hamilton), Grone and Stratton, New York.

Schwartz, R. and Lehman, A.F. (1995) Overview of treatment principles. In *Double jeopardy: chronic mental illness and substance abuse* (ed. A.F. Lehman and L.B. Dixon), Harwood Academic Publishers, Baltimore.

Scott, H., Johnson, S., Menezes, P., Thornicroft, G., Marshall, J., Bindman, J., *et al.* (1998) Substance misuse and risk of aggression and offending among the severely mentally ill, *British Journal of Psychiatry*, 172, 345–50.

Segal, H. (1983)Some clinical implications of Melanie Klein's work. Emergence from narcissism, *International Journal of Psychoanalysis*, 64:3, 269–80.

Sensky, T., Hughes, T., and Hirsch, S. (1980) Compulsory psychiatric treatment in the community. I. A controlled study of compulsory community treatment with extended leave under the Mental Health Act: special characteristics of patients treated and impact of treatment, *British Journal of Psychiatry*, 158, 792–9.

Shearin, E.N. and Linehan, M.M. (1994) Dialectical behavior therapy for borderline personality disorder: Theoretical and empirical foundations, *Acta Psychiatrica Scandinavica Supplement*, 379, 61–8.

Simpson, G.M. and Angus, J.W. (1970) A rating scale for extrapyramidal side effects, *Acta Psychiatrica Scandinavica Supplement*, 212, 11–19.

Siris, S.G. (2000) Depression in schizophrenia: perspective in the era of atypical antipsychotic agents, *American Journal of Psychiatry*, 157:9, 1379–89.

Slade, M., Thornicroft, G., Loftus, L., Phelan, M., and Wykes, T. (1999) *Camberwell assessment of need*, Gaskell, London.

Smith, A. (1987) Quality-adjusted life-years, *Lancet*, 2:8549, 46–7.

Smyth, M.G. and Hoult, J. (2000) The home treatment enigma, *BMJ*, 320: 7230, 305–9.

Solomon, P. and Draine, J. (1995*a*) The efficacy of a consumer case management team: 2-year outcomes of a randomized trial, *Journal of Mental Health Administration*, 22:2, 135–46.

Solomon, P. and Draine, J. (1995*b*) One-year outcomes of a randomized trial of case management with seriously mentally ill clients leaving jail, *Evaluation Review*, 19, 256–73.

Soni–Raleigh, V. and Balarajan, R. (1992) Suicide and self-burning among Indians and West Indians in England and Wales, *British Journal of Psychiatry*, 161, 365–8.

Steadman, H.J., Mulvey, E.P., Monahan, J., Robbins, P.C., Appelbaum, P.S., Grisso, T., *et al.* (1998) Violence by people discharged from acute psychiatric inpatient facilities and by others in the same neighbourhoods, *Archives of General Psychiatry*, 55:5, 393–401.

Stefansson, C.G. and Cullberg, J. (1986) Introducing community mental health services. The effects on a suburban patient population, *Acta Psychiatrica Scandinavica*, 74:4, 368–78.

Stein, L.I. and Santos, A.B. (1998) *Assertive community treatment of persons with severe mental illness*, W.W. Norton & Company Inc, New York.

Stein, L.I. and Test, M.A. (1978) An alternative to mental hospital treatment. In *Alternatives to mental health hospital treatment* (ed. L.I. Stein and M.A. Test), Plenum Press, New York.

Stein, L.I. and Test, M.A. (1980) Alternative to mental hospital treatment. I. Conceptual model, treatment program, and clinical evaluation, *Archives of General Psychiatry*, 37:4, 392–97.

Steinwachs, D.M., Kasper, J.D., and Skinner, E.A. (1992) *Family perspectives on meeting the needs for care of severely mentally ill relatives: a national survey. Final report.* Center of the Organisation and Financing of Care for the Severely Mentally Ill, John Hopkins University, Baltimore.

Swanson, J.W., Estroff, S.E., Swartz, M.S., Borum, R., Lachicotte, W., Zimmer, C., *et al.* (1997) Violence and severe mental disorder in clinical and community populations: the effects of psychotic symptoms, comorbidity and lack of treatment, *Psychiatry*, 60, 1–22.

Swartz, M.S., Swanson, J.W., Hiday, V.A., Borum, R., Wagner, H.R., and Burns, B.J. (1998) Violence and severe mental illness: the effects of substance abuse and nonadherence to medication, *American Journal of Psychiatry*, 155:2, 226–31.

Szymanski, S., Lieberman, J.A., Alvir, J.M., Mayerhoff, D., Loebel, A., Geisler, S., *et al.* (1995) Gender differences in onset of illness, treatment response, course, and biologic indexes in first-episode schizophrenic patients, *American Journal of Psychiatry*, 152:5, 698–703.

Talbott, J.A., Clark, G.H.J., Sharfstein, S.S., and Klein, J. (1987) Issues in developing standards governing psychiatric practice in community mental health centers, *Hospital & Community Psychiatry*, 38:11, 1198–202.

Tarrier, N., Barrowclough, C., Vaughn, C., Bamrah, J.S., Porceddu, K., Watts, S., *et al.* (1989) Community management of schizophrenia. A two-year follow-up of a behavioural intervention with families, *British Journal of Psychiatry*, 154, 625–8.

Tarrier, N., Yusupoff, L., Kinney, C., McCarthy, E., Gledhill, A., Haddock, G., *et al.* (1998) Randomised controlled trial of intensive cognitive behaviour therapy for patients with chronic schizophrenia, *BMJ*, 317: 7154, 303–7.

Taylor, D. (1997) Pharmacokinetic interactions involving clozapine, *British Journal of Psychiatry*, 171, 109–12.

Taylor, P.J. and Gunn, J. (1999) Homicides by people with mental illness: myth and reality, *British Journal of Psychiatry*, 174, 9–14.

Teague, G.B., Drake, R.E., and Ackerson, T.H. (1995) Evaluating use of continuous treatment teams for persons with mental illness and substance abuse, *Psychiatric Services*, 46:7, 689–95.

Teague, G.B., Bond, G.R., and Drake, R.E. (1998) Program fidelity in assertive community treatment: development and use of a measure, *American Journal of Orthopsychiatry*, 68:2, 216–32.

Telles, C., Karno, M., Mintz, J., Paz, G., Arias, M., Tucker, D., *et al.* (1995) Immigrant families coping with schizophrenia. Behavioural family intervention v. case management with a low-income Spanish-speaking population, *British Journal of Psychiatry*, 167:4, 473–9.

Test, M.A. (1992) Training in community living. In *Handbook of psychiatric rehabilitation* (ed. R.P. Lieberman), Macmillan, New York.

Test, M.A. and Stein, L.I. (1980) Alternative to mental hospital treatment. III: social cost, *Archives of General Psychiatry*, 37:4, 409–12.

Thornicroft, G. and Tansella, M. (1999) *The mental health matrix: a manual to improve services*, Cambridge University Press, Cambridge.

Thornicroft, G., Strathdee, G., Phelan, M., Holloway, F., Wykes, T., Dunn, G., *et al.* (1998*a*) Rationale and design. PRiSM psychosis study 1, *British Journal of Psychiatry*, 173, 363–70.

Thornicroft, G., Wykes, T., Holloway, F., Johnson, S., and Szmukler, G. (1998b) From efficacy to effectiveness in community mental health services. PRiSM psychosis study 10, *British Journal of Psychiatry*, **173**, 423–427.

Thornley, B. and Adams, C. (1998) Content and quality of 2000 controlled trials in schizophrenia over 50 years, *BMJ*, **317**, 1181–4.

Tuckett, D., Boulton, M., Olson, C., and Williams, A. (1985) *Meetings between experts—an approach to sharing ideas in medical consultations*, Tavistock Publications, London.

Tyrer, P. (1998) Whither community care?, *British Journal of Psychiatry*, **173**, 359–60.

Tyrer, P. (2000a) The future of the community mental health team, *International Review of Psychiatry*, **12**, 219–25.

Tyrer, P. (2000b) Effectiveness of intensive treatment in severe mental illness, *British Journal of Psychiatry*, **176**, 492–3.

Tyrer, P., Morgan, J., Van Horn, E., Jayakody, M., Evans, K., Brummell, R., *et al.* (1995) A randomised controlled study of close monitoring of vulnerable psychiatric patients, *Lancet*, **345:8952**, 756–9.

Tyrer, P., Coid, J., Simmonds, S., Joseph, P., and Marriott, S. (1999) Community mental health team management for those with severe mental illnesses and disordered personality. In *Schizophrenia module of the Cochrane database systematic reviews* (ed. C.G. Adams, L. Duggan, and J. de Jesus Mari), Update Software, Oxford.

UK700 Group: Burns, T., Fahy, T., Thompson, S., Tyrer, P., and White, I. (1999a) Intensive case management for severe psychotic illness (authors' reply), *Lancet*, **354**, 1384–6.

UK700 Group: Burns, T., Creed, F., Fahy, T., Thompson, S., Tyrer, P., and White, I. (1999b) Intensive versus standard case management for severe psychotic illness: a randomised trial, *Lancet*, **353**, 2185–9.

UK700 Group: Byford, S., Fiander, M., Torgerson, D.J., Barber, J.A., Thompson, S.G., Burns, T., *et al.* (2000) Cost-effectiveness of intensive versus standard case management for severe psychotic illness, *British Journal of Psychiatry*, **176**, 537–43.

UK700 Group: Creed, F., Burns, T., Butler, T., Byford, S., Murray, R., Thompson, S., *et al.* (1999) Comparison of intensive and standard case management for patients with psychosis. Rationale of the trial., *British Journal of Psychiatry*, **174**, 74–8.

UK700 Group: Laugharne, R., Byford, S., Barbour, J., Burns, T., Walsh, E., and Holme, S. (in press) The effect of alcohol consumption on cost of care in severe psychotic illness.

UK700 Group: Tyrer, P., Hassiotis, A., Ukoumunne, O., Piachaud, J., and Harvey, K. (1999) Intensive case management for psychotic patients with borderline intelligence, *Lancet*, **354:9183**, 999–1000.

UKCC (1996) *Position statement on clinical supervision*, United Kingdom Central Council for Nursing, Midwifery, and Health Visiting, London.

Vaccaro, J.V., Pitts, D.B., and Wallace, C.J. (1992) Functional assessment. In *Handbook of psychiatric rehabilitation* (ed. R.P. Liberman), MacMillan, New York.

Vaughan, K., Doyle, M., McConaghy, N., Blaszczynski, A., Fox, A., and Tarrier, N. (1992) The Sydney intervention trial: a controlled trial of relatives' counselling to reduce schizophrenic relapse, *Social Psychiatry & Psychiatric Epidemiology*, **27:1**, 16–21.

Vaughan, K., McConaghy, N., Wolf, C., Myhr, C., and Black, T. (2000) Community treatment orders: relationship to clinical care, medication compliance, behavioural disturbance and readmission. *Australian and New Zealand Journal of Psychiatry*, **34**, 801–808.

Vaughn, C. and Leff J. (1976) The measurement of expressed emotion in the families of psychiatric patients, *British Journal of Social Clinical Psychology*, **15:2**, 157–65.

Wall, S., Buchanan, A., Hotopf, M., Wessely, S., and Churchill, R. (1999) *A systematic review of data pertaining to the Mental Health Act (1983). Report to the Department of Health*, HMSO, London.

Weisbrod, B.A., Test, M.A., and Stein, L.I. (1980) Alternative to mental hospital treatment. II: economic benefit-cost analysis, *Archives of General Psychiatry*, **37**:4, 400–5.

Weissman, M.M., Bland, R.C., Canino, G.J., Faravelli, C., Greenwald, S., Hwu, H.G., *et al.* (1996) Cross-national epidemiology of major depression and bipolar disorder, *Journal of the American Medical Association*, **276**:4, 293–9.

White, E. (1991) *The 3rd quinquennial national community psychiatric nursing survey*, University of Manchester, Department of Nursing, Manchester.

White, E. (1999) The 4th quinquennial national community mental health nursing census of England and Wales, *Australian & New Zealand Journal of Mental Health Nursing*, **8**:3, 86–92.

White, R., Tata, P., and Burns, T. (1996) Mood, learned resourcefulness and perceptions of control in type 1 diabetes mellitus, *Journal of Psychosomatic Research*, **40**:2, 205–12.

Wig, N.N., Menon, D.K., Bedi, H., Leff, J., Kuipers, L., Ghosh, A., *et al.* (1987) Expressed emotion and schizophrenia in north India. II: distribution of expressed emotion components among relatives of schizophrenic patients in Aarhus and Chandigarh, *British Journal of Psychiatry*, **151**, 160–5.

Wilkinson, G. (1994) Can suicide be prevented? Better treatment of mental illness is more appropriate aim, *BMJ*, **309**:6958, 860–1.

Williams, H., Clarke, R., Fashola, Y., and Holt, G. (1998) Diogenes' syndrome in patients with intellectual disability: 'a rose by any other name'?, *Journal of Intellectual Disability Research*, **42**:4, 316–20.

Wing, J., Curtis, R.H., and Beevor, A. (1999) Health of the nation outcome scales (HoNOS). Glossary for HoNOS score sheet, *British Journal of Psychiatry*, **174**, 432–4.

Wing, J.K. (1968) Social treatments of mental illness. In *Studies of psychiatry* (ed. M. Shepherd and D.L. Davies), Oxford University Press, London.

Wing, J.K. and Brown, G.W. (1970) *Institutionalism and schizophrenia*, Cambridge University Press, Cambridge.

Wing, J.K., Cooper, J.E., and Sartorius, N. (1974) *The measurement and classification of psychiatric symptoms: an instruction manual for the PSE and the Catego program*, Cambridge University Press, Cambridge.

Wolff, G., Pathare, S., Craig, T., and Leff, J. (1996) Community knowledge of mental illness and reaction to mentally ill people, *British Journal of Psychiatry*, **168**:2, 191–8.

Wood, H. and Carr, S. (1998) *Locality services in mental health, developing home treatment and assertive outreach: the North Birmingham experience*, Sainsbury Centre for Mental Health/North Birmingham MHT.

Wooff, K., Goldberg, D.P., and Fryers, T. (1986) Patients in receipt of community psychiatric nursing care in Salford 1976–82, *Psychological Medicine*, **16**:2, 407–14.

Wooff, K., Goldberg, D.P., and Fryers, T. (1988) The practice of community psychiatric nursing and mental health social work in Salford. Some implications for community care, *British Journal of Psychiatry*, **152**, 783–92.

World Health Organisation (1992) *The ICD-10 classification of mental and behavioural disorders*, World Health Organisation, Geneva.

Yerkes, R.M. and Dodson, J.D. (1908) Relation of strength and stimulus to rapidity of habit-formation, *Journal of Comparative Neurology & Psychology*.

Zigmond, A.S. and Snaith, R.P. (1983) The hospital anxiety and depression scale, *Acta Psychiatrica Scandinavica*, **67**:6, 361–70.

Zisook, S., McAdams, L.A., Kuck, J., Harris, M. J., Bailey, A., Patterson, T. L., *et al.* (1999) Depressive symptoms in schizophrenia, *American Journal of Psychiatry*, **156:11**, 1736–43.

Zubin, J. and Spring, B. (1977) Vulnerability—a new view of schizophrenia, *Journal of Abnormal Psychology*, **86:2**, 103–26.

Index